ROUTLEDGE LIBRARY EDITIONS: LITERARY THEORY

Volume 18

NATURE AND LANGUAGE

NATURE AND LANGUAGE
A Semiotic Study of Cucurbits in Literature

RALF NORRMAN AND JON HAARBERG

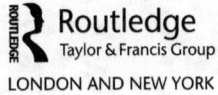

LONDON AND NEW YORK

First published in 1980 by Routledge & Kegan Paul Ltd

This edition first published in 2017
by Routledge
2 Park Square, Milton Park, Abingdon, Oxon OX14 4RN

and by Routledge
711 Third Avenue, New York, NY 10017

Routledge is an imprint of the Taylor & Francis Group, an informa business

©1980 Ralf Norrman and Jon Haarberg

All rights reserved. No part of this book may be reprinted or reproduced or utilised in any form or by any electronic, mechanical, or other means, now known or hereafter invented, including photocopying and recording, or in any information storage or retrieval system, without permission in writing from the publishers.

Trademark notice: Product or corporate names may be trademarks or registered trademarks, and are used only for identification and explanation without intent to infringe.

British Library Cataloguing in Publication Data
A catalogue record for this book is available from the British Library

ISBN: 978-1-138-69377-7 (Set)
ISBN: 978-1-315-52921-9 (Set) (ebk)
ISBN: 978-1-138-68339-6 (Volume 18) (hbk)
ISBN: 978-1-138-68341-9 (Volume 18) (pbk)
ISBN: 978-1-315-54451-9 (Volume 18) (ebk)

Publisher's Note
The publisher has gone to great lengths to ensure the quality of this reprint but points out that some imperfections in the original copies may be apparent.

Disclaimer
The publisher has made every effort to trace copyright holders and would welcome correspondence from those they have been unable to trace.

Ralf Norrman and Jon Haarberg

Nature and Language
A semiotic study of cucurbits in literature

Routledge & Kegan Paul
London, Boston and Henley

*First published in 1980
by Routledge & Kegan Paul Ltd*

*39 Store Street, London WC1E 7DD,
9 Park Street, Boston, Mass. 02108, USA, and
Broadway House, Newtown Road,
Henley-on-Thames, Oxon RG9 1EN*

*Set in IBM Journal by
Hope Services, Abingdon, Oxon*

© *Ralf Norrman and Jon Haarberg 1980
No part of this book may be reproduced in
any form without permission from the
publisher, except for the quotation of brief
passages in criticism*

British Library Cataloguing in Publication Data

Norrman, Ralf
   Nature and language.
   1. Cucurbitaceae in literature
   2. Semiotics and literature
   I. Title   II. Haarberg, John
   809'.933'6   PN56.C/

ISBN 0 7100 0453 2

T.N. *altipetaci*

Naturam expelles furca, tamen usque recurret

(Hor. *Ep.* I.10.24)

Contents

Foreword	xi
Acknowledgments	xiii
Introduction	1
Part 1: 'Pregnant Gourds' and 'Delirious Pumpkins': The Semiotic Matrix of Cucurbits	11
Part 2: Implications	81
1 Is a literary work written by the author or by the readers?	83
2 Does a literary work write itself?	94
3 Sign and signification	124
4 Independent creation versus tradition	149
5 On the nature of signs used in cucurbitic metaphors	154
Conclusion	169
Notes	172
Works cited	209
Translations	220
Index	224

Plates

between pages 80 and 81

I   Juan Sánches Cotán, Still Life
II Frans Floris, *Adam and Eve*
III Ferdinando Maria Campani, *The Temptation of Adam*
IV Lambert Doomer, *Hirtenstück*
V   Lambert Doomer, *Distelstaude*
VI Albrecht Dürer, *St. Jerome in His Study*
VII Giuseppe Archimboldo, *Vertumnus-Rudolf II*
VIII Drawing by W. Miller
IX American comic postcard
X   Faustino Bocchi, *Bambocciate*
XI Giant cucurbits

Foreword

From the very moment we had decided, in the spring of 1977, to write this book, we realized that the subject was one that many would not have touched with a barge pole. In wading through numerous – sometimes rather undignified – texts in quest of evidence for or against the hypothesis, it was good for each of us to know from the start that there was at least one other person who believed unreservedly in the idea. During our work on the manuscript, however, we were later pleased to find that after all a great number of people were willing to give us generous assistance and encouragement.

Mrs. Eva-Liisa Norrman was an instant convert, whose zeal was not diminished during the work. We wish to thank her for her interest and for many helpful comments and ideas, as well as for typing and proof-reading.

We are greatly indebted to Professor H.W. Donner, whose generous support made the book possible.

A large number of people have given their valuable help in one way or another. Dan Holm, of Åbo Akademi, was our knowledgeable guide when we first tried to find our way through the history of cucurbits in pictorial art; and he called our attention to several of the pictures used as illustrations in this book. Larzer Ziff, of the University of Pennsylvania, read an early version of Part 1, and we are grateful to him not only for his useful comments but also for encouraging us to go on. John Bamborough, Principal of Linacre College, Oxford, Ruth Gounelas, St Anne's College, Oxford, Demetrios Gounelas, King's College, London, Sixten Ringbom, Åbo Akademi, Nils Erik Enkvist, Åbo Akademi also all read the manuscript in one version or another. We are grateful to them for their pertinent remarks and suggestions. There are many more people who have helped in various ways – by reading parts of the manuscript, discussing its contents with us, or

FOREWORD

acting as our informants or experts in one way or another (in alphabetical order): Paul Foote, Joe Garver, Warwick Goymer, Auli Hakulinen, Jim Haynes, Fred Karlsson, Harold Kolb, Rolf Lindholm, Märta Malmström, Joseph Millichap, Jean-Luc Oulhen, Michael Winterbottom. To all these and many others who are not mentioned here our sincerest thanks are due. From all we have learnt much – yet should have learnt more.

We are grateful to Linacre College, the Queen's College and Wadham College, Oxford, and to the Finnish Academy.

Oxford, December 1978
Ralf Norrman   Jon Haarberg

Acknowledgments

Grateful acknowledgment is made to the San Diego Museum of Art for permission to reproduce the Cotán Still Life in Plate I; to the Cognac Museum for permission to reproduce Floris's *Adam and Eve* in Plate II; to the Ashmolean Museum, Oxford, for permission to reproduce Campani's *The Temptation of Adam* in Plate III; to the Landesmuseum für Kunst und Kulturgeschichte, Oldenburg, for permission to reproduce Doomer's *Hirtenstück* in Plate IV; to the Statens Museum for Kunst, Copenhagen, for permission to reproduce Doomer's *Distelstaude* in Plate V and Albrecht Dürer's copper engraving *St Jerome in His Study* in Plate VI; to the Nationalmuseum, Stockholm, for permission to reproduce Arcimboldo's *Vertumnus – Rudolf II* in Plate VII; to the *New Yorker* magazine for permission to reproduce W. Miller's drawing in Plate VIII; to Professor J. Stanley Lemons for permission to reproduce the postcard (Plate IX) from the J. Stanley Lemons collection; to the Direzione Musei Civici di Brescia for permission to reproduce the detail from Bocchi's *Bambocciate* in Plate X; to Mr Ed Weeks and Mr Grover P. Hopkins, North Carolina, for permission to reproduce the picture of Mr Weeks and his monster watermelon, and to Mr Colin Bowcock and Mel Grundy Photographic Agency, Chester, for permission to reproduce the picture of Mr Bowcock's record pumpkin.

Some of the material in Chapters 1, 2 and 5 has been dealt with previously: in Ralf Norrman, 'On the Semiotic Function of Cucurbits', *Scripta Instituti Donneriani Aboensis,* Vol. 10, Uppsala and Stockholm: Almqvist & Wicksell, 1979, pp. 126–38; 'Valsituationen i konsten: Två exempel', *Horisont,* no. 5, 1978, pp. 1–9; 'On the Degree of Motivation in Signs Used in Metaphors Involving Plant Symbolism', in Jan-Ola Östman (ed.), *Reports on Text Linguistics: Semantics and Cohesion*; publications of the Research Institute of the Åbo Akademi Foundation, no. 41, Åbo, 1979, pp. 35ff. We are grateful to the editors for permission to reprint certain sections of these essays.

Nature and Language

Introduction

This study, as the title suggests, is on the semiotic role of cucurbits in literature. Even before the book was published it had already become the inevitable fate of the authors to experience, again and again, how this simple statement unfailingly caused some consternation and much hilarity.

Know then, that precisely that consternation, and precisely that hilarity, are the subject of this work.

Pumpkins are ridiculous and funny, and as such they evoke matching responses. Laughter and derision are natural human reactions to pumpkins, and far be it from us to deny our readers the right to be human – we have laughed often enough ourselves while working on this study.

But our reaction did not stop at this. Curiosity prompted us to ask 'why do we laugh?' and with the detachment of the inquisitive to try to determine the causes of laughter, and analyse its function, even while indulging in it. We hope that our readers will transcend their automatic – and quite legitimate – initial reactions to cucurbits in the same way. Doubtless there is a section of the public who are not capable of this; who will let their reactions to pumpkins colour their relation to a work on pumpkins. Nevertheless we hope that such readers will be only a tiny minority.

Cucurbits are a taboo subject not only because of their ridiculous connotations but also because of their association with sex. Needless to say, the passages illustrating this aspect were chosen only for their value as examples of a major part of the semiotic role of cucurbits. Neither literary quality nor sensationalist value was a criterion in our sampling of this area of cucurbitic literature.

Although readers may at first find the subject of this book unusual, we hope that on closer inspection, and in retrospect, it will seem different. So far as the subject is concerned there is, therefore, no

INTRODUCTION

need for further preliminaries. As to methodology, however, we should say a few words, since there are some organizational features of the text that the reader may wish to be prepared for. There are, in particular, three aspects of our methodology that have given the text its character: our study is paradigmatic, panchronic and, to some extent, interdisciplinary. Let us look briefly at each of these.

A paradigmatic study

Two basic ways of approaching an element in a literary text are the syntagmatic and the paradigmatic. In order to gain a fuller understanding of the nature and function of the textual element one can study either its relation to the other elements, and particularly the neighbouring ones, in the same text (its syntagmatic relations); or its relation to elements that are the same, or similar, or likely to occur in a corresponding position, in other texts (its paradigmatic relations).

Our study will be paradigmatic. In Part 1 we shall lay bare the language of cucurbits by presenting a number of literary passages where they occur and comparing and analysing the similarities and differences between these occurrences. In this way our implicit reactions as readers will be made explicit. We believe that in order to understand the function of metaphors and similes that make use of things taken from nature (such as plants, animals, vegetables, metals, liquids, etc.) as signs, one must first become consciously aware of one's reactions to the literary passages in which such signs occur.

Paradigmatic studies are comparatively rare in literary scholarship at the moment. The schools of thought that have dominated the scene in literary criticism during the last few decades have practically all favoured other approaches. New criticism, for example, was syntagmatically oriented; its aim was to explicate texts, often the whole text, in its variety of aspects.

For a semiotic study such as ours, however, a paradigmatic approach is the most practical and also the most natural. We believe that literature can be regarded as a kind of language. In order to establish the meanings of this language, make the code explicit and put it on record we decided to do what any compiler of a dictionary does, i.e. to collect a number of instances of use and then analyse the material.

The paradigmatic method is routine with scholars trying to decipher words in a dead language. These scholars collect as many as possible –

preferably all – of the contexts in which a word occurs, and by studying these they can gradually establish the semantic matrix of the word. We, too, shall collect a number of passages, compare and contrast them and thus establish the semiotic matrix, in literature, of the cucurbits.

To master the language of cucurbits is to know the elements of that language and above all their relations to each other. In language, as Saussure insisted, everything is connected with everything else. This means that the learner of a language – whether the symbolic language of cucurbits or language in the sense of a natural language like French – may well long for an ideal situation in which he could learn everything at once and not have to pass painfully through various stages of interlanguage; that he could skip the equivalents of the mother's 'baby-talk', the accommodating 'foreigner-talk' of the native or the simplifications of the textbook texts that are so odious to the adult learner.

For practical reasons, however, this is impossible. One has to begin somewhere, and proceed somehow, and some simplification at the beginning is inevitable. In foreign-language textbooks the first texts are usually completely artificial; verbs are used only in the present tense; cases are introduced one at a time and so on. We, too, shall simplify at the beginning of this study. But we beg the reader to bear in mind that this is only a presentational device. Just as 'textbookese' is spoken nowhere in the world, neither are cucurbits used anywhere in literature in such a simple fashion as the first few pages of this book may seem to suggest. In order to get into a system in which everything is connected with everything else one has to take a plunge, and swim, to begin with, as best one can. We wanted to provide some help by simplifying, by dealing with cucurbitic connotations one at a time and refraining from comments on more than one aspect of a symbol the first time it is introduced. It must be remembered, however, that there is no intrinsic merit in these arrangements. The organization exists only as a presentational device and should be forgotten once it has served its purpose. We wanted to write Part 1 of this book in such a way that it could become a heuristic ladder for us and the readers to climb together; to reach, we hope, at the end of it a level of awareness of cucurbitic language from which we can draw the ladder up after us.

In Part 1 we usually proceed from one example to the next by means of transitional links based on abstract principles such as similarity or oppositeness. These relations naturally exist as real relations between the elements of the language of cucurbits; but they should be perceived as existing simultaneously at the same level. We think that no

INTRODUCTION

other order should be imposed. We have, therefore, programmatically refrained from chapter division in Part 1. For a referential guide we hope readers will consult the Index.

The reason for our insistence on this point is our conviction that the best way for the reader to gain an understanding of the linguistic phenomena with which we are concerned is for him to share a *process* with the authors, rather than to be handed a *product*. The insight into the semiotic function of naturally motivated signs that is to be gained from an understanding of the semiotic role of the cucurbits will be lost or obscured if the thought is separated from the act of its discovery. It is our opinion that categorization or hierarchization would give a false impression of what we take to be the way that cucurbitic symbols work.

The unpopularity of paradigmatic studies is particularly evident in the cases when these studies take 'real-world knowledge' into account. In his *Aspects of the Novel*, a book that has been read by generations of undergraduates, E.M. Forster has a passage in which he ridicules a literary study which, among other things, classifies works according to their use of 'the weather'.[1] We have not seen this study and it may deserve everything it got and more besides; but we suspect that such works attract hostile reactions not only for being badly done, but because of their nature. There is a strong latent aversion to any work that deals with things, objects, *realia*.

Resistance against paradigmatic studies is not so strong if they deal with matters of technique, such as, for instance, rhetorical devices. A study of irony in Roman literature needs no apology for its existence. It is easy to see that something could be learnt about irony, and especially about its function in Roman literature, from a comparison and analysis of a number of passages of Roman literature in which it occurs. In contrast, a study on 'pumpkins in Roman literature' (or in literature in general) will arouse suspicion and elicit negative and hostile reactions.

It is easy to see why there should be this aversion to subject-matter. The purpose of intellectual speculation is to transcend the earth-bound and physical. There is more glory in sorting out abstract ideas than in studying earthly and embarrassingly everyday subject-matter. Man should aspire to 'fruit spiritual and celestial' which are 'far beyond the merely pumpkinish and grossly terrene', as Carlyle would have put it.[2] Therefore a study of cucurbits will be suspect and will be regarded as a subversive attempt to pervert linguistic and literary studies into botany.

This suspicion does not disappear entirely, though it is clear to everyone that a study of 'roses in literature' does not deal with roses as plants but as symbols, just as our study will deal with cucurbits not as such but as signs, particularly as used in metaphors, similes and figurative language.

Though the legitimacy of a literary study on the symbolic use of a plant can hardly be in dispute, yet a work such as the present will be controversial because it cannot escape the taint of dealing with the grossly terrene world of real-life things. During our research, we have become convinced that a study of the cucurbits as signs cannot ignore the non-literary aspects of cucurbits – their biology, economy etc. – because the former is influenced by the latter to such a degree as to be almost entirely determined by it.

We are moving in the area of overlap where language and nature meet, and neither can be studied in isolation from the other. The relation between language and the world is usually a referential one which poses none of the problems encountered in understanding the function of metaphors. If there are two real-world objects, a pumpkin and a man, and there is in language a word 'pumpkin' that can be used to refer to the former, and a word 'man' that can be used to refer to the latter, when this happens the case is unproblematical and language and reality can largely be studied separately. *But when a man is called a pumpkin* in a metaphor of abuse, the case is radically altered. 'Pumpkin', in shifting its reference to a man, is no longer language characterized by arbitrariness of the sign. *Nature has become language,* or is being used as language, and this means that the sign 'pumpkin' in the pumpkin metaphor (sign being used here in a wide sense) preserves its *pumpkinness,* which again means that to understand its meaning it is necessary not only to study language but to study reality as well. Otherwise it will be impossible to understand the most fascinating aspect of the phenomenon of metaphor, which is the interpretability of new metaphors the first time they are used.[3]

For a comprehensive explanation of language linguistic theories must ultimately take into account not only a set of rules governing the relations between linguistic units ('grammatical rules') but also, eventually, the relations between whatever these units refer to ('real-world rules').

Relations between referents – that is, relations between, for example, physical objects – are sometimes thought to be outside the realm of linguistics. But at least in the study of plant symbolism they cannot be ignored. As to the necessity of taking 'real-world relations' into account, metaphors, similes and figurative language are a special case, because these signs are not arbitrary. The classification of signs varies with the classifier, but most taxonomies recognize at least three categories: icons (real likeness between the sign and what it stands for); indices (a causal or contiguous relationship); and 'signs proper'. The characteristic feature of the last category is their arbitrariness – as in the Morse code, for instance, the 'b' sign could just as well stand for 'a' if only everyone agreed on the change. This standard classification is difficult in that it seems to classify several things at once, and it has turned out more practical for us to think of signs as having iconic, indexical or sign-proper aspects to a varying degree, many signs often partaking of the nature of all three.[4] The essential question, however, concerns the degree of arbitrariness. It is of fundamental importance to anyone trying to understand its nature and function to know whether a sign is arbitrary or not.

The literary symbols that authors use are often arbitrary and vary with the culture and period of the text. Authors are in one sense free to choose any element they like for a particular place in the text and invest this element with any meaning they like through manipulation of the context, since lability or malleability is one-half of the dual nature of language – the half that permits us to use language the way a sculptor uses wet clay, making of it whatever we wish.

But the opposite force, stability, is also at work in language; and because of that force speaking or writing is on the other hand like shopping in a linguistic supermarket, where the user of language chooses from the shelves, among stable linguistic elements, the particular one that will suit his communicative need at the moment.

One of the features distinguishing the former half from the latter is the degree of natural motivation in the literary signs. If something is used as a sign because of its intrinsic appropriateness for the task, this tends to reinforce stability rather than lability; and then the relations of the element to the same, or similar, elements in other texts will be more important than its relations to other elements in the same text.

Thus, although literary symbols may be fairly arbitrary, there are some cases when the symbols are very stable. Plant or animal symbolism – when man uses something from nature to express some idea about himself, or to define somehow his own position – is such a case, and plant and animal symbolism is often very stable. 'Goose' as a sign of stupidity is used not only because it is agreed that this should be its role in the code; ultimately it is used because geese really are stupid (or, to put it more precisely, because they seem stupid to humans – whether geese, cows and donkeys are stupid from an animal point of view is irrelevant).[5] 'Goose' as a sign of stupidity is not arbitrary. If language had been characterized only by its malleability one could also have expected 'intelligent' birds to be used as a sign of stupidity, since in principle it should be possible to invest any linguistic element with any meaning through manipulation of the context. But this does not seem to happen – at least, it is rare. 'Goose' as a sign of stupidity is superior because the sign preserves a link with its origin. Every user of the sign can get at its meaning not only through his knowledge of the code (which could have been arbitrary tradition) but also by deducing on his own the meaning of the sign through observation of that part of nature from which it is taken.

In their symbolic use in literature the various plants and animals are thus often given their semiotic role because of intrinsic suitability for it.

This has many consequences. One obvious corollary is that the study of plant or animal symbolism has to take 'real-world knowledge' into account. If a passage likens a man to a lion it is necessary to know that lions are brave in order to understand the point of the comparison. When a man is called a pumpkin there is a bisociation of two elements, each belonging to a different system, and an allegation of similarity between the two, despite the definitional dissimilarity. It is alleged that the man is to other men as pumpkins are to other fruit. In order to understand the sign we must know how pumpkins differ from other fruit.

The sentence 'the cat barks' could be condemned as unacceptable either through an appeal to real-world rules ('cats do not bark') or grammatical rules ('one does not say that cats bark'). The words 'cat' and 'bark', or the real-world referents *cat* and *barking*, are incombinable, and maybe it does not matter which level of incompatibility one takes notice of.

This is not the case with the signs under consideration. They come into use because of qualities in the nature they are borrowed from, and the history of their birth influences their life.

A panchronic study

Another consequence of the stability of these signs is that in studying them one can by and large ignore chronology. When we note in a certain culture or period that a plant from the family *Cucurbitaceae* occurs in connection with a narrative element depicting abundance, vitality and fertility, and then find that the plant occurs in a similar context in a later culture, we need not automatically assume an influence from the earlier culture to the later. In order to understand the semiotic role of the plant it may be much more important to study its physiology (fertility, fast growth, abundant harvest) and its special status in the flora. These signs tend to remain the same, provided the nature they refer to remains the same and provided human thought remains essentially the same – which in this context is a reasonable assumption.

Our study is therefore neither synchronic, in the sense of studying the cucurbits at one single time, nor diachronic, in the sense of taking history into account. Our study ignores time; it is 'achronic', or 'panchronic' – though panchronic in the sense of dealing with all times or none, instead of panchronic in the sense of uniting a synchronic and a diachronic perspective. History is relatively unimportant in comparison with the relations between the different elements within the system – irrespective of time. Naturally it would have been interesting to investigate the development of cucurbitic imagery through the ages, but such a study and our present work are two distinctly separate things.

An interdisciplinary study

Semiotic studies often tend to sprawl across many traditional disciplines, like the cucumber in Matron's *Parodies*, which lay extended over nine tables. If it is true in language that 'tout se tient' it is not surprising that everything should become connected with everything else for anyone who accepts the idea that literature is a kind of language.

All through the text we have tried not to branch out into pictorial art, anthropology, etc. Nevertheless, it soon became obvious that for our purposes some borders between traditional disciplines were rather artificial. We have, therefore, allowed some references to cucurbitic material in anthropology, the history of pictorial art, folklore, folkmedicine, etc.

Because the explanation of the semiotic role of the cucurbits is mainly to be sought in the physiology of the plant, it was necessary to include comments on the size, shape, smell, taste, price, etc., of cucurbits. To understand the symbolic use of the plant in literary texts it is necessary to know these things – an absolute minimum is to know as much as the users of the signs. Apart from a knowledge of literature, and in addition to dabbling in linguistics (particularly semantics), anthropology, art history, folklore, etc., the cucurbitologist should therefore preferably have a smattering of botany as well – even if the knowledge be extracted from such undignified sources as, for instance, the *Guinness Book of Records.*

Translations

For the convenience of readers who are primarily interested in the general drift of the argument, rather than in detailed and meticulous scrutiny of each example, we have provided an appendix with translations of all quotations in languages other than English. References to the appendix will be in small Roman numerals. All translations are our own unless otherwise stated.

Part 1: 'Pregnant gourds' and 'delirious pumpkins': the semiotic matrix of cucurbits

> tortusque per herbam
> cresceret in ventrem cucumis...
>
> Virgil, *Georgics*
>
> Est quaedam Proarche, regalis, proanennoetos, proanhypostatos virtus, procylindomene. Cum illa autem est virtus, quam ego cucurbitam voco: cum hac cucurbita autem est virtus quam et ipsam voco perinane. Haec cucurbita et perinane, cum sint unum, emiserunt, cum non emisissent, fructum, in omnibus visibilem, manducabilem, et dulcem, quem fructum sermo cucumerem vocat. Cum hoc cucumere est virtus eiusdem potestatis ei, quam et ipsam peponem voco. Hae virtutes, cucurbita et perinane, et cucumis et pepo, emiserunt reliquam multitudinem Valentini deliriosorum peponum.
>
> Interpres Irenaei, *Adversus haereses*

The family *Cucurbitaceae*, of the order *Cucurbitales*, comprises more than ninety genera and 700–900 species. This study will deal primarily with some well-known cucurbits such as cucumber (*Cucumis sativus*), melon (*Cucumis melo*), watermelon (*Citrullus lanatus*, formerly *Citrullus vulgaris*), pumpkin (*Cucurbita pepo* and *Cucurbita maxima*), gourd (*Cucurbita pepo* and *Cucurbita ficifolia*) and calabash (*Lagenaria siceraria*); but often our arguments concerning these are extendable by analogy to other cucurbits. It should also be remembered that there is extreme confusion in the terminology both at present and during earlier

PART ONE: 'PREGNANT GOURDS' AND 'DELIRIOUS PUMPKINS'

periods of history.[1] The same species often has several names; or several species have the same name. The same name in different languages need not designate the same species; nor, obviously, do differing names in different languages guarantee that different plants are referred to.

The history of cucurbits in connection with human culture goes back at least several thousand years. Remains of cucurbits and numerous and detailed pictures have been found in ancient Egyptian sepulchres.[2]

The cucurbits are important to man for a variety of reasons. Some provide food: cucumbers, gherkins (*Cucumis anguria*), musk-melons, watermelons, pumpkins, squash (*Cucurbita mixta*), etc. Some serve as raw material in certain branches of industry or manufacture: sponges and cloths from *Luffa cylindrica* and *Luffa acutangula*, and particularly bottles, containers, floats, cutlery, rattles (and other types of musical instruments) from the *Lagenaria siceraria*.[3] Several varieties have been used as medical plants since antiquity (particularly the *Ecballium elaterium*). Some gourds, notably the *Cucurbita pepo*, are widely used in ornamental gardening, to cover stone walls or fences and to form roofs that provide shadow and shelter. Of the incidental uses of cucurbits one could mention their significance to archaeologists, who, for example, derive valuable information from the remains of household gourds.[4]

In the history of art cucurbits are enormously important. There are few plants that can compete with them although, of course, the grape-vine has a lead because of its connection with alcohol and intoxication.[5] Cucurbits are found in literature, in the myths, in pictorial art and in ornamental gardening. In order to understand their semiotic role in literature one must study the anatomy of the plant on the one hand, and cucurbitic tradition on the other.

It is hardly surprising that man should be fascinated by this plant. The life of cucurbits is spectacular. From a small seed they grow in an exceedingly short time to a decorative plant with enormous fruit.[6] The associations one should look for first of all would then be associations with summer, sunshine, wellbeing, vitality, fertility, rejuvenation, luxury and abundance.

The cucurbits are tropical plants, requiring warmth and humidity to thrive and develop. Thus in the temperate zones of the earth, where summer is something precious, the cucurbits acquire positive connotations from being associated with the summer season. Cucurbits symbolize the best of summer: warmth, peace and rural life. That melons are dependent on honeybees for their pollination ties this species to

PART ONE: 'PREGNANT GOURDS' AND 'DELIRIOUS PUMPKINS'

another summer motif – the life of insects who gather nectar and produce honey, a theme that has fascinated man since antiquity.

In the northern countries of Europe it is a common habit among amateur gardeners to plant a pumpkin on the compost heap of their garden in the spring. The warmth of the rotting compost gives the plant the good start it needs (all cucurbits require a warm soil) and the explosive growth of the vines, leaves and fruit covers the least attractive spot in the garden. But the fruit of the pumpkin is not particularly savoury and maybe in the act of planting the pumpkin there is a ritual element, a gesture in recognition of summer, rejuvenation and fertility. In that case the act of doing homage to life at the same time takes death into account, since the pumpkin grows on the compost heap. On the rotting remains of last year's life new life grows, and thus the eternal cycle of life and death is symbolized. Since cucurbits grow so fast and die so easily (none can tolerate frost) they are symbolic in that they stand for an acceleration of the life cycle.[7]

The associations with wellbeing are of two kinds. One is the wellbeing that we know the dainty plant requires to produce its decorative vines and delicious fruit. Thus one finds expressions such as 'thrive like cucumbers in a frame'.[8] Second, we are also influenced by the idea of the wellbeing that the cucurbits offer our own tired senses: the lush green of the leaves, the delicious taste and smell of musk-melons, the cool refreshing watermelon, taken from the shadow and eaten to quench one's thirst on a hot day, the shadow of the gourd foliage on a fence or a roof. When Eve in Milton's *Paradise Lost*, 5.326-9, wants to offer her angel guest the very best that earth can produce (in order to show that God has bestowed his bounties on Earth as well as in Heaven) she goes to pick the 'juiciest Gourd':[9]

> But I will haste and from each bough and break,
> Each plant & juiciest Gourd will pluck such choice
> To entertain our Angel guest, as hee
> Beholding shall confess that here on Earth
> God hath dispenst his bounties as in Heav'n.

Since the cucurbits, particularly the melon, are very delicious they are often found in literature in connection with gluttons and gourmands. Several Roman emperors (above all Clodius Albinus and Carinus) were very fond of cucurbits. This weakness became fatal for a Chinese emperor who was so partial to musk-melons that he actually died of over-eating them.[10]

Generally the connotations of melons have developed most markedly

PART ONE: 'PREGNANT GOURDS' AND 'DELIRIOUS PUMPKINS'

as a positive and approving sign of social status in the colder regions of the world. In these parts the cucurbits require the intensive care of growers with considerable knowledge of horticultural techniques and ample time to apply them. They are therefore seasonal, expensive and scarce, with all the symbolic development that a commodity with such characteristics usually goes through. They are regarded as something of a luxury and are grown not by people whose immediate concern is mere subsistence but by people with an abundance of leisure such as the rich, the endowed (monks), or those who command other people's time (the aristocracy). To go as high as we can in the social scale, apart from the emperors already mentioned, there is Tiberius, who, according to Columella and Pliny, was exceedingly fond of cucumbers. He put his cucumber cultures on wheels so as to be able to move them indoors during cold weather and thus have an uninterrupted supply of his favourite delicacy through the whole year.[11]

In tropical regions, where cucurbits are cheap and grow easily, part of the reason for a positive semiotic development in terms of class status is absent. Thus melons do not conjure up the same mental image to the southerner in the United States as to a Yankee. To grow melons in the climate of New England is if not a challenge at least an art, and as such is held in esteem and considered a fit occupation for anybody, without the potential danger to one's dignity that is sometimes thought to come from manual work. Poets have often grown melons, and the New Englanders are no exception. Hawthorne, we believe, grew melons. But the most famous melon-grower was certainly Henry David Thoreau, whose love of nature is well symbolized by his skill in growing them. He grew new varieties of melons and he kept an eye on children to prevent them from eating watermelons before they were ripe. On 29 August 1839 Thoreau gave one of the first of the melon parties that later became a social tradition in Concord, and to which everyone tried to secure an invitation.[12]

Some authors have used cucurbits to symbolize artistic creative power. In the poem 'Kurbitsmålning' (gourd painting) by the Swedish poet Karlfeldt, the plant symbolizes the work of art, the fruit of the artist's efforts.[13]

> Men se min kurbits,
> dess resning och snits!
> Allt högre den gror,
> blir kunglig och stor,
> en alla gurkornas gurka
> från landen där solen bor. [i]

PART ONE: 'PREGNANT GOURDS' AND 'DELIRIOUS PUMPKINS'

The poem includes several familiar elements: the reference to sunshine, the rise of the *kurbits* (with symbolic overtones ranging from ambition to power), the size. But when Karlfeldt improves on the idea of royal ('kunglig') - the pumpkin is commonly regarded as the king of the garden — and uses a *Verstärkungsgenitiv* (the biblical construct state), in 'cucumber of cucumbers', the praise of artistic creative power verges on the burlesque. Nevertheless the poet, who takes his image from folk-painting, feels sympathy for the tradition and a strong sense of affinity with its artists.

In painting and other pictorial art cucurbits have as rich a history as in literature. They occur, for instance, in paintings on mythological themes of abundance.[14] Cucurbits suggest a paradisiacal opulence and a carefree existence, and in a painting aiming to present a picture of total rural bliss it helps to put in a few. Cucurbits go well with naked nymphs and chubby infants. If the cucurbits are not in the picture itself they are sometimes found in ornaments in the frame.[15]

That cucurbits symbolize opulence even in a concrete, pecuniary sense can be seen in the American expression 'to cut the melon', which means divide the loot.[16] In a growth of this image, if you get a bad deal in a sharing of something you 'get the rind'. It is no coincidence that Robert Browning in his poem 'Soliloquy of a Spanish Cloister' has his protagonist express his dissatisfaction, envy and hatred starting from the unfair division of a melon:[17]

> Oh, those melons? If he's able
>   We're to have a feast! so nice!
> One goes to the Abbot's table,
>   All of us get each a slice.
> How go on your flowers? None double?
>   Not one fruit-sort can you spy?
> Strange! – And I, too, at such trouble,
>   Keep them close-nipped on the sly!

That melons should undergo this development could be expected, but that pumpkins, whose taste is after all rather prosaic, should as well is more surprising. Naturally the size of the pumpkin fruit may contribute, since size means food value; cf. Leitch Ritchie (1833):[18]

> If at any time the garden vegetables were scarce, there was plenty of sorrel growing on the hills, and this, it is well known, is an excellent substitute: but indeed there was little risk of a truly rich man – that is, a propriétaire – being at a loss, since *a single pumpkin could furnish a forthnight's pottage.* [our italics]

PART ONE: 'PREGNANT GOURDS' AND 'DELIRIOUS PUMPKINS'

But another word that is persistently applied to pumpkins may hint at another aspect: 'gold'. Obviously it is the yellow colour of the pumpkin (and some other cucurbits, such as certain musk-melons) that is associated with gold; cf. the following example from *London Gazette* (1691): 'A piece of pure Gold in form of a Mellon'.[19]

But since fertility is the force that creates riches in a rural society, and most societies have a rural past, the reason for choosing the pumpkin may be double, yellow being associated with gold and the species being associated with fertility. The Franco-American word for dollar, *gourde*, is relevant in this context.[20]

Grapes and cucurbits (usually the melon or watermelon) fairly predictably occur at the top in any hierarchy of fruit.[21] Next one often finds figs – a fruit rich both in positive class connotations and in association with sex, particularly in connection with femaleness.[22] On the 'Isle of Fruits' in Tennyson's poem 'The Voyage of Maeldune', grapes, melons and figs occur in that order:[23]

> And we came to the Isle of Fruits: all round from the cliffs and the capes,
> Purple or amber, dangled a hundred fathom of grapes,
> And the warm melon lay like a little sun on the tawny sand,
> And the fig ran up from the beach and rioted over the land,
> [VI, ll. 54–8]

Later on come plums, pears etc. In symbolic passages in literature melons can also be antithetically contrasted with low-status fruit such as the banana.[24] In his book, *The White Pumpkin*, Denis Hills is somewhat disillusioned with Uganda, particularly after Idi Amin's *coup d'état*, and he expresses his feelings in fruit symbolism: 'Uganda has the banana; but grapes and melons do not grow here'.[25]

The ancient authors often dwelt on the positive connotations of cucurbits. The very names of the plants were thought to reveal vitality and fertility. Athenaeus mentions that 'Demetrius Ixion, in the first book of the "Etymologumena", says that the word σίκυος comes from σεύομαι (burst forth) and κίω (move), for it is a stimulating plant.' His statement is a significant testimony indicating how the plant was looked upon in his time.[26] Athenaeus also calls attention to the rapid growth of the plant: 'αὔξονταιδ᾽ ἐν τοῖς κήποις οἱ σίκυοι κατὰ τὰς πανσελήνους καὶ φανερὰν ἴσχουσι τὴν ἐπίδοσιν, καθάπερ καὶ οἱ θαλάττιοι ἐχῖνοι.'[27] [ii]

The growth of the cucumber plant is so extraordinarily fast that it really has no other worthy competitor than itself. Therefore it is possible to say, in a modern Greek proverb, that the cucumber plant has over-

PART ONE: 'PREGNANT GOURDS' AND 'DELIRIOUS PUMPKINS'

taken the cucumber fruit: '*ἔφτασε ἡ ἀγγουριὰ τ' ἀγγούρια*'.[28]

The growth of cucurbits is actually quite phenomenal. To be in a watermelon patch on a hot summer night in the tropics is a strange experience. The air is filled with whispers and noises; the melons grow not only visibly but audibly, creating noise as the vines creep over the ground. It seems that the Greeks used the vitality of cucurbits proverbially: '*ὑγιώτερόν θήν ἐστι κολοκύντας πολύ*[29]'[iii]. This, in our view, should be interpreted as meaning something very good, pumpkins being the best imaginable and the subject better still, i.e. better than the best.

Important evidence of the semiotic role of cucurbits can be found in such occurrences in literature where cucurbits are part of an antithesis or a juxtaposition of opposites. The lily for the Greeks was the flower of death. The proverbial juxtaposition '*ἢ κολοκύντη ἢ κρίνον*' (i.e. either a pumpkin or a lily) is preserved in fragments by the comic poets Diphilus and Menander.[30] Since the lily stands for death, the antonymic symbol, the pumpkin, must stand for life.

Tennyson contrasted lily ('lily-handed') and cucurbit in his poem 'The Princess' in order to convey the idea that the English upper class are so robust and healthy that the revolutions on the Continent cannot be repeated in England.[31]

> In such discourse we gained the garden rails,
> And there we saw Sir Walter where he stood,
> Before a tower of crimson holly-hoaks.
> Among six boys, head under head, and looked
> No little lily-handed Baronet he,
> A great broad-shouldered genial Englishman,
> A lord of fat prize-oxen and of sheep,
> A raiser of huge melons and of pine,
> A patron of some thirty charities,
> A pamphleteer on guano and on grain,
> A quarter-sessions chairman, abler none;
> Fair-haired and redder than a windy morn;

Assuming that cucurbits stand for luxury, fertility and abundance, it should be possible to predict the type of literary passages in which cucurbits are likely to appear. One such place is Numbers, Chapter 11. The Jews have been trekking through the Sinai Desert for ages and discontent flares up regularly. In Num. 11:5-6, the immediate source of discontent is the diet. Having eaten mostly the same food for forty years the Jews get sick and tired of manna for breakfast, lunch and dinner; and being in the sterile Sinai their thoughts antithetically

PART ONE: 'PREGNANT GOURDS' AND 'DELIRIOUS PUMPKINS'

go to the fertile Goshen, where the menu was more varied [NEB]:

> Will no one give us meat? Think of it! In Egypt
> we had fish for the asking, cucumbers and
> water-melons, leeks and onions and garlic. Now
> our throats are parched; there is nothing
> wherever we look except this manna.

Predictably, two cucurbits are introduced in the passage. Eating 'the bread of the angels' has become monotonous and the Jews recall the taste of the two primary dishes for the main course (meat and fish), nice desserts (cucumbers and melons) and spices (leeks, onions and garlic). Of course, one reason why these vegetables are mentioned is that, presumably, they were grown in Goshen; but this, although (possibly) a necessary explanation, is not a sufficient or exhaustive one, since one may assume that hundreds of plants were grown there. The additional, specific explanation is that cucumbers and melons had such a strong symbolic value in the semiotic fruit-lexicon of the people who were to read the text that they were symbolically appropriate. It was precisely the longing for those things symbolized by melons and cucumbers that Moses had to combat if he was ever to lead the Jews to their destination, since those are the products of a stationary life, and to give in to one's longing for them could have led to being stuck in the Sinai for ever.

Another antithetical relationship may be found in the story of an early Christian hermit who hung a tempting cucumber in front of himself.[32] What is the monk castigating? His gluttonous desire for a fruit which, with its 98 per cent water content, must be a delicacy in the desert? Certainly, but the monk, living his celibate, sterile life in the sterile wilderness, uses a memento that is the symbol of fertility. Perhaps the monk is also reminding himself of his chastity vow, and the cucumber is a visual instrument to conquer his lust.[33]

Throughout history melons are often associated with monks. The explanations for this could be several. The monks were learned and had the necessary knowledge and horticultural skill; they had the necessary time, and perhaps the inclination, since monks as gourmands is a popular cliché. But one should not rule out the possibility that the preoccupation with a plant that is so closely connected with reproduction is some kind of harmless vicarious compensation for the sacrifice of their own reproductive role.

The symbolism of Num. 11:5, and of a passage in Jonah which we shall return to later, may have served as a model for later writers,

PART ONE: 'PREGNANT GOURDS' AND 'DELIRIOUS PUMPKINS'

influencing the development of stock expressions that illustrate the contrast barren-fertile. A typical case is Petter Dass, a prominent Norwegian baroque poet and a parish pastor in the unfruitful Nordland. In *Nordlands Trompet* he invites his countrymen to a dinner party (an allegory for the reading of his poem, which is a description of northern Norway). The poet tells his guests not to expect 'Peponer' or similar fare. In a device typical of baroque literature, he extends the antithesis from a mere rhetorical device to a basic principle which structures the entire opening poem.[34]

One of the most conspicuous examples of the cucurbit representing abundance and fertility is given by Virgil, in *Georgics* IV, in the vivid praise of gardens and gardening. The poem is an optimistic poetic vision of the times to come: of rebirth, peace and fertility. It is the Augustan concept of 'the golden age'. After stating that he will sing about 'rich gardens' and 'twice-blooming Paestum', Virgil incarnates the idea of fertility in the shape of a cucurbit (vv. 121-2): 'tortusque per herbam/cresceret in ventrem cucumis. . . .' [iv]The commentators (including Servius), in interpreting this passage, have tried to determine 'to which species this *cucumis* belongs'.[35] However, the question here is not of *Cucumis melo* or *Cucumis sativus*, but of a fruit swelling of fertility – though Conington is of course right in explaining that 'Virgil does not talk of growing the *cucumis* amid the grass, but it is spreading so far from the place where the root is, as to ramble anywhere beyond bounds.'[36] Propertius' *Elegiae* IV.2.43 has often been cited as a parallel to this passage – 'caeruleus cucumis tumidoque cucurbita ventre' – but even closer is *Moretum* 78 (in the *Appendix Vergiliana*): 'et gravis in latum demissa cucurbita ventrem'. To say that the cucurbit in these contexts represents abundant nature is, however, in our opinion only half the truth. Virgil does not say that the cucurbit develops a round shape like that of a belly.[37] He says: 'It swells into a belly'. The pregnancy connotation is evident.[38] Livy uses the expression 'ventrem ferre' (I.34.3), i.e. to be pregnant. Ovid (*Met.* XI.311), by the expression 'maturus venter', denotes the unborn child. In *Moretum*, directly modelled on the Virgilian passage, the case is even clearer. Like 'venter', 'gravis' is also ambiguous. The equation of 'gravis' with 'gravida' is common.[39]

That this deeper implication has not always been missed is evident from the history of the transmission of the text. We may imagine the associations of the medieval copyist who emended 'ventrem' to 'Venerem'.[40] The conclusion suggests itself: The fruit's bulging shape and the

PART ONE: 'PREGNANT GOURDS' AND 'DELIRIOUS PUMPKINS'

general concept of cucurbitic lushness together relate the cucurbit not only to fertility, but to the female sex.

Pliny provides direct support here. In book XX.3.6 he states: 'putant conceptus adiuvari adalligato semine (cucumeris), si terram non adtigerit'. [v] The fertility symbolism in this usage is blatant. As the cucumber seed longs to be planted in the earth and grow and produce fruit, so the body of the woman will analogically long for conception. Columella, in book XI.3.50, warns that 'custodiendum est, ut quam minime ad eum locum, in quo vel cucumeres vel cucurbitae consitae sunt, mulier admittatur. Nam fere contactu eius languescunt incrementa virentium. Si vero etiam in menstruis fuerit, visu quoque suo novellos fetus necabit.' [vi] Not only by touching, but even by looking at cucurbit patches will a woman attract all of its fertile potentiality. That her periods of menstruation are especially dangerous comes as no surprise.

A presumably not uncommon medieval sense of the word 'cucurbitare' (and correspondingly 'cucurbita', 'cucurbitatio') throws some bright light on this relation to femininity. DuCange's *Glossarium Mediae et Infimae Latinitatis* (1678)[41] provides us with the following information: 'cucurbitare, uxorem alterius adulterio polluere; proprie de vasallo, qui domini uxorem adulterio polluit, et eius ventrem instar cucurbitae inflat, i.e. impraegnat'. [vii] On this usage DuCange gives references to medieval legislation and didactic literature, proving that it was not restricted to slang.[42] Do we not dimly see 'Peter, Peter, pumpkin-eater' looming not too far off on the horizon?

The comic poet Theopompus in one of his plays used the word melon to describe a beloved woman who is softer than a melon: 'μαλθακωτέρα πέπονος σικυοῦ μοι γέγονε'.[43] [viii] Cf. also G.F. Ruxton: 'Afore I left the settlements I know'd a white gal, and she was some pumpkins. I have never seed nothing as 'ould beat her. Red blood won't 'shine' any way you fix it. . . .'[44] When a girl in Ben Jonson's *Volpone* is 'lustie and full of juice', the epithet echoes a long adjectival tradition which still continues.[45]

In this context we may also mention the Greek proverb quoted by Athenaeus: 'σικυὸν τρώγουσα, γύναι, τὴν χλαῖναν ὕφαινε'.[46] [ix] We would imagine that the proverb manifests a spirit that might nowadays be described as male chauvinist. The sense of the proverb is probably that a woman should stick to a woman's tasks, i.e. childbearing, symbolized by the cucumber, and household work, represented by the weaving. Weaving is used in a similar sense in Aristophanes' *Lysistrata*

PART ONE: 'PREGNANT GOURDS' AND 'DELIRIOUS PUMPKINS'

586. The proverb again testifies to the connection cucumber–woman.

The Virgilian passage with its Augustan parallels standardized the rhetorical cliché of 'locus amoenus', a well-known topos in medieval literature. The cucurbit does not, however, seem to be a stock ingredient in these miniature garden paradises, either in antiquity or in the Middle Ages. Therefore, when Priapus, the phallic garden-god of fertility, specifically brings forth cucurbits as representatives of his garden and says 'cucurbitarum ligneus vocor custos' [x], his statement becomes ambiguous and may well be interpreted as a pun.[47]

However that may be, the Carolingian poet Walafrid Strabo's poem *Hortulus* yields first-class evidence that the plant was not forgotten altogether in the Middle Ages. Walafrid's poetic praise of the 'cucurbita' is something unique in literature.[48] He wrote his hexametric poem with both a real and a literary model: his own monastery garden (he was abbot in the monastery of Reichenau, an island in the Boden Sea), and the literary topos of garden praise. The poem abounds in classical allusions throughout and borrows in particular from the Augustans Virgil and Ovid.

What is remarkable about the poem is the prominent position given to cucurbits. Out of 444 verses altogether, 152 deal with 'cucurbita' and 29 with 'pepo'; i.e., cucurbits make up two-fifths of the whole poem. The 'cucurbita' is made the chief representative of the garden; its complex cucurbitic qualities make it serve as the embodied idea of the nature of gardens: peace, beauty, shadow, lushness.[49] The poem is no mere horticultural description. To Walafrid, the abbot, growth in nature also means spiritual growth. The symbolism becomes clear from the first line (vv. 99–100):

> 'Haud secus altipetax semente cucurbita vili
> assurgens, parmis foliorum suscitat umbras
> ingentes, ...' [xi]

The parallel to the parable of the Kingdom of Heaven and the insignificant mustard seed suggests itself.[50] 'Altipetax' suggests something more. The Carolingian Virgil links the 'cucurbita' to two other plants in this passage: the ivy and the vine. These plants have several botanic and symbolic traits in common. They are all trailing plants with tendrils, and need a tree or a prop to climb on. Thus all three by their inseparable clinging symbolize friendship.[51] But most importantly they all signify fertility, resurrection and eternity – not only because of their common feature, the spiralling, aspiring growth[52] – but because of the peculiar characteristics of each one. Ivy is evergreen and is usual both

PART ONE: 'PREGNANT GOURDS' AND 'DELIRIOUS PUMPKINS'

in weddings and in funerals; without the vine there would be no 'eau de vie'; and Jesus called himself 'the real vine'.[53] Even if the vine was also Dionysus' sacred plant, his thyrsus was wound with ivy, and thus the two plants have always been intimately related. However, Walafrid's 'altipetax' here overshadows both of them. We have reasons to believe that the poet combines two cucurbitic traditions: the tradition of fertility painted in Virgilian colours, and the Christian tradition originating from the Book of Jonah to which we shall return later. To Walafrid the cucurbitic tradition is not twofold, but a unity. The poem has sprung up from the nature of the plant and the poet's love for it with all its different aspects working together (vv. 126-7):

> Iam quis poma queat ramis pendentia passim
> mirari digne? [xii]

In this context we may also consider a problem of textual scholarship in Milton. The original printed text of *Paradise Lost,* book VIII, lines 320-1, reads: 'forth crept/The smelling Gourd, . . .' Richard Bentley, in an edition of the poem in 1732, changed 'smelling' to 'swelling'.[54] Other editions have variously printed 'swelling' or 'smelling', and among editors of annotated editions a controversy has arisen over the question whether 'swelling' should be accepted as a reasonable emendation or not.[55] We wish to make a contribution to this debate here, since an understanding of the lexicon-role of cucurbits in symbolism is relevant to the choice between 'smelling' and 'swelling'.

Bentley explains the reasons for his decision as follows:[56]

> V. 321. *Forth crept The* smelling *Gourd.*] A mere
> Mistake of the Printer: The Author gave it,
> > *Forth crept The swelling Gourd.*
>
> As Propertius;
> > *Caeruleus Cucumis,* tumidoque Cucurbita *ventre.*
>
> Those that stiffly maintain, that *smelling* was *Milton's* Word, and interpret it the *Melon,* seem not to attend that he had the Word *Smelling* two lines before, and would not have doubled it so soon again: and that he does not name here any particular Plant, but whole Tribes and Species; the Vine, the Gourd, the Reed, the Shrub, the Bush, the Tree. *Gourds* are as numerous a Family, as most of the other; and include the Melon within the general Name; which though it smells, it swells likewise.

Bentley's first point is the observation that smelling occurs two lines before and this favours the reading 'swelling'. One modern editor presents a diametrically opposite argument from the same fact:[57]

PART ONE: 'PREGNANT GOURDS' AND 'DELIRIOUS PUMPKINS'

> 321. *smelling*: emended by Bentley to swelling, but 'smelling sweet' occurs two lines above, and G. McColley notes, 'we have ... a pungently smelling gourd in the East Indian pepper of DuBartas'.

In our opinion the principles of textual criticism should in this case favour Bentley's line of argument. In the tradition in which Milton wrote, repetition was either avoided or used in a pointedly artistic way. In this passage there is no rhetorical reason for a repetition; thus the normal instinct to avoid repetition would be at work. It is not as if we needed to note that the word 'smelling' existed in Milton's vocabulary. Therefore the reference to the 'pungently smelling gourd in the East Indian pepper of Dubartas' is not relevant, because, if we wish to read 'smelling', the odorous species of the melon are much closer at hand than the East Indian pepper.

Bentley's second argument concerns the level of taxonomic abstraction, and he makes the important point that Milton mentions wide generic names rather than particular: vine, gourd, reed, shrub, bush, tree. 'Swelling' is an adjective of the whole gourd family, whereas 'smelling' is not. 'Smelling' here almost has a tinge of a contrastive epithet, 'the smelling gourd [as distinguished from other gourds]', which is totally inappropriate in the context. (In botanical modern Latin nomenclature smell is one of the characteristics whereby varieties of melons are distinguished from each other.) All the other adjectives in the passage are such as could be typically applied to their entire class.

Further, we may add that the passage is about *action*, and that 'smelling' would be too weak, whereas 'swelling' is entirely appropriate.

> Forth flourish't thick the clustering Vine, forth crept
> The smelling Gourd, up stood the cornie Reed
> Embattell'd in her field: ...

Each of the three sentences begins with an adverb denoting direction of movement, continues with a verb (the predicate) and ends with a noun (the subject). The subject is characterized by some generic epithet – the vine is thick and clustering, the gourd is swelling, the reed is corny – and, by extension, the vine is flourishing, the gourd creeping, the reed standing (upright). The verb 'swell' is much more in keeping with the character of 'flourish', 'cluster', 'creep' and 'stand up' than is 'smell'.

Of classical parallels Bentley mentions Propertius. But, as other commentators have noted, Virgil is even more important, and against the background of our discussion of Virgil above we submit that Milton's line is directly modelled on Virgil's passage in the *Georgics*.

PART ONE: 'PREGNANT GOURDS' AND 'DELIRIOUS PUMPKINS'

In exactly the same way, in both poets, two characteristics of the plant, creeping and swelling, are curiously telescoped so that they refer primarily to the plant as a whole, though one of them (creeping, *torquere*) is primarily a characteristic of the vine and the other (swelling, *crescere*) is a characteristic of the fruit (although both in Virgil and in Milton *torquere* and 'creeping' respectively are ambiguously referable both to the fruit and the whole plant). The subject of the corresponding passages in the *Georgics* and *Paradise Lost* is the same. There are numerous other allusions or parallels specifically to the *Georgics* elsewhere in Milton's poem.

Finally, we may note that the subject at this point in *Paradise Lost* is the Creation (cucurbits occur regularly in cosmogonies; in Burmese and Laotian mythology the creation of man started from a cucurbit[58]), and the specific function of the passage where the gourd occurs is the fertility and abundance of the world after the latest stage of God's creation compared with the as-yet barren land of the situation immediately before.

> *He scarce had said, when the bare Earth, till then*
> *Desert and bare, unsightly, unadorn'd,*
> Brought forth the tender Grass, whose verdure clad
> Her Universal Face with pleasant green,
> Then Herbs of every leaf, that sudden flour'd,
> Op'ning their various colours, and made gay
> Her bosom smelling sweet: and these scarce blown,
> Forth flourish't thick the clustering Vine, forth crept
> The smelling Gourd; . . . [our italics]

In the antithetical contrast to the previous barrenness it would be bad semiotic economy to assign the role of smelling to the gourd when there are available for the purpose herbs, flowering, of various colours, which are far better at smelling than the gourd and have just been mentioned as making gay her bosom smelling sweet.

Against the background of this our decided opinion is that Bentley's emendation should be accepted, and 'smelling' considered an error by the compositor. And indeed, it is a common error among compositors to substitute for a word a similar word that occurs two lines previously.

Since the cucurbits are such distinguished fruit, one could expect them to play a part in the ritual life of societies. Certainly harvest feasts are enhanced if cucurbits are included in the range of produce displayed. There is, for example, a suspiciously large number of pumpkin societies in Oxfordshire compared with clubs dedicated to competition in growing other plants.[59] The Oxford English Dictionary (OED) defines

PART ONE: 'PREGNANT GOURDS' AND 'DELIRIOUS PUMPKINS'

a melon feast as 'a rustic gathering at which prizes were offered for the finest melons' and cites an example from 1826, but the phenomenon is probably far older than that.[60] In America pumpkin pie is considered especially appropriate on Thanksgiving day; cf. Whittier, 'The Pumpkin', 1844: 'Ah! on Thanksgiving day, . . . What calls back the past, like the rich Pumpkin pie?'[61] The Fête du Potiron (Festival of King Pumpkin) used to be celebrated in the Halles Centrales in Paris in September. A large pumpkin, decked out as a king, was carried about and all made obeisance. Of the elements of this rite the idea of the pumpkin as king may have its origin in an idea of the grotesque and absurd; or it may be in keeping with the pattern of other fertility rites; or it may be a dramatization of the name of the pumpkin – the idea that cucurbits are the leading produce of a garden. In China the pumpkin, symbol of fruitfulness, health and gain, is called the 'Emperor of the Garden'.[62]

To Benjamin Tompson (1676), opposing the imposition of royal authority in New England, and lamenting the earlier days of lost simplicity in true classical Roman strains, the pumpkin is more than a king; it is a saint:[63]

> The times wherein old *Pompion* was a Saint,
> When men far'd hardly yet without complaint
> On vilest *Cates*; the dainty *Indian Maize*
> Was eat with *Clamp-shells* out of wooden Trayes
> Under thatcht *Hutts* without the cry of *Rent*,
> And the best *Sawce* to every Dish, Content.

If your ideal is simplicity, as was the case with Tompson in 1676, and you want to elevate and do homage to it, you must choose a suitable symbol of noble simplicity; the pumpkin. Parallel to the development away from simplicity towards artifice has been the decline in the status of the pumpkin – it is no longer a saint, but a term of abuse.[64]

It is necessary to be aware of the positive connotations of the cucurbits in order to understand the vehement controversy that has long raged over the translation of Jonah 4:6. Which plant was it that grew up and gave Jonah shelter? Was it a cucurbit? By now the debate is so old that the English Revised Standard Version has resigned and translates the word as 'plant', leaving speculation to a footnote:[65]

> And the LORD god appointed a plant[b], and made it come up over Jonah, that it might be a shade over his head, to save him from discomfort. So Jonah was exceedingly glad because of the plant.[b]
>
> [The footnote]: [b]Heb. *qiqayon*, probably *the castor oil plant*.

PART ONE: 'PREGNANT GOURDS' AND 'DELIRIOUS PUMPKINS'

To this oriental 'plant', in Hebrew ק׳קיון, translators have had difficulties finding a more European equivalent. The Septuagint uses the word κολοκύντη, and this served as a model for the early Latin translations which have the corresponding Latin: 'cucurbita'. But in the Vulgate St Jerome replaces cucurbita with 'hedera': 'Et praeparavit Dominus Deus hederam, et ascendit super caput Ionae, ut esset umbra super caput eius, et protegeret eum (laboraverat enim); et laetatus est Ionas super hedera laetitia magna.' This met with strong protest, and thus soon after, in the *Commentarii in Ionam*,[66] St Jerome has to defend his decision:

> In hoc loco quidam Cantherius de antiquissimo genere Corneliorum, sive, ut ipse iactat, de stirpe Asinii Pollionis dudum Romae dicitur me accusasse sacrilegii, quod pro cucurbita hederam transtulerim: timuit videlicet, ne si pro cucurbitis hederae nascerentur, unde occulte et tenebrose biberet, non haberet. [xiii]

Some years later he is also attacked by St Augustine, who begs him not to follow the Hebrew in translating the Old Testament. St Augustine's attack is backed by vivid illustration of the violent feelings the problem gave rise to. He tells the story of an African parish that was scandalized and almost broken up when the bishop read the prophet Jonah in Jerome's new version. When the bishop reached the word *hedera* in the last chapter, the people rose and shouted *cucurbita,* and finally the bishop had to give in and return to the old translation. Jerome replied:[67]

> Super qua re in commentario Ionae prophetae plenius respondimus hoc tantum nunc dixisse contenti, quod in eo loco, ubi septuaginta interpretes 'cucurbitam' et Aquila cum reliquis 'hederam' transtulerunt, id est ק׳קיון, in Hebraeo volumine 'ciceion' scriptum habet, quam vulgo Syri 'ciceiam' vocant; est autem genus virgulti lata habens folia in modum pampini, cumque plantatum fuerit, cito consurgit in arbusculam absque ullis calamorum et hastilium adminiculis, quibus et cucurbitae et hederae indigent, suo trunco se sustinens. Hoc ergo verbum de verbo edisserens si 'ciceion' transferre voluissem, nullus intellegeret, si 'cucurbitam', id dicerem, quod in Hebraico non habetur; 'hederam' posui, ut ceteris interpretibus consentirem. [xiv]

As the debate raged back and forth St Jerome took advantage of the situation to play on another connotation of the word 'cucurbita' or κολοκύντη, i.e. stupidity, and hint at the idea that anyone who is such a fanatic supporter of cucurbitae must be a pumpkin-head himself.[68]

The debate on this lower level, however, was carried on not only by St Jerome but by his adversaries as well. Rufinus, in the *Apologia contra Hieronymum*, asks whether we should now go down into the

PART ONE: 'PREGNANT GOURDS' AND 'DELIRIOUS PUMPKINS'

graves and inform the dead of the changes, all according to the latest whims of the law-giving translator:[69]

> Modo ergo nobis post quadringentos annos legis veritas empta pretio de synagoga procedit. Posteaquam senuit mundus et cuncta perurguentur ad finem, scribamus etiam in sepulchris veterum, ut sciant et ipsi qui hic aliter legerant, quia Ionas non habuit umbram cucurbitae sed hederae; et iterum, cum voluerit legislator, nec hederae, sed alterius virgulti. [xv]

To understand the context of Rufinus' comment we must note that Jonah and the fish and Jonah under the plant were two of the most popular motives in early Christian art.[70] The problem of the representation of the plant in the sepulchres, which was raised by Rufinus in a spirit of mockery, turned out to be a real one. Evidently the learned debate confused the artists to such a degree that they tried not only both 'cucurbita' and 'hedera', but even some bastard versions – ivy leaves with cucurbita fruit[71] – but it is worth noting that for a long time after the Vulgate came into use the plant still appeared as the old cucurbit with large leaves and bottle-shaped fruit hanging down, an interpretation supporting the Septuagint and the Vetus Latina versions.

This violent resistance against the new translation cannot be explained as mere conservative stubbornness alone. The text itself gives excellent evidence of this. Jerome did not only change 'cucurbita' to 'hedera'; he also made another change. The old version(s), and thus the Septuagint, all gave the inhabitants of Niniveh a period of three days before the destruction. Jerome followed the Hebrew and gave forty. No one, so far as we know, took any sort of notice of this discrepancy. But to the 'cucurbita versus hedera' issue people reacted, and reacted very strongly. It is clear that to a certain cast of mind there were factors involved that made only the cucurbit acceptable. With the aid of the examples of cucurbit connotations mentioned above we may make a guess as to why the cucurbit was preferred by some people.

We have already seen that cucurbits are characterized by their rapid growth and sudden death. In Jonah the plant grows in a day and dies the next. It is therefore, as we have already noted, the epitome of the life cycle, a highlighting of vitality and death, and is easily equated with life itself.

Why, as a textual unit, is the plant there in Jonah in the first place? To answer this we must look at the larger context of the whole episode. Jonah has been sent to Niniveh to tell the inhabitants that, because of their sinful way of life, destruction will be upon them in forty days. On hearing this, however, the inhabitants of Niniveh regret their

PART ONE: 'PREGNANT GOURDS' AND 'DELIRIOUS PUMPKINS'

sins, lament and do penance; and seeing this, God in turn repents and decides to spare them. Though this should not concern Jonah, he is a little disposed to sulk. The reason for his moroseness is the crucial theological question of the book. In any case it seems obvious that Jonah feels deluded. To Jonah the inhabitants' repentance comes as an anticlimax.

This is where the plant comes in. God lets it grow and Jonah is 'delighted with a great delight', if we may imitate the figure of the Hebrew and the Vulgate. Then the Lord lets it die and Jonah is sorry. At this point Jonah is ripe for the moral lesson which God teaches him with the use of a parallel or analogy.

What the exact allegorical meaning of the text is is difficult to make out, but one could guess at something like the following. When the plant thrives, Jonah is happy. When it withers, Jonah feels depressed; he is 'dead'. 'In the same way,' God says, 'I am happy when my creatures prosper, and when they perish I feel depressed.'

Thus the plant is employed as a symbolic device to teach a lesson about mercy and the saving of life. Doubtless this could be one reason why some translators preferred κολοκύντη or 'cucurbita'. The seventy were in this case concerned with Language in a wide sense, including the 'fictional language' of a 'grammar of symbols'. They translated, like King Alfred, sometimes word by word and sometimes according to the sense; and apparently in this case it was their opinion that the idiomatic sense of the passage demanded κολοκύντη. Though St Jerome was not anti-allegorical, he was also interested in accuracy (he follows the original), and possibly even in geography. One of his reasons for choosing 'hedera' may have been that hedera is a familiar European plant whereas qiqayon is not. Jerome himself states in his commentary (loc.cit.) that 'sermo Latinus hanc speciem arboris non habebat'. But the philosophy of translation that 'translates' phenomena geographically has always been controversial. In replacing a foreign phenomenon (a thing, a plant, a deity) with a native one you can make any number of mistakes. In exchanging 'cucurbita' for 'hedera' Jerome shed most of the symbol value that the Septuagint and Vetus Latina translation had had. It is difficult to assess the original symbolic potential of 'qiqayon', but in a European context the qiqayon was hardly symbolic at all. Even though he does not say so himself, Jerome's reason for choosing 'hedera' may have been that his theological disposition led his thoughts to the New Testament 'sign of Jonah', a sign of resurrection. The chief symbolic function of the

PART ONE: 'PREGNANT GOURDS' AND 'DELIRIOUS PUMPKINS'

evergreen ivy has always been to signify eternity. As Jonah was linked to Christ, the ivy would naturally be linked to Jonah.[72]

Two reasons for choosing cucurbita have been mentioned: the rapid growth and decay and the symbolic equation with life. A third reason may have been the connection between the idea of wellbeing and cucurbits. As we have seen a cucurbit is the perfect contrast to a desert. A shadow-casting, refreshing plant to 'save Jonah from discomfort' in the desert – certainly, if the choice were free, who would not pick the likeliest candidate: the cucurbit? [73]

As to the later history of the tradition it seems that both the cucurbita side and the hedera side got support from the Christian idea, which took Jonah to be a foreshadowing of Christ, who in turn is to bring universal renewal. Apparently the Christian concept favoured the use of cucurbita or hedera, but not the qiqayon, as a symbolic parallel to the hope for an eventual universal rebirth.[74]

Important and widespread texts influence the development of symbolic tradition. The Old Testament is such a text in the Jewish and Christian world, and the gourd passage in Jonah stabilized the role of gourd as symbol of something fast-growing and short-lived. Through the centuries authors invented new variations on the theme, using the Jonah passage as a model. These authors usually not only expected readers to understand the symbolism in the allusions but to be familiar with the model as well.

The Jonah tradition is rich.[75] To begin with, there are the translations, and though some have ivy or other translations of hedera, many have gourd.[76]

To symbolize fast growth the gourd in English competes with mushrooms. E.M. Clowes writes in 1911: 'I found myself receiving the odd impression that all the lodging-houses had sprung up, gourd-like, to their present proportions the very night after the lease had been signed.'[77] The Syrian Church Father Ephraem also seems to have used the plant proverbially: 'Youths have lately made themselves disciples; they have blossomed like Jonah's gourd.'[78] In Coleridge's translation of Schiller the image is used to depict the capriciousness of court favour:[79]

> [Countess:]
> Well now, what then? Duke Friedland is as others,
> A fire-new Noble, whom the war hath raised
> To price and currency, a Jonah's Gourd,
> An over-night creation of court-favour,

PART ONE: 'PREGNANT GOURDS' AND 'DELIRIOUS PUMPKINS'

> Which with an undistinguishable ease
> Makes Baron or makes Prince.

In Tennyson's 'The Princess' two cases of friendship are contrasted; one grows slowly but is real, whereas the fast growth of the other suggests that it will suffer the same destiny as Jonah's gourd - to grow quickly but die as quickly: (ll. 290-3; Ricks, p. 793):

> and thus a noble scheme
> Grew up from seed we two long since had sown;
> In us true growth, in her a Jonah's gourd,
> Up in one night and due to sudden sun:

The life of some insects is thought to be very short, sometimes only a day. Cucurbits are therefore mentioned together with these insects in cases where the author doubles his symbolism. But naturally an allusion to Jonah's gourd is usually sufficiently suggestive on its own:[80]

> who is so blind as not to see that the hand of the Almighty is upon Us, and that his Anger waxes hotter and hotter against Us? How have our hopes been blasted? how have our Expectations been disappointed? how have our ends been frustrated? All those pleasant Gourds, under which We were sometimes solacing and caressing our selves, how are they perish'd in a moment? how are they wither'd in a Night? how are they vanish'd, and come to nothing?

If you wish to depict destruction and death the most dramatic way is to show the *Vergänglichkeit* of the symbol of life itself, the cucurbit. This explains why the withered gourd is such a fitting image in literary works describing destruction and death, as in the following passage from Blake:[81]

> He chokes up the paths of the sky; the Moon is leprous as snow,
> Trembling & descending down, seeking to rest on high Mona,
> Scattering her leprous snows in flakes of disease over Albion.
> The Stars flee remote; the heaven is iron, the earth is sulphur,
> And all the mountains & hills shrink up like a withering gourd
> As the Senses of Men shrink together under the Knife of flint
> In the hands of Albion's Daughters. . . .

Since, on the one hand, the cucurbit is a symbol of life, and since blood, on the other, is the vital fluid of human beings, authors see the shedding of blood and the shedding of the juice of watermelons as analogous activities. See for instance William Styron's *Lie Down in Darkness*: 'A railroad trestle arched over the creek nearby, and long tables had been set up in its shadow: they sagged with food, and around them the juice from discarded melon rinds ran like blood in the sand.'[82]

Furthermore, since the melon is a symbol of life it follows that a destroyed melon becomes an appropriate symbol of destroyed life. In the final scene of *Lie Down in Darkness* Styron uses a melon rind to recall to mind the lost life of the female protagonist Peyton who has committed suicide (p. 400):

> La Ruth let the melon rind drop from her fingers and began to moan. 'I don't know,' she said, 'comin' around to thinkin' about all dat time an' ev'ything, po' Peyton, po' little Peyton. Gone! Gone!' She thrust her head in her hands and spread out her legs, snuffling into the wet sleeves of her robe. 'God knows, I don't know....'

In an article on Styron's literary technique, William J. Scheick argues, at length, that the action of dropping the melon rind 'contributes to Styron's rainbow motif and climactically illustrates his aesthetic practice' (p. 253):[83]

> Like the crumpled, brightly-colored Christmas wrapping in an earlier scene, the discarded melon rind, with its rainbow-like arc of colors, objectifies the beauty of fleeting loveliness intrinsic to the destruction of aspiration or hope – a fragile sail torn or collapsed by the wind, a kite caught in a tree, a bird entangled and flightless, a frozen moment of insight shattered by the resurgence of reality.... The novel is a rainbow of decay, crumpled Christmas wrapping, a discarded watermelon rind – a fleeting glimpse of the sadly beautiful ascent of human hope or aspiration in lives discarded, decaying, and crushed by the inevitable deluge that is the increasing dispersion of reality, both in man's mind and in the manifestation of that mind in such technological developments as the atomic bomb.

This is possible. Staying, however, for the moment within the realm of the demonstrable, it is obvious that the melon rind symbolizes Peyton's lost life. It occurs in the passage where La Ruth is overcome by grief thinking of Peyton's death. The action of dropping the rind is on the one hand, looking back, an epi-action to Peyton's killing herself, apparently by jumping from a height, when her own life has outlasted its meaningfulness to her; and it symbolizes simply 'loss of life'. Looking forward, La Ruth's action of dropping the melon rind symbolizes her final attempt to forget Peyton's death and take part in the rejoicing after the baptizing – at the end of the scene (the last paragraph of the novel) she repeatedly shouts that she has seen Jesus. She is supposed by the others to be finding comfort in the thought of Jesus and to be forgetting her grief. In this direction (pointing forward)

PART ONE: 'PREGNANT GOURDS' AND 'DELIRIOUS PUMPKINS'

the action of dropping the rind means La Ruth's attempt to forget Peyton's destroyed life (symbolized by the destroyed melon); i.e., Peyton has to die again when she dies in La Ruth's memory, and that ultimate death is also prefigured and symbolized by the dropping of the watermelon rind – the act has a dual symbolic function.

Apart from being a symbol of destroyed life the cucurbit also has other connotations here. There are the associations with sex – Peyton's problems were of that nature – and associations with the Negro; since watermelons, like 'chicken' (p. 399), are Negro food.

In Sembène Ousmane's novel, *Les bouts de bois de Dieu*, a passage in which a woman is killed compares her breasts to calabashes that have been left for too long in the sun during the hot season:[84]

> Houdia M'Baye n'eut pas la même présence d'esprit et le jet l'atteignit au visage et, tel le coup de point d'un géant, lui rejeta la tête en arrière. Elle ouvrit la bouche pour crier, l'eau s'y engouffra. Dans le giclement brutal on n'entend pas le petit bruit dérisoire des cartilages brisés. Houdia M'Baye battit des bras comme pour s'accrocher à l'air ainsi que font les noyés, puis ses mains s'agrippèrent à sa camisole qu'elles déchirèrent, elle tomba sur le côté à moitié nue, ses maigres seins semblables à des gourdes oubliées au soleil pendant la saison chaude. [xvi]

Once the idea had been firmly connected with the plant it was possible for the image to grow and the meaning nevertheless remain, though the subject was extended to the fruit as in the last few examples. See also OUIDA's *Pascarèl*:[85]

> And the old King would speak sadly aright; for his name is almost emptiness, and his earth-swaying orb is but now an empty gourd in which the shrivelled beans of the world's spent pleasures are shaken in fruitless sport and sound.

In this image the writer has gained more associations by transferring interest from the vine to the dried calabash fruit: first the idea of emptiness and shrinkage, and second the associations with rattles, which as instruments carry some ridiculous associations.[86]

In the following example from 1660, there is almost more emphasis on sudden death than on fast growth: 'Yet we have lived to see many *short-lived Gourd-Lords*, created in a chaos of times from very small principles or pre-existency of birth....'[87]

In the light of this tradition, and assuming that the dictionary entries on Franco-American 'gourde' are reliable, we can assess the full significance of the expression. In addition to the symbolization of

PART ONE: 'PREGNANT GOURDS' AND 'DELIRIOUS PUMPKINS'

abundance and the green colour of the paper dollar bill, there is a third reason for 'gourde'. The saying 'easy come, easy go' is used about money in several European languages. It seems obvious that there is a similar allusion to the short-lived joy of the possession of easily earned money in the Louisiana expression. The reasons for the use of the word 'gourde' should not be looked for only in the connotations of the cucurbit but also in the character of money. Money, like crime or sex, is a taboo subject, a thing that must be joked about and be referred to by humorous terms. Therefore many words for money, in various languages, contain phonetic features that are thought to be intrinsically funny. The explanation of the relation between cucurbits and money in the word 'gourde' is dependent not only on the positive connotations of the cucurbits, with which we have been concerned until now, but also on the negative or ridiculous connotations, to which we shall shortly proceed.

These two are not mutually exclusive, even though they are each other's opposites. What gourds and money share in particular is their paradoxical nature. Money can be associated with a sudden growth of riches, similar to the sudden growth of the gourd. But the history of the monetary system of the United States during past centuries is replete with instances of galloping inflation, worthless paper money (e.g. continentals), bank crashes and forgeries, which have made a lasting impression on the imagination of the Americans.[88] Thus the disasters connected with the history of money are as much part of its image as the cases of sudden success, and it may be that a green plant that grows quickly but dies as quickly is used in the word 'gourde' to hint at the worthlessness of greenback dollars and thereby indirectly of other kinds of money. But we think that the basic connotation is positive. Other cucurbits can also be used to symbolize money and this usually positively – even though jocosely.[89]

The cucurbits have not acquired only positive connotations. A semiotic development in the opposite direction has also taken place. To some people the vitality and fertility of the plant must have associated with something primitive, something they wished to repress in themselves and in society. Accordingly cucurbits have come to stand for anything close to nature; hence antithetical to urban culture and therefore fit to be despised.

The explosive growth of the cucurbits can easily become too much for the imagination. There may be a slightly surrealistic aspect to this growth, and instances abound where the growth is perceived as riotous.

PART ONE: 'PREGNANT GOURDS' AND 'DELIRIOUS PUMPKINS'

Cucurbit vines (like the beanstalk) often appear in fantastic tales of plants that run totally amok, engulfing everything in sight. There is a slight absurdity in a fruit that can grow to a weight of 100 kilos or more (*Cucurbita maxima*)[90] and a length of several metres (various cultivars of the *Lagenaria siceraria* and the *Cucumis melo*). Matron, in his *Parodies* says: 'καὶ σικυὸν εἶδον, γαίης ἐρικυδέος υἱόν,/κείμενον ἐν λαχάνοις· ὃ δ᾽ ἐπ᾽ ἐννέα κεῖτο τραπέζας'[91] [xvii] By using, in a totally new and inappropriate context, the same expression as Homer, who names the giant Tityus the real son of Earth, and by substituting cucumber for Tityus, the writer tips the sublime into the ridiculous, which has always been one of the favourite techniques of parodists.[92] The intrinsic symbolic properties of the cucurbits made him pick on a cucumber. We find this tendency again and again among parodists.

From the idea of riotous growth there is a short step to the idea of diseased or cancerous growth; and thus 'gourding' is a medical term for swellings, particularly in the legs of horses.[93] It is possible that the disease hydrocephalus has contributed to the development of the word 'pumpkin-head' (there is often a connection between cucurbits and water).[94]

Another aspect of the negative symbolic value of cucurbits is tied up with the idea of insensitivity. Pumpkins are seen as thick, insensitive and immovable. By extension the term can then be applied also to a person who shares these characteristics.

Insensitivity need not be entirely negative; a related idea could be self-control or self-possession, as in the expression 'cool as a cucumber', which is almost always a term of praise. Heat is associated with violence, movement, ardent feelings (heat makes even atoms move faster; coldness induces slowness and repose), whereas someone who is self-possessed or unaffected is cold, or 'cool'. But on a hot day the cucumber is also cool in the sense of refreshing, the fruit having stored water under its skin. Two senses of the word 'cool' thus coincide conveniently so that the associations mutually support one another.[95] But usually the basic sense is negative.

In Stephen Crane's short story, 'The Blue Hotel', when the Swede is murdered the author says the knife cuts his body as it would have a melon:[96]

> There was a great tumult, and then was seen a long blade in the hand of the gambler. It shot forward, and a human body, this citadel of virtue, wisdom, power was pierced as easily as if it had been a melon. The Swede fell with a cry of supreme astonishment.

PART ONE: 'PREGNANT GOURDS' AND 'DELIRIOUS PUMPKINS'

A melon, like a man, is a prominent example of life; but a melon is insensitive.

Actually, the very act of cutting a melon appeals to the imagination. In Mabbe's 1622 translation of Aleman's *The Rogve* one's thoughts are led to an image of fatalistic arbitrariness.[97]

> There are not wanting in *Rome* as good, and better ware than she, which may be had with lesse danger, at an easier rate, and giue your Lordship more content, and lesse trouble. I know not how it is with others, but my loue is not so feruent, as to loue for loue, but for fashion sake to laugh and be merry, and to make sport, as they vse to doe in my countrie. I am like a Melon-mongers Knife, cutting here a slice and there a slice, now at this corner, then at that, changing and altering my markes, rouing sometimes at one, sometimes at another, here to day (as they say) and to morrow in *France*. I take thought for nothing, nor am I wedded to my will in any thing, nor am I constant in my purposes, especially in matters of loue.

Pumpkin, in its negative use, can stand for the body of a stupid or conceited person; cf. Galt (1830): ' "If that ben't particular," replied he, "Squire Lawrie, I'm a pumpkin, and the pigs may do their damnest with me. But I ain't a pumpkin, the Squire he knows that".'[98] In the next example an insurgent captured by the authorities realizes that his body has become only an encumbrance. He decides to confess so as to be executed more quickly: 'Summary justice meanwhile was being dealt in Florence. Jacopo da Diacceto, on being put to the torture, unhesitatingly confessed: "I wish to rid myself of this pumpkin of a body: we intended to kill the Cardinal." '[99] But pumpkin can also stand for part of the body to suggest something negative about the usual function of that part.

Aristophanes uses pumpkins in such a sense in connection with eyes. In *The Clouds*, when Strepsiades cannot see what the philosopher sees in the sky, Socrates says: 'νῦν γέ τοι ἤδη καθορᾷς αὐτάς, εἰ μὴ λημᾷς κολοκύνταις'[100] [xviii]

The fatal resemblance of the human head[101] to a pumpkin is a fundamental cause of the expression 'pumpkin-headed', but is by no means the whole explanation. 'Wooden-headed', as in Ger. *Holzkopf*, Sw. *träskalle*, Fi. *puupää*, suggests stupidity through impenetrability – no ideas can get into a wooden head. But the opposite quality, softness, which would be close at hand in 'pumpkin-headed', is negative as well.

Another element at work in 'pumpkin-headed' is the idea of size.[102]

PART ONE: 'PREGNANT GOURDS' AND 'DELIRIOUS PUMPKINS'

Anything extreme arouses suspicion, and thus in American English you can express the same idea (stupidity) through an allusion to smallness ('pin-headed') or largeness ('pumpkin-headed'). In northern Europe one finds a saying 'big head, little sense', which suggests that the growth of the brains have not kept up with the growth of the skull. The standard retort, 'small head, no sense at all' is a parallel to the American idea in 'pin-headed'.

As to the growth of the brains not keeping pace with the growth of the skull, this gives rise also to another idea: 'hollowness', i.e. empty-headed, cf. Ger. *Hohlkopf*. In Swabia there is a saying: 'Der hat'n Kopf wie eine Kürbis, vornen sind Kerne und hinten is nix'.[103] The idea of the presence of the seeds within the empty shell is a great improvement because it provides a possibility of demonstrating audibly the emptiness of a vessel. Recall here the 'shrivelled beans' of the world's spent pleasure in an earlier quotation.

Calabashes being of the gourd family, and being used for musical instruments throughout history (the *OED* mentions rattles in America in 1624), the *Lagenaria siceraria* fruit provides the link that ties the symbolic aspects together. Calabash too is used for head: (*OED*) 'humorous name for the head'.

Various art forms such as painting and films sometimes take up a linguistic cliché and dramatize it. In his book *Language of Fiction*, David Lodge has commented on Henry James's method of 'heightening clichés'.[104] In the engravings of Hogarth, some verbal cliché is often expressed in pictorial terms. Such series as *Harlot's Progress* and *Industry and Idleness* can be 'read' in quite a verbal sense.

In the early cinema the process of communication between filmmaker and audience was seriously hampered by poor sound and the unnatural speed of movements. But also the theory was that everything should be twice as obvious as life; the ruling ideology was one of semiotic over-kill. Some of the memorable products of that era are heightenings of verbal clichés, and we submit here that one of the ideas the early movies dramatized was the word 'Kürbiskopf'. When the big Hardy shakes the small Laurel by the throat a rattling sound is heard (does not the same thing happen in Chaplin's early movies?) This is a heightening of the cliché *Kürbiskopf* - you know the head is empty, because you hear the rattling of the seeds. In addition Mr Laurel has a haircut that most people instinctively regard as funny. It is similar to the stump of a *Kürbis* (the haircut is a stock-in-trade of comic cartoonists, and it might not be too much to suggest that one can trace

PART ONE: 'PREGNANT GOURDS' AND 'DELIRIOUS PUMPKINS'

its roots to the idea of the cut-off stump of the stem of a vegetable).[105]

Pumpkin, melon and gourd may quite neutrally or only semi-humorously mean the head, as in the example: 'Nimm dich in acht, dass dir nicht etwas auf den Kürbis fällt.'[106] In slang the word 'head' can be replaced by the name of any vegetable or fruit. In P.G. Wodehouse's *Joy in the Morning*, 'head' is variously replaced by 'coconut' (pp. 158, 207), 'bean' (p. 243), 'nut' (p. 41), 'lemon' (p. 242) and 'pumpkin' (pp. 9, 20). But there is a clear gradation in the pejorative value of the different uses. Bean, coconut, nut and lemon are only jocose synonyms; but 'pumpkin-head' is reserved for the villain of the story, and it is only with pumpkin that the vegetable humour is connected with other humorous elements in the novel as in the following dialogue:[107]

> 'Was Nobby alone?'
> 'No, sir. There was a gentleman with her, who spoke as if he were acquainted with you. Miss Hopwood addressed him as Stilton.'
> 'Big chap?'
> 'Noticeably well developed, sir.'
> 'With a head like a pumpkin?'
> 'Yes, sir. There was a certain resemblance to the vegetable.'

The comedy depends on a contrast between the stilted language of the butler and the colloquial style of his employer. The biggest test of Jeeves's capacity for formality comes in the pumpkin passage, where, naturally, the tension is greatest and the humour best.

Apart from the fact that 'pumpkin' may carry the most negative connotations of all vegetables, we have to take into account, after all, that often the replacing of head with any vegetable is a pejorative substitution. The caricaturist Charles Philippon, who replaced the head of a French king, Louis-Philippe, with a pear, hardly did it to commend the royal intellect (note that a pear is calabash-shaped). There is a wealth of abusive words in many languages involving the idea of vegetable-heads; e.g., It. *testa di cavolo* (cabbage-head), head of *rapa* (turnip), *carciofo* (artichoke); Sw. *kålrot* (turnip); substandard metropolitan Finnish *pottupää* (potato-head; also used in American).

But cucurbits certainly do the best work after all: Ger. *Kürbiskopf*; Croatian *tvrda tikva*; Bulgarian likewise тиква or кратуна; It. *cocomero, zucca, zuccone, peponella, mellone, citrullo*; Fr. *melon, citrouille, gourde, cornichon*; Sp. *calabaza, sandio*.[108] In modern Greek there is a rather clear hierarchy, so that κολοκυϑοκέφελος (pumpkin-headed) is the most negative; καρπουζοκέφαλος (watermelon-headed) is slightly milder; and πεπονοκέφαλος (melon-headed) may even imply cleverness.

PART ONE: 'PREGNANT GOURDS' AND 'DELIRIOUS PUMPKINS'

If heads are likened to a cucurbit in a passage in which the author has no specific intention to hurt, the cucurbit is usually the melon:[109]

> One doubts if this tribal remnant of some 1,500 Teuso (they are also known as Ik), whose origins the anthropologists have not yet cleared up, will survive. One wonders for how long they will continue to squat round their tiny fires, eating baked tortoise, skinny, chattering, and cheerful, their small heads bunched together like black melons in the starlit nights.

In an early Greek example in Hermippus the idea is likewise primarily only a comparison, 'τὴν κεφαλὴν ὅσην ἔχει·/ὅσην κολοκύντηο'.[110] [xix] The subject is presumably merely the external aspect of Pericles' (?) head – not the internal qualities, or lack of them. But Hermippus is after all a comic poet, so the tendency is clear.

In the *Metamorphoses* Apuleius used the word 'cucurbita' twice. One of the passages, 'cucurbitae caput non habemus', has given rise to the assumption that the phrase was a Latin proverb.[111] The idea of the passage, one would assume, is simply stupidity. But one commentator argues that the association is with baldness.[112] It is of course correct that a pumpkin can associate with baldness.[113] Cf. Baker (1867):[114]

> Beating his own head and tearing his hair were always the safety valves of Mahomet's rage, but as hair is not of that mushroom growth that reappears in a night, he had patches upon his cranium as bald as a pumpkin shell, from the constant plucking, attendant upon losses of temper. . . .

The other passage in Apuleius, 'maritum cucurbita calviorem', obviously signifies a bald husband. But in the light of the evidence of the material collected in this study the interpretation of 'cucurbitae caput habere' as 'bald' seems far-fetched.

Tertullian provides two very interesting examples on the use of pumpkin. In *De Anima* he explicitly describes Empedocles as a 'pepo, tam insulsus', thus corroborating our present sense of the word in an interpretative comment.[115] The other example, a passage in *Adversus Marcionem*, on the incarnation, 'Cur autem panem corpus suum appellat, et non magis peponem, quem Marcion cordis loco habuit?' [xx] is significant, because it shows that one should not make too much of the connection between pumpkin and head, but rather, specifically, between pumpkin and intellect.[116] Marcion does not have a pumpkin for a head but a pumpkin for a heart; which is appropriate, if pumpkin is to signify stupidity, since not only the head but the heart was regarded as the seat of the intellect in antiquity.

PART ONE: 'PREGNANT GOURDS' AND 'DELIRIOUS PUMPKINS'

We already touched upon the idea of cucurbits and a swelling growth in connection with associations with pregnancy. But naturally it is not only childbearing that causes rotundity in persons. Cucurbits can also be associated with ordinary obesity. During a long period of history laboratory vessels were made of gourds.[117] Even after they began to be made of other materials they kept their name so that for instance in England in the sixteenth or seventeenth century you find phrases such as a gourd of glass or a gourd of iron. But they not only kept their name; like rattles and other musical instruments (the lute, for instance) and bottles, they also kept their shape. This is common cultural conservatism – for decades after the motorcar was introduced it looked like the horse-drawn vehicle. From 1600 we have this sentence in a chapter on distilling: 'the one of them is properly called the containing vessell, because it receiueth and containeth the matter that you would distill, some call it the body or corpulent vessel, or the gourd: . . .'[118] Corpulence is obviously also implied in the following example (1819): 'Her melon-formed head and double chin were lost in what she called a quimpe; . . .'[119] How else do you get double chins except by being fat, and again a cucurbit (melon) and bigness are coupled.[120] In a culture where slim is beautiful the symbolic value of cucurbits tends to develop in the negative direction. In a baroque culture, or any culture that likes swelling forms, the opposite is true. One should be able to find lots of cucurbits in the paintings of the colleagues of Rubens.

With the established negative content of cucurbits anything that is regarded as ridiculous magnetically attracts cucurbits. Crooked legs are ridiculous, and since the description of something ridiculous is aided if the descriptive epithets are ridiculous in their own right, we find expressions like the following in Washington Irving's *Salmagundi Papers* (1807):[121]

> Such breadth of nose, such exuberance of lip! his shins had the true cucumber curve, – his face in dancing shone like a kettle; and, provided you kept to windward of him in summer, I do not know a sweeter Youth in all Hayti than Tucky Squash.

In the following medical comment it is explicitly stated that the expression is a popular saying: 'Again, it has been supposed that the Negro races are characterised by that peculiar curved form of the bones of the leg, which gives rise to what is popularly designated as the "cucumber-shin;" also by. . . .'[122] A related idea can be found in the comic poet Plato:

PART ONE: 'PREGNANT GOURDS' AND 'DELIRIOUS PUMPKINS'

$$\text{οὐχ ὁρᾷς ὅτι}$$
$$\text{ὁ μὲν Λέαγρος, Γλαύκονος ὢν μεγάλου γένους,}$$
$$\text{ἀβελτεροκόκκυξ ἠλίθιος περιέρχεται}$$
$$\text{σικυοῦ πέπονος εὐνουχίου κνήμας ἔχων,}\ [\text{xxi}]$$

and Anaxilas: 'τὰ δὲ σφύρ' ᾦδει μᾶλλον ἢ σικυὸς πέπων.'[123] [xxii] We shall return below to the connection between Negroes and cucurbits, but first let us look at some exemplifications of cucurbitic stupidity.

In George Washington Harris' *Sut Lovingood's Yarns* there is one yarn, 'Blown Up With Soda', in which the narrator-character George fails to understand what Sut means with the phrase 'the huggin place':[124]

> 'She cudent crawl thru a whisky barrel wif bof heads stove out, nur sit in a common arm-cheer, while y cud lock the top hoop ove a chun, ur a big dorg collar, roun the huggin place.'
> 'The *what*, Sut?'
> 'The *wais*' yu durn oninishiated gourd, yu!'

Though one should not squeeze too much significance out of the fact that the field in which George shows a lack of initiation is love-making, the piece does fit the puzzle. The author is playing not only on the connotations of stupidity but, unconsciously at least, on the sex connotations as well.

A similar connection between 'pumpkin-headed' and another dumb animal, the sheep (cf., e.g., Sw. *fårskalle*) is found in Jerome K. Jerome's *Novel Notes* (1893): 'Surely as to a matter of this kind, I, a professed business man, must be able to form a sounder judgment than this poor pumpkin-headed lamb.'[125] The man referred to is professedly stupid and keeps asking the narrator for advice, which he gives, but which later always turns out to have been unsound.

There is something grotesque and absurd about pumpkins. When American children make preparations for Halloween they cut out a grotesque mask from a pumpkin shell. The witchcraft connected with Halloween originated in old heathen beliefs. The Celtic festival of Samhain was observed on 31 October and coincided with the Christian All Saints' Day. During that night the dead revisited their homes; the world was full of witches and sprites, and bonfires were lit on hilltops to scare the evil spirits away. The pumpkin shell mask no doubt served the same purpose. When a candle was put inside a pumpkin shell, making it a jack-o'-lantern masque, the two elements – fire and mask – were combined, and the effect was doubled.

One reason why pumpkins were used is of course that they are available at that time of the year (in Scotland turnips were substituted for the cucurbits) and that they are easy to cut (cf. Crane) but undoubtedly other cucurbitic characteristics – particularly their tremendous growth – also make them suitable for use in magic.[126] In the subconscious of American children pumpkins still stand for something grotesque.

After one has been alerted to the grotesque connotations of cucurbits it is not surprising to find that pumpkins occur in scholarly treatises on the grotesque as a literary mode (and particularly in the examples), as in Philip Thomson's book *The Grotesque*, where a pumpkin passage from Browning's *Caliban upon Setebos* is quoted in a discussion of the essential nature of the grotesque:[127]

> Will sprawl, now that the heat of day is best,
> Flat on his belly in the pit's much mire,
> With elbows wide, fists clenched to prop his chin.
> And, while he kicks both feet in the cool slush,
> And feels about his spine small eft-things course,
> Run in and out each arm, and make him laugh;
> And while above his head a pompion-plant,
> Coating the cave-top as a brow its eye,
> Creeps down to touch and tickle hair and beard,
> And now a flower drops with a bee inside,
> And now a fruit to snap at, catch and crunch....

Similarly predictable is the occurrence of cucurbits in nonsense literature. In the works of the British laureate of nonsense, Edward Lear, for instance, cucurbits figure extensively. For a sample let us take the opening stanza of 'The Courtship of the Yonghy-Bonghy-Bò':[128]

> On the Coast of Coromandel
> Where the early pumpkins blow,
> In the middle of the woods
>   Lived the Yonghy-Bonghy-Bò.
> Two old chairs, and half a candle, –
> One old jug without a handle, –
>   These were all his worldly goods:
>   In the middle of the woods,
>   These were all the worldly goods,
>   Of the Yonghy-Bonghy-Bò,
>   Of the Yonghy-Bonghy-Bò.

Apart from the humour, there is the predictable connection with courtship and later in the poem there are references to Yonghy's big head, etc. It is obvious that such 'nonsense' as this is not at all as devoid of sense as the label seems to claim.

PART ONE: 'PREGNANT GOURDS' AND 'DELIRIOUS PUMPKINS'

In some literary passages where cucurbits occur one gets the feeling that again antithesis is involved though this time cucurbits stand for the negative or ridiculous extreme. Wodehouse, in *Right Ho, Jeeves* (1934), writes:[129]

> An eerie stillness seemed to envelop the room like a linseed poultice. I happened to be biting on a slice of apple in my fruit salad at the moment, and it sounded as if Carnera had jumped off the top of the Eiffel Tower on to a cucumber frame.

Certainly cucumber frames qualify as noise-making apparatuses if fallen upon and thus one prerequisite for the role is taken care of, but there are many other things one could let someone jumping from the Eiffel Tower fall on to. Obviously the idea of the elevated (the Eiffel Tower is an absurdification of the idea of height through exaggeration) needed an antithetical extreme idea of the low, and cucumber frames are appropriate because cucurbits are bathetic (cf. the following example to suggest total boredom: Cowper, 1728):[130]

> *My dear Friend,* – Having thanked you for a barrel of very fine oysters, I should have nothing more to say, if I did not determine to say every thing that may happen to occur. The political world affords us no very agreeable subjects at present, nor am I sufficiently conversant with it to do justice to so magnificent a theme, if it did. A man that lives as I do, whose chief occupation, at this season of the year, is to walk ten times in a day from the fireside to his cucumber frame and back again, cannot show his wisdom more, if he has any wisdom to show, than by leaving the mysteries of government to the management of persons, in point of situation and information, much better qualified for the business.

In Browning's poem 'The Melon-Seller' the cucurbits play a role in an antithetical juxtaposition of high and low in terms of social class. The melon-seller is a former prime minister; i.e., he has fallen from a very prestigious position to a very low one.[131]

> *Going* his rounds one day in Ispahan, –
> Half-way on Dervishhood not wholly there, –
> Ferishtah, as he crossed a certain bridge,
> Came startled on a well-remembered face.
> 'Can it be? What, turned melon-seller – thou?
> Clad in such sordid garb, thy seat yon step
> Where dogs brush by thee and express contempt?
> Methinks, thy head-gear is some scooped-out gourd!
> Nay, sunk to slicing up, for readier sale,
> One fruit whereof the whole scarce feeds a swine?

PART ONE: 'PREGNANT GOURDS' AND 'DELIRIOUS PUMPKINS'

Wast thou the Shah's Prime Minister, men saw
Ride on his right-hand while a trumpet blew
And Persia hailed the Favourite? Yea, twelve years
Are past, I judge, since that transcendency,
And thou didst peculate and art abased;
No less, twelve years since, thou didst hold in hand
Persia, couldst halve and quarter, mince its pulp
As pleased thee, and distribute – melon-like –
Portions to whoso played the parasite,
Or suck – thyself – each juicy morsel. How
enormous thy abjection, – hell from heaven.
Made tenfold hell by contrast! Whisper me!
Dost thou curse God for granting twelve years' bliss
only to prove this day's the direr lot?'
Whereon the beggar raised a brow, once more
Luminous and imperial, from the rags.
'Fool, does thy folly think my foolishness
Dwells rather on the fact that God appoints
A day of woe to the unworthy one,
Than that the unworthy one, by God's award,
Tasted joy twelve years long? Or buy a slice,
Or go to school!'
     To school Ferishtah went;
And, schooling ended, passed from Ispahan
To Nishapur, that Elburz looks above
– Where they dig turquoise: there kept school himself,
The melon-seller's speech, his stock in trade.
Some say a certain Jew adduced the word
Out of their book, it sounds so much the same,
את־הטוב נקבל מאת האלהים
ואת־הרע לא נקבל: In Persian phrase,
'Shall we receive good at the hand of God
And evil not receive?' But great wits jump.

Wish no word unspoken, want no look away!
What if words were but mistake, and looks –
    too sudden, say!
Be unjust for once, Love! Bear it – well I may!

Do me justice always? Bid my heart – their shrine –
Render back its store of gifts, old looks and words of thine
– Oh, so all unjust – the less deserved, the
    more divine?

In the literary version of the folktale Cinderella, created by Perrault, the carriage that the good fairy supplies Cinderella with is created from a pumpkin. Tradition is strong and may account for much – pumpkin is a common means of transport among fairies (cf. Whittier, 'The

PART ONE: 'PREGNANT GOURDS' AND 'DELIRIOUS PUMPKINS'

Pumpkin', 1844: 'Telling tales of the fairy who travelled like steam,/In a pumpkin-shell coach, with two rats for her team!'[132]) – but there is also the idea of contrast. The magic of the transformation is enhanced when the transformation starts from the least changeable that Gallic and Anglo-Saxon minds can imagine – a pumpkin. The principle involved is the same as when you prefer to have kings as protagonists in tragedies, because, tragedies being stories of the fall of great men, and kings being the greatest of all men, it is best to have them because their fall will be greatest; or, when the Salvation Army calls forth the worst exrabble to testify, because the miracle of their conversion will be greater than that of a character who was well on his way to righteousness already.[133] One must also observe that the elevation of the lowly pumpkin to a splendid carriage is a parallel to the elevation of the humble Cinderella to the Prince's wife.

Maybe it is significant that the pumpkin grows on a vine like the grape. In Hawthorne's novel *The Scarlet Letter* a pumpkin is made symbolic of the whole poverty of puritan culture and the pumpkin is contrasted with more sophisticated European forms of ornamental gardening. Governor Bellingham's garden is described as follows:[134]

> Pearl, accordingly, ran to the bow-window, at the farther end of the hall, and looked along the vista of a garden-walk, carpeted with closely shaven grass, and bordered with some rude and immature attempt at shrubbery. But the proprietor appeared already to have relinquished, as hopeless, the effort to perpetuate on this side of the Atlantic, in the hard soil and amid the close struggle for subsistence, the native English taste for ornamental gardening. Cabbages grew in plain sight; and a pumpkin vine, rooted at some distance, had run across the intervening space, and deposited one of its gigantic products directly beneath the hall-window; as if to warn the Governor that this great lump of vegetable gold was as rich an ornament as New England earth would offer him.

The garden symbolizes both the material and spiritual poverty of the New World. The grass is cropped as close as the hair of the puritans, the 'attempt' at shrubbery is rude and immature, and cabbages – rude, prosaic and proletarian – are indecently visible.[135]

The word 'rich' is there in the text to suggest its opposite 'poor'. It is tied to the word 'gold' through the colour of the pumpkin; the phrase, 'this great lump of vegetable gold', contains mutually contradicting tendencies. The sound of 'lump' is unpleasant (coincides partially with pumpkin); a very valuable thing would not be described as a lump. The combination 'vegetable gold' is oxymoronic, vegetable

PART ONE: 'PREGNANT GOURDS' AND 'DELIRIOUS PUMPKINS'

being a negative word and gold a positive. Symbolic vines in the New World carry no riches. The passage brings out the absurdity of the picture in its tone and its choice of words, e.g. 'deposited' rather than 'left'.

Pumpkins and New England go together not only in the sense that strangers connect the two but also in the sense that New England seems fairly rich in pumpkin lore. The New England poet Whittier once wrote a poem called 'The Pumpkin'. It is full of clichés in the manner of many Victorian poems, and since it seems that Whittier tried to give as full a cucurbitic picture as possible (at least of the positive associations) we may quote the entire poem here as a demonstration of what connotations the word 'pumpkin' had for a cultured Yankee at the middle of the nineteenth century:[136]

> *O, Greenly* and fair in the lands of the sun,
> The vines of the gourd and the rich melon run,
> And the rock and the tree and the cottage enfold,
> With broad leaves all greenness and blossoms all gold,
> Like that which o'er Niniveh's prophet once grew,
> While he waited to know that his warning was true,
> And longed for the storm-cloud, and listened in vain
> For the rush of the whirlwind and red fire-rain.
>
> On the banks of the Xenil the dark Spanish maiden
> Comes up with the fruit of the tangled vine laden;
> And the Creole of Cuba laughs out to behold
> Through orange-leaves shining the broad spheres of gold;
> Yet with dearer delight from his home in the North,
> On the fields of his harvest the Yankee looks forth,
> Where crook-necks are coiling and yellow fruit shines,
> And the sun of September melts down on his vines.
>
> Ah, on Thanksgiving day, when from East and from West,
> From North and from South come the pilgrim and guest,
> When the gray-haired New-Englander sees round his board
> The old broken links of affection restored,
> When the care-wearied man seeks his mother once more,
> And the worn matron smiles where the girl smiled before,
> What moistens the lip and what brightens the eye?
> What calls back the past, like the rich Pumpkin pie?
>
> O, – fruit loved of boyhood! – the old days recalling,
> When wood-grates were purpling and brown nuts were falling!
> When wild, ugly faces we carved in its skin,
> Glaring out through the dark with a candle within!
> When we laughed round the corn-heap, with hearts all in tune
> Our chair a broad pumpkin, our lantern the moon,
> Telling tales of the fairy who travelled like steam,

PART ONE: 'PREGNANT GOURDS' AND 'DELIRIOUS PUMPKINS'

> In a pumpkin-shell coach, with two rats for her team!
> Then thanks for thy present! – none sweeter or better
> E'er smoked from an oven or circled a platter!
> Fairer hands never wrought at a pastry more fine,
> Brighter eyes never watched o'er its baking, than thine!
> And the prayer, which my mouth is too full to express,
> Swells my heart that thy shadow may never be less,
> That the days of thy lot may be lengthened below,
> And the fame of thy worth like a pumpkin-vine grow,
> And thy life be as sweet, and its last sunset sky
> Golden-tinted and fair as thy own Pumpkin pie!

That pumpkins are so closely connected with Yankees (the inhabitants of New England) in the minds of others is due to a number of circumstances. Pumpkins and melons have always been popular in New England, and pumpkin pie is a famous Yankee dish.[137] In ethnic vituperation it is common to give peoples names after what you take to be their staple diet; to call Italians 'spaghetti' and Germans 'Kraut'. When the southern alpine Germans call the northern Germans 'Kartoffeldeutschen' the pejorative sense is helped by the intrinsic low value of potato ('tater-eatin Irishmen' often suffer the same fate). But for particularly aggravating circumstances you should unmask your enemies as cabbage-eating or pumpkin-eating. Such abuse need not necessarily have any foundation in truth; it is just a convenient element to put into any string of invective, as in the following diatribe against a tailor who wants to be mayor: 'this cross-legged cabbage-eating son of a cucumber'.[138] Compound epithets, with '-eating' as the second part and 'pumpkin' (or 'cabbage') as the first are very popular in America. They are presumably favoured not only for semic but also for rhythmic reasons. In the following German example the ending is an adoneus: 'Das war der "principe tedesco" von dem man so viel hörte? Dieser langweilige, grosse, phlegmatische Kürbis?'[139] The ending need not be a hexameter ending, however; any sort of rhythm that highlights the last element will do, as long as a pumpkin is included and the last element carries some weight – cf. Haliburton (1835–40): 'They ain't got two ideas to bless themselves with – the stupid, punkin-headed, consaited blockheads!'[140] The Americans are particularly fond of this kind of rhythmic stringing together of invectives, and apart from being a semantically appropriate expression 'pumpkin-eating' is also rhythmically suitable.

Once the connection between Yankees and pumpkins is established it is enough for satiric authors to bring in a mere reference to pumpkins

PART ONE: 'PREGNANT GOURDS' AND 'DELIRIOUS PUMPKINS'

and Yankees to remind the readers of the whole symbolic complex. In Washington Irving's story 'The Legend of Sleepy Hollow' the Dutch hero Brom Bones frightens the superstitious Ichabod Crane away by making him think he sees a headless ghost. The head that Brom Bones throws at Ichabod is a pumpkin. Ichabod is ridiculous in many respects: his name is ridiculous; his looks are ridiculous; his behaviour is ridiculous and his voracious imagination is ridiculous. It serves him right that he should be scared away by a pumpkin. But another very strong theme that Irving dwelt on in 'The Legend of Sleepy Hollow', like Cooper in *Satanstoe*, is ethnic antagonism between Yankees and New Yorkers. Ichabod is sent packing by a pumpkin not only as an individual but as the representative of a hateful pumpkin-eating neighbouring nation in the north.[141]

In Nathaniel Hawthorne's 'The Maypole of Merry Mount' (1836), the puritans are in conflict with an alien culture closer to their homeland. Hawthorne contrasts the stern, serious, joyless puritans with the riotous inhabitants of Merry Mount, not entirely to their disadvantage, but in the main so, in order to reinforce the idea of puritan dullness and intolerance. The puritans subjugate the inhabitants of Merry Mount and destroy the symbols of their way of life one by one. The maypole is cut down; the tame bear (a symbol of the ability of fertility religions to live in harmony with nature) is shot; and then, predictably, captain Endicott fixes his attention on the locks of the Lord of the May. Long hair is anathema to the puritans. When one of the puritans points out the pernicious hair style of the Lord of the May to Endicott the captain says: 'Crop it forthwith, and that in the true pumpkin-shell fashion.'[142] Conformistic societies, such as armies, often make their members cut their hair. For people who do not go along with the conformism the hair style becomes a central symbol of what is hateful about such societies. The opponents of right-wing extremists in America in the 1950s and 1960s made much of the uniform crew-cuts of many of their adversaries.

For the enemies of the puritans the standardized haircut became an epitome of the procrustean intolerance of variety and individualism that they saw as a characteristic feature of puritanism. Thus the 'haircut' aspect of 'pumpkin-head' came into existence, and 'pumpkin-head' partly became a synonym for round-head, i.e. puritan. In S. Peter's *A General History of Connecticut* a factualistic interpretation of the origin of the term is presented:[143]

PART ONE: 'PREGNANT GOURDS' AND 'DELIRIOUS PUMPKINS'

> Newhaven is celebrated for having given the name of pumkin-heads to all the New-Englanders. It originated from the Blue Laws, which enjoin every male to have his hair cut round by a cap. When caps were not to be had, they substituted the hard shell of a pumkin, which being put on the head every Saturday, the hair is cut by it all round the head.

This must not be taken too literally. The central idea is the authorities' refusal to admit any individual variation and the arbitrary nature of the standard that everyone was supposed to conform to. As sleepers in the procrustean beds were stretched if they were too short and cut shorter if too long, in a similar way the cap sets an arbitrary standard; what is above is left, what is below is cut off, and the operation takes place with arbitrary regularity every Saturday.

The idea of arbitrariness is funny in itself. It falls under Henri Bergson's definition of the comic as the mechanical superimposed on the living. But for those people who saw the phenomenon not only as funny but as hateful, or for those who wanted to make fun of people with such a culture as the round-head culture, it was obvious that the instrument should be changed in the myth from a cap to a pumpkin shell. A cap is not intrinsically funny; a pumpkin is. We need not assume that a pumpkin shell was ever actually employed as a barber's tool; it is necessary only for the myth. Where pumpkins are scarce the same story can be told with a substitution of chamberpot for pumpkin shell. The reason for picking on a chamberpot to replace pumpkin shell is of course that chamberpots are intrinsically funny because they are associated with a taboo subject. Symbols tend to cluster and interrelate and seek companions that are in keeping with the semiotic drift of the passage in which they occur.

We do not know how the business of seventeenth-century male coiffure, and the cucurbitic slinging match connected with it, started between puritans and cavaliers, but fairly soon the length of male hair was such a central issue that the two antagonistic groups were named and abused after their hair style, the puritans being called round-heads and the cavaliers long-haired rattle-heads. We may guess that the short hair of the puritans offered too inviting a temptation for the cavaliers to be able to resist and soon the hints of pumpkin-headism are rampant. This incensed the puritans beyond imagination. William Prynne in 1644 (or 1643?) published '*A Gagge* for *Long-Hair'd Rattle-Heads* who revile all civill *Round-heads*', which is a very extraordinary document indeed. Prynne sets forth in couplets for three pages the view that short hair is associated with everything that is best in the universe.

PART ONE: 'PREGNANT GOURDS' AND 'DELIRIOUS PUMPKINS'

New-born and re-born are round-heads; the celestial sphere resembles a round-head. Prynne enumerates an endless number of prominent short-haired people from history; and exhibits a monumental learning in backing up his knowledge. Rattle-heads, on the other hand, have more hair than wits; they are effeminate; long hair induces lewdness, so that, after the pox has made them bald, the cavaliers are rattle-heads in day-time (wigs) but round-heads at night (whores having made them round-heads); long hair gives the devil a better grip; long hair is a badge of shame; etc. All the learned support for short hair is very effective, but equally effective is the turning of the tables on the cucurbitic issue. The puritans throw the name pumpkin-head back at the cavaliers. 'Rattle-head' is a variation of the *Kürbiskopf* from Swabia which we analysed above, and it suggests emptiness. The cavaliers were precursors of Mr Laurel and Mr Chaplin and this sense was very widespread in the seventeenth century.[144]

Emptiness very easily suggests lightness. The New England author Nathaniel Ward, in *The Simple Cobler,* uses the word 'feather-headed'[145] He also speaks out violently against long hair (pp. 30–1):

> If those who are tearmed Rattle-heads and Impuritans, would take up a Resolution to begin in moderation of haire, to the just reproach of those that are called Puritans and Round-heads, I would honour their manlinesse, as much as the others godlinesse, so long as I knew what man or honour meant: if neither can finde a Barbours shop, let them turne in, to *Psal.* 68.21 *Jer.* 7.29 I *Cor.* 11.14, if it be thought no Wisdome in men to distinguish themselves in the field by the Scissers, let it bee thought no Injustice in God, not to distinguish them by the Sword.

In this passage, full of antitheses, Ward's typical love of word-play comes out in the word 'Impuritans'.

But apparently Ward made a mistake elsewhere in the work when he wrote about an imaginary adversary (p. 63):

> If he fears any such thing, that he would come over to us, to help recruite our bewildred brains: we will promise to maintain him so long as he lives, if he will promise to live no longer than we maintain him.

The first two editions read 'our pumpkin blasted brains' instead of 'our bewildred brains'. Apparently Ward then realised that it was a superfluous act to apply to the puritans the epithet used by the enemy – it was unnecessary to speak too convincingly from the enemy point of view – so he changed the expression to 'bewildred' for the third and fourth editions.

PART ONE: 'PREGNANT GOURDS' AND 'DELIRIOUS PUMPKINS'

Hawthorne, who used the Puritans as material for his fiction, continues the tradition of 'light-headed'. He wrote an allegorical story called 'Feathertop: A Moralized Legend', in which 'top' stands for the shrivelled, shrunken, withered, empty, light, pumpkin-head of a scarecrow.[146] The story is a variation of the Hans Christian Andersen tale of the emperor's new clothes. A New England witch makes a scarecrow of a broomstick for a backbone, a meal-bag stuffed with straw for a body and a pumpkin for a head; infuses life into it, and sends it into human society, where it does very well, except with some clear-eyed observers such as children. Hawthorne's allegory is explicit (p.420):

> It was really quite a respectable face.
> 'I've seen worse ones on human shoulders, at any rate,' said Mother Rigby. 'And many a fine gentleman has a pumpkin-head, as well as my scarecrow.'

Again in this case we have a literary text in which the intrinsic negative value of pumpkin is used in auxiliary symbolism. It is absurd to be taken in by appearances and not see through to reality, but twice as absurd if the reality is an absurd pumpkin. In that case you must be a pumpkin-head yourself and your brains light as a feather. A rule of semiotic economy thus seems to say that you should not waste any stretch of a story by having any element that does not carry a symbolism that supports the whole or opens up secondary symbolism of the same tendency.[147] Replace 'cap' with 'pumpkin'; it is an improvement![148]

But of course 'pumpkin' is capable of standing on its own. In particular, when your enemies get high-falutingly sublime you must bring in cucurbits to take them down to earth. Athenaeus refers to a comedy by Epicrates where Plato and some fellow-philosophers are having a debate, making definitions about nature, trying to determine which species the pumpkin belongs to.[149] They are sitting with their heads bowed in deep silence until an impertinent Italian physician snaps his fingers at them, naming them lunatics. Strangely enough none of the philosophers get angry, but continue their research as if nothing had happened. It is no coincidence that cucurbits are the debated topic. In Aristophanes' Socrates-ridiculing tradition Plato and his followers are eclipsed by their topic. The contrast between the wise men and the pumpkins is evident.[150] Practical people consider it just as futile to spend time on theoretical speculation as to contemplate vegetables. If you ask too many metaphysical 'warum?'s in German you get the impatient answer: 'Warum? Warum? Warum ist die Banane krumm?'[151]

PART ONE: 'PREGNANT GOURDS' AND 'DELIRIOUS PUMPKINS'

In Dickens's *The Mudfog Papers,* in the 'Report of the Second Meeting of the Mudfog Association' a certain Professor Pumpkinskull takes part in the proceedings. The names of his colleagues too, as of the association itself, reveal the same discrepancy between supposed and actual learning:[152]

> *The* number and rapidity of the arrivals are quite bewildering. Within the last ten minutes a stage-coach has driven up to the door, filled inside and out with distinguished characters, comprising Mr. Muddlebranes, Mr. Drawley, Professor Muff, Mr. X. Misty, Mr. X. X. Misty, Mr. Purblind, Professor Rummun, The Honourable and Reverend Mr. Long Eers, Professor John Ketch, Sir William Joltered, Doctor Buffer, Mr. Smith (of London), Mr. Brown (of Edinburgh), Sir Hookham Snivey, and Professor Pumpkinskull. The ten last-named gentlemen were wet through, and looked extremely intelligent.

Apart from the obvious allusion to stupidity there may be a secondary allusion to baldness, because Professor Pumpkinskull's remark in the debate concerns the prevalent taste for bears' grease as a means of promoting the growth of hair. (Professor Pumpkinskull thinks that the use of bears' grease has imperceptibly infused in the youth something of the nature and quality of the bear[153]).

A similar passage in Irenaeus' *Adversus haereses*, preserved in the Latin translation only,[154] yields a most striking example of the whole set of cucurbits being used in a pejorative sense – to ridicule the gnostic Valentinus' 'absurd' cosmological structures. According to Irenaeus, Valentinus' terminology is nothing but empty words; his 'aeons' and different emanations could just as well be replaced by pumpkins, cucumbers and melons![155]

> Est quaedam Proarche, regalis, proanennoetos, proanhypostatos virtus, procylindomene. Cum illa autem est virtus, quam ego cucurbitam voco: cum hac cucurbita autem est virtus quam et ipsam voco perinane. Haec cucurbita et perinane, cum sint unum, emiserunt, cum non emisissent, fructum, in omnibus visibilem, manducabilem, et dulcem, quem fructum sermo cucumerem vocat. Cum hoc cucumere est virtus eiusdem potestatis ei, quam et ipsam peponem voco. Hae virtutes, cucurbita et perinane, et cucumis et pepo, emiserunt reliquam multitudinem Valentini deliriosorum peponum. [xxiii]

In the next paragraph the author, in a term of abuse, develops this metaphoric use of cucurbits: 'O pepones, sophistae vituperabiles, et non viri,' while the Greek text has only got 'Ὦ ληρολόγοι σοφισταί.'

53

PART ONE: 'PREGNANT GOURDS' AND 'DELIRIOUS PUMPKINS'

[xxiv] The model is probably Homer, *Iliad* II.235: 'Ὦ πέπονες, κάκ' ἐλέγχε', Ἀχαιΐδες, οὐκέτ' Ἀχαιοί'.[156] [cxxv] However, the epic ὦ πέπονες has nothing to do with the fruit: it is the old adjective in Homer being used to characterize a person either positively (sing.) or, as in this context, negatively (pl.): 'weaklings'. In line with the above pumpkinification of terminology, the author interprets the adjective as the noun, the fruit – parodying the Homeric line.[157] In Latin, as we have seen, cucurbits very readily take connotations of stupidity and femininity and both are present here.

The aspect of absurdity, so often implied in cucurbitic passages, must also be the basis for the expression 'cucumber-time', which is found in several languages, e.g. Ger. *Gurkenzeit* or *Sauregurkenzeit* (of which latter word the *Saure*- is probably folk-etymology); Dutch *komkommertijd*; Norwegian *agurktid*. The expression denotes the summer holiday, the dead summer season when there is a lull in the public and political calendar; and it seems in particular to be used for the difficult situation faced by newspapers at this time of year. 'Cucumber-time' is not primarily the season when the cucumbers are ripe, but rather the time when events of public importance are rare, and substantial news is replaced by empty talk, flatulent dilettantisms and cucurbitic embroideries. The *OED* notes that cucumber is used in slang 'with some obscure reference to a tailor', and cites several examples; e.g. *Pall Mall Gazette* (1865): 'Tailors could not be expected to earn much money "in cucumber-season". . . . Because when cucumbers are in, the gentry are out of town.'[158] The basic mechanism of the sense of the expression 'cucumber-time' or 'cucumber-season', whether it refers to tailors or to newspapers, thus seems to be the same, i.e. lack of material. The tailors lack orders from their customers – largely the same people who provide most of the subjects for the newspapers.

Seneca's infamous satire on the emperor Claudius' death, the *Apocolocynthosis*, has in translations generally been known as 'the pumpkinification of Claudius', a coinage meant to render the emperor's mock-deification as metaphoric transformation into a pumpkin, which, as we have seen, is a handy symbol of stupidity. Otto Weinrich, in his commentary on the satire, says:[159]

> statt einer Apo-theosis gibt Seneca eine Apo-colocynthosis, statt einer Vergottung eine Verkürbsung. Das heisst nicht Claudius werde in einem Kürbis verwandelt – er wird ja auch gar nicht Theos! Sondern: Apocolocynthosis ist reiner Titelscherz. Κολοκύντη heisst Kürbis. Und im Altertum wie im modernen Volkstum nahezu

PART ONE: 'PREGNANT GOURDS' AND 'DELIRIOUS PUMPKINS'

> jeder Nation empfand man die fatale Ähnlichkeit eines mennschlichen Hohlkopfes mit dem Rund eines Kürbis.

However, many commentators have not found this a satisfactory account. There is no trace of the title pun in the satire itself. The feeling of uneasiness has also been fed by the well-known fact that we do not know for certain that this is the satire Seneca wrote and named *Apocolocynthosis*; and its finale seems unexpectedly abrupt, so that one could suspect it to be incomplete.

We do not intend to solve this hoary old riddle here. We would, however, like to suggest in what directions an interpretation should be looked for.

We assume that when Seneca coined this apparently new word, he wanted it to be understood by as wide an audience as possible. The rather rude, mocking spirit of the satire suggests that this is not the kind of literature in which occult subtleties are likely to appear. The question we must ask then is: what kind of associations would a κολοκύντη be apt to call forth in Seneca's audience? An answer to this question should be sought in the manifold aspects of the cucurbitic tradition and the general and well-known features of the plant.

That the pumpkin implied stupidity is certain. We know how Claudius' physical defects were an easy target of mockery and ridicule, and we know that in classical Greek and Roman tradition as well as in modern times cucurbits have been used in connection with bodily defects (see above: cucumber shins, double-chin, swollen legs, etc.).

It is on the other hand clear that cucurbits had not only a high horticultural status, but also intrinsically a prominent value in human thought. We already mentioned the Chinese ranking of them as Emperors of the Garden, and Karlfeldt's poem where he names the cucumber 'royal'. Recall also St Augustine, who asked the Manicheans: 'Cur de thesauris Dei melonem putatis aureum esse?'[160] Melons also grow in the Islamitic paradise.[161] The cucurbits are inherently of high status, and thus use of a cucurbit in connection with an emperor is most appropriate. Its positive value does not lessen the effect of ridicule; both effects coexist. The pumpkin is a vegetable king: to be a pumpkin (or vegetable) is bad; to be a king is good; it is therefore a complex symbol. For his purpose Seneca paradoxically needed something not only with as low a semiotic value as possible but with as high a semiotic value as possible at the same time; something capable of remaining ridiculous even while being elevated.

The *Apocolocynthosis* relates a deification even though it is a deification that fails. It is striking in connection with deification to see how the plant in several cultures, through the ages, has been associated with immortality. The step from the cyclic fertility that we have seen demonstrated in the Augustan poets to eternal life is a small one. In Indian myth Triçanku uses a cucurbit to ascend to heaven.[162] Above we had Walafrid Strabo's 'altipetax' and the biblical 'sign of Jonah'. We may also add old Germanic seed rites on Annunciation Day and Ascension Day.[163]

However, in Imperial Rome the allusions to femaleness and fertility (cf. above) were possibly the most immediate. It is therefore difficult to believe that it could have been possible for Seneca to mention the pumpkin without evoking such associations. Claudius was recognized among his fellow-Romans as the limping and snuffling emperor. But he was also commonly known as a 'vir uxorius'. Was it possible for the satirist to use a cucurbitic word without hinting at the usual subject, sex? The text provides no clue, no definite trace of mocked sexuality. Nevertheless, several speculations have been put forward.

Here we may look briefly at the so-called Oxford fragment in Juvenal's sixth satire. It is generally agreed that the couple presented in v. 6 are in some way sexually deviant, though precisely how is a moot point:

> his violare cibos sacraeque adsistere mensae
> permittunt, et vasa iubent frangenda lavari
> cum colocyntha bibit vel cum barbata chelidon.[164] [xxvi]

'Barbata chelidon' is undoubtedly feminine, the epithet semantically masculine. Applying our cucurbitic insight, we do not hesitate to determine 'colocyntha''s sex as feminine. To make the couple fit, both mutually and in the context, we assume the character to be an emasculated male. Feminine nicknames for men (and of course masculine names for women) have always been popular and immensely useful. Additionally, to consider physiological matters, we know that a eunuch, who would indeed be appropriate in the context, loses his growth of beard and becomes smooth as a pumpkinish woman.

In a passage in Procopius' *Anecdota*, chapter 9,[165] we have the same possible ambiguity as in Seneca's satire. Justinian's 'praefectus urbis', Theodotus, is named 'Pumpkin'. We are given no direct hints on how to understand the nickname, perhaps because it was obvious to Procopius' contemporary readers. Or did he intentionally leave it ambiguous? From the context we may guess that Theodotus was labelled 'Pumpkin'

PART ONE: 'PREGNANT GOURDS' AND 'DELIRIOUS PUMPKINS'

by Justinian's mistress and later empress Theodora, who was a nymphomaniac, and we have just got a vivid and slightly resentful description of her peculiar sexual insatiability when we meet the sober prefect in conflict with the unrestrained lady and her friends. Theodotus is obviously not affected by Theodora's special attractions. Does the nickname suggest anything to describe Theodotus' sexual (in-?) abilities? We are inclined to believe so, because the actual form of the nickname could favour this interpretation. Κολοκύντιος is hypocoristic: my dear little pumpkin.

Of the various cucurbits the cucumber most readily takes 'male' indecent connotations because of its shape. In television comedies in England in which humour is dependent on *double entendre* and a willing mind, cucumbers occur frequently. Nevertheless, such words as modern Greek ἀγγούρι, stiff, and the saying 'to collect ἀγγούρια', be a prostitute, should not be explained by shape alone. We must note that the subject is the same as we could expect with cucumbers, i.e. sex; or conversely that, if the subject is sex, surely enough cucumbers crop up.[166] The use of cucumber directly in connection with the sexual organ is very old. In Plautus' comedy *Casina* there is a conversation between Olympio servus and Cleostrata matrona in which the use can be studied in an amusing context where the bawdy expression fits the general style of burlesque humour in this playwright:[167]

> Ol: ferrum ne haberet metui; id quaerere occepi
> dum gladium quaero, ne habeat, arripio capulum.
> sed cum cogito, non habuit gladium, nam esset frigidus.
> Cl: Eloquere.
> Ol: At pudet.
> Cl: Num radix fuit.
> Ol: Non fuit.
> Cl: Num cucumis?
> Ol: Profecto hercle non fuit quicquam holerum,
> nisi quidquid erat, calamitas profecto attigerat numquam
> ita, quidquid erat, grande erat. [xxvii]

The explanation of Olympio's consternation here is that, in the dark room, instead of the bride, he started to fondle the male slave dressed up as a woman that had been sent as a substitute, and in his attempt at love-making he encountered some anatomical surprises.

Actually all the cucurbits are often connected with sex, or various aspects of it.[168] During permissive periods of history the sex connotations are taken up joyfully and added to the other features that give the fruit a positive character. During periods of repression and prudery

57

PART ONE: 'PREGNANT GOURDS' AND 'DELIRIOUS PUMPKINS'

on the other hand the cucurbits are looked upon with suspicion and the sex connotations tend to reinforce the negative symbolic value. The Victorian period is well known for its prudery, and accordingly the cucurbits occur as sinful plants in Tennyson's poem 'The Vision of Sin':[169]

> I had a vision when the night was late:
> A youth came riding toward a palace-gate.
> He rode a horse with wings, that would have flown,
> But that his heavy rider kept him down.
> And from the palace came a child of sin,
> And took him by the curls, and led him in,
> Where sat a company with heated eyes,
> Expecting when a fountain should arise:
> A sleepy light upon their brows and lips –
> As when the sun, a crescent of eclipse,
> Dreams over lake and lawn, and isles and capes –
> Suffused them, sitting, lying, languid shapes,
> By heaps of gourds, and skins of wine, and piles of grapes.

Apart from the gourds and the wine and the grapes being sinful in themselves there is also sin in the lack of moderation. Tennyson seems to be saying that if you must have these sinful things, at least you ought not to have 'heaps', 'skins' and 'piles' of them.

Any poem with the word 'pumpkin' in it invites parody because of the ridiculous connotations of pumpkins; but it invites indecent parodies in particular, because of the sexual connotations of pumpkins. The American popular poet James Whitcomb Riley wrote a poem, 'When the Frost is on the Punkin', which became widely read in the United States. The first stanza goes:[170]

> WHEN the frost is on the punkin and the fodder's in the shock,
> And you hear the kyouck and gobble of the struttin' turkeycock
> And the clackin' of the guineys, and the cluckin' of the hens,
> And the rooster's hallylooyer as he tiptoes on the fence;
> O, it's then's the times a feller is a-feelin' at his best,
> With the risin' sun to greet him from a night of peaceful rest,
> As he leaves the house, bareheaded, and goes out to feed the stock,
> When the frost is on the punkin and the fodder's in the shock.

There is a widespread parody of this poem which goes as follows:

> When the weather's hot and sticky,
> that's no time to dunk the dicky;
> But when the frost is on the punkin,
> that's the time for dicky-dunkin. [anon.]

PART ONE: 'PREGNANT GOURDS' AND 'DELIRIOUS PUMPKINS'

We assume that the parodist started out with a general wish to ridicule Riley's poem – a wish that may have been triggered by the presence in the poem of that intrinsically ridiculous thing, the pumpkin. But given the idea of parody, it was predictable that the parody would be indecent because the idea of pumpkin furthermore guided the thoughts of the parodist to sexual matters.

Conversely, of course, it is also true that if the language in some literary passage is already heavily sexual in tone then cucurbitic terminology is likely to creep in. This can be exemplified with a passage from John Updike's novel *Couples*, from one of the scenes – so exceedingly numerous in this book – where the subject of drunken talk is sex:[171]

> 'You know, honey, you're a fantastic piece – I say this as a disinterested party, girl to girl – and you don't have to wear all those flashy clothes to prove anything. Just you, fat or skinny, Janet Applesauce, that's all we want for dessert; we *love* you, stop worrying. As I say, you're all gorgeous women. It killed me tonight, it really tumified me, seeing old Terry Tightcunt sitting there with her legs spread and her hair down jerking off that poor melon. Have you ever noticed her mouth? It's enormous. Her tongue is as big as a bed. Every time I work on her molars I want to curl up in there and go to sleep.'
> 'Freddy, you're drunk,' Marcia said.

Thus cucurbits bring in sex, and sex brings in cucurbits, especially in texts like these.

Either cucurbitic symbolism comes particularly easily to Updike's mind, or else the frequent occurrence of cucurbits in his books merely testifies to the fact that usually one of their main themes is sex. A few pages earlier in *Couples*, Updike reinforces a thematic complex of women–music–love-making with an observation on the gourd-like shape of the musical instrument (pp. 162–3):

> Marcia was listening to Matt Gallagher explain the Vatican's likely verdict, now that the ecumenical council was adjourned, on artificial birth control: 'Nix. They won't give us sex, but they may give us meat on Fridays.' Marcia nodded understandingly – having a lover deepened her understanding of everything, even of Matt Gallagher's adherence to the letter of an unloving church – and glanced toward Terry. Terry, sitting cross-legged on the floor in black stretch pants, carefully picked through a chord sequence on her lute; it was a gourd-shaped, sumptuous instrument, whose eight strings produced a threadbare distant tone. Matt had bought it for her for Christmas, in line with the policy of conspicuous consumption

> that had led to the Mercedes, and perhaps with a more symbolic in-
> tent, for its blond lustre and inlaid elegance seemed sacramental,
> like their marriage. Piet lay beside her on the rug gazing at the taut
> cloth of her crotch. The seam had lost one stitch.

Associating the feminine form of instruments such as the guitar or the lute with women is of course a commonplace in literature; here the concept of femininity is furthermore reinforced by a reference to the feminine fruit, the cucurbit (– from which, by the way, some instruments appear to derive their origin).

Since the rule is, then, that cucurbits bring in sex and sex brings in cucurbits, we believe that Seneca's use of κολοκύντη would have led the thoughts of his audience to sexual matters, in addition to stupidity, bodily defects, ridiculousness, etc. It is furthermore likely that Seneca would have realized that the word would be thus understood.

Like the Bible, the works of the classical authors were widespread and influential texts during many centuries in the Western world. The apocolocynthosis therefore influenced European literary cucurbitic tradition strongly, and with little exaggeration one can say that Seneca stabilized one aspect of the negative connotations of pumpkin the same way as the Book of Jonah stabilized one of the positive. In the seventeenth century pumpkin symbolism seems very important. This is also the century when in England and France authors began to turn away from Cicero as a model for prose writers and instead began to read, admire and imitate Seneca.

In addition to the continued reading of the Latin itself, the apocolocynthosis tradition is carried on in historical writings on the Roman Empire in English; cf. Bridges (1885): 'I'll let Rome know how pumpkin Claudius died';[172] or Merivale (1856):[173]

> There is no more curious fragment of antiquity than the Vision of Judgment which Seneca has left us on the death and deification of Claudius. The traveller who has visited modern Rome in the autumn season has remarked the number of unwieldy and bloated gourds which sun their speckled bellies before the doors, to form a favourite condiment to the food of the poorer classes. When Claudius expired in the month of October, his soul, according to the satirist, long lodged in the inflated emptiness of his own swollen carcass, migrated by an easy transition into a kindred pumpkin. The senate declared that he had become a god; but Seneca knew that he was only transformed into a gourd. The senate decreed his divinity, Seneca translated it into pumpkinity; and proceeded to give a burlesque account of what may be supposed to have happened in heaven on the appearance of the new aspirant to celestial honours.

PART ONE: 'PREGNANT GOURDS' AND 'DELIRIOUS PUMPKINS'

Also 'the unhappy Emperor Claudius, who has gone down to posterity as mercilessly "pumpkinified" by Seneca'.[174]

Apart from the fairly clear tradition arising out of comments and translations of this kind, words like 'pumpkinify' or 'to pumpkinize', meaning 'extravagant or absurdly uncritical glorification' (*OED*), also came into use. Some examples: 'The writer ... has ... given us, not an apotheosis, but a pumpkinification of the Emperor William II';[175] also, 'The phrases whereby the pumpkinifier constructs his pumpkin';[176] finally, 'There will be an outpouring of spirit of Pumpkinism upon me the moment I get back, and I shall not have half the pleasure in seeing you there amidst the interruptions we generally have. . . .'[177]

It is sometimes difficult to decide whether a modern writer or artist is consciously working in the Seneca tradition when he replaces the head of a ruler with a vegetable, or whether the apocolocynthosis tradition is so diffused that the symbolic act is used even by people who are not directly aware of Seneca. Above all it is often difficult to decide whether an occurrence is due to tradition at all or whether the writers independently create the same image as Seneca out of the material of the negative connotations of cucurbits, and the sought-for antithesis between high and low.

Stephen Crane, like so many naturalists, often took a rather pessimistic and bitter view of the actions of mankind. His pessimism comes over particularly starkly in his poems. In one of these he describes a newspaper in the following contradictory or negative terms:[178]

> A newspaper is a collection of half-injustices
> Which, bawled by boys from mile to mile,
> Spreads its curious opinion
> To a million merciful and sneering men,
> While families cuddle the joys of the fireside
> When spurred by tale of dire lone agony.
> A newspaper is a court
> Where every one is kindly and unfairly tried
> By a squalor of honest men.
> A newspaper is a market
> Where wisdom sells its freedom
> And melons are crowned by the crowd.
> A newspaper is a game
> Where his error scores the player victory
> While another's skill wins death.
> A newspaper is a symbol;
> It is fetless life's chronicle,
> A collection of loud tales
> Concentrating eternal stupidities,

PART ONE: 'PREGNANT GOURDS' AND 'DELIRIOUS PUMPKINS'

> That in remote ages lived unhaltered,
> Roaming through a fenceless world.

The phrase, 'melons are crowned by the crowd', involves the idea of elevation (though in Crane's poem from melon to emperor, whereas in Seneca from emperor to god), but whether Crane was conscious of what he was doing is difficult to determine. The likelihood is that Crane's use is an independent creation and the similarity between the passage and the apocolocynthosis cliché is accidental. Nevertheless, one need not see the problem as a choice between either a direct influence or a totally independent construction of the same image, starting from the intrinsic properties of the fruit and the antithesis high–low. There is much in between. This type of tradition spreads easily; even when the source is forgotten the semiotic idea travels. Like dirty jokes, which are so often global, traditions like the indecent or negative connotations of cucurbits travel far and wide, undergo local adaptation and go through variations (like all narrative art, which is mainly oral). In the end, however, in most cases like this, independent creation seems more probable than borrowing.

Cucurbits used for words of abuse can be fairly general or include several negative connotations. Goethe uses Kürbis as a straightforward term of abuse in *Claudine von Villa Bella*: 'Wer glaubst denn du zu sein,/dass du mich schelten willst, du Kürbiss?'[179] The Roman imperial architect, Apollodorus, in Dio's *Roman History*, tells Hadrian: 'ἄπελθε καὶ τὰς κολοκύντας γράφε· τούτων γὰρ οὐδὲν ἐπίστασαι.'[180] The author adds in an explanatory note: 'ἐτύγχανε δὲ ἄρα τότε ἐκεῖνος τοιούτῳ τινὶ γράμματι σεμνυνόμενος.' [xxviii] However that may have been, one should be wary of calling the high and mighty cucurbitic names. They may not appreciate the message. Apollodorus was executed not many years afterwards.

One aspect of the anatomy of the plants of the *Cucurbitaceae* family that surprisingly has been neglected is the trailing growth of the vines, and their clinging, clutching and climbing propensity which one would have expected to be taken over into symbolic use to stand for dependence or parasitic clinging. The ideas do occur in overtly symbol-hunting works, but sparsely. The idea of parasitic existence, however, is probably behind the nickname 'Σικύα' in Athenaeus. One of the participants in the party of the *Deipnosophistae*, Clearchus, tells a story about a free-loader who is called 'cucumber' (σικύα) from the way he clings to parties.[181]

The word 'pompeon' seems to have been a fairly common word

PART ONE: 'PREGNANT GOURDS' AND 'DELIRIOUS PUMPKINS'

of abuse during the Elizabethan period: cf. Fletcher (1623):[182]

> O here's another pumpion,
> Let him loose for luck sake, the cram'd son
> Of a stav'd Usurer, *Cacafogo*, both their brains butter'd,
> Cannot make two spoonfulls.

and Fletcher and Massinger (?) (1625):[183]

> Thou Dog-whelp, thou, pox upon thee what
> Should I call thee, Pompion,
> Thou kiss my Lady? Thou scour her chamber-pot;
> Thou have a Maiden-head? a mottly Coat,
> You great blind fool, farewell and be hang'd to ye.

In a somewhat later example pumpian is used to denigrate excessive rhetoric:[184]

> But can that Nation pass over such a Triumph as this Entertainment, without Pumpian Words, and ruffling Grandiloquence? 'tis impossible. Therefore one *Andres de Mendoza* wrote a Relation of all these Passages, which he dedicated to *Don Juan de Castilià*, wherein he pities us poor English, that we had seen nothing but Country Wakes, or Popit-Plays, compared with these Rarities, which were the seven Wonders of Bravery.

In Shakespeare's *Merry Wives* the most prominent feature of the cucurbit is its water content. 'We'll use this unwholesome humidity, this grosse watery pumpion. . . .'[185] The connection between cucurbits and water has usually[186] resulted in positive uses.[187] Water is closely connected with life and fertility. In some American and African religions the medicine-men have used rattles to produce music for the dance that was meant to entice forth life-giving rain. The gourd instrument was entirely appropriate here since there is a symbolic triangle: water (rain), gourds and fertility; cf. the English word 'gourder', which used to mean a sudden flooding of rain, a spate. In many cosmogonies where cucurbits occur water also appears. In Milton's *Paradise Lost*, book VII, both water and the gourd are mentioned, and shortly after the gourd a life-giving dewy mist. In an American version of the story of the creation the following episode involves both water and cucurbit. A man had a child that died. He took the body to the foot of a mountain and put it in a large, hollow gourd. Later when he returned the body was gone and the gourd was full of water with fishes and whales in it. The villagers lifted the gourd, the father surprised them, they dropped the gourd, it cracked, the water spilt and ran down the slope, and thus rivers and seas were created.[188]

PART ONE: 'PREGNANT GOURDS' AND 'DELIRIOUS PUMPKINS'

This story of the creation views life as cyclical and takes death into account. Life arose out of death. This idea recurs in many parts of the world. In those parts where people hold a belief in some kind of resurrection cucurbits thus come to stand for the hope of a new life. Gourds have been found in graves, e.g. in Germany.[189] The reason for giving gourds to the dead is not only that gourds are good food to have on a journey, or good containers, but surely also that gourds symbolize the hope for resurrection. Note how well this idea fits in with other parts of cucurbitic tradition. When cucurbits in early Christian Rome were used in ornaments in the graves, the artists may have picked the Jonah tradition because of the cucurbits.

There is a triangular relationship between water, cucurbits and the moon. Cucurbits and the moon are connected; so are the moon and water (the moon rules the tide) and cucurbits and water. In addition there is a connection between cucurbits and women and the moon and women.

The water aspect of cucurbits is used very wittily in the *Cena Trimalchionis*, where it is stated that 'copones et cucurbitae' are born under the sign of Aquarius. Cucurbita meaning a stupid person, the copones (landlords at inns) are stupid too, being born under the same sign. But since the sign is Aquarius, and the pumpkin is watery, surely there is a connection with copones here as well, and the passage probably hints at the practice of unscrupulous and dishonest landlords to dilute the wine.[190]

In the English rhyme

> Peter, Peter, Pumpkin eater,
> Had a wife and couldn't keep her.
> He put her in a pumpkin shell
> And there he kept her very well

pumpkins are perhaps linked to yet another ridiculous subject: the cuckold. In the early 1960s Penelope Mortimer published a novel called *The Pumpkin Eater* where the rhyme was used as motto.[191] Predictably, the subject of unfaithfulness is an important theme in the novel. But many other themes easily associated with cucurbits figure prominently as well. Fertility versus sterility is one issue. The female protagonist has an indefinite number of children, a great horde that she has accumulated through the years with her various husbands; and the great betrayal in the book is the chapter where the husband convinces the wife that she should let herself be sterilized, and then goes off and makes another woman pregnant. The mood of the novel is slightly

PART ONE: 'PREGNANT GOURDS' AND 'DELIRIOUS PUMPKINS'

absurdistic which fits in well with the pumpkin theme; and a woman (connection to cucurbits) wrote it, which fits in with the fashion of female collective introspection in the 1960s. Cucurbits used in connection with unfaithfulness is an old idea; cf. the passage on the medieval 'cucurbitare' above.

With the basis of positive connotations on the one hand, and this wealth of possibilities for negative connotations on the other, it is hardly surprising that authors should begin to use cucurbits as an ambiguous symbol. Emily Dickinson's poems are often extremely subtle, full of ambiguities and multiple layers of meaning. She therefore made a much more sophisticated symbolic use of the pumpkin than many other New England authors:[192]

> 'Twas just this time, last year, I died.
> I know I heard the Corn,
> When I was carried by the Farms -
> It had the Tassels on -
>
> I thought how yellow it would look -
> When Richard went to mill -
> And then, I wanted to get out,
> But something held my will.
>
> I thought just how Red-Apples wedged
> The Stubble's joints between -
> And Carts went stooping round the fields
> To take the Pumpkins in -
>
> I wondered which would miss me, least,
> And when Thanksgiving came,
> If Father'd multiply the plates -
> To make an even Sum -
>
> And would it blur the Christmas glee
> My Stocking hang too high
> For any Santa Clause to reach
> The Altitude of me -
>
> But this sort, grieved myself,
> And so, I thought the other way,
> How just this time, some perfect year -
> Themself, should come to me -

The basic thematic structure of this poem is the opposition between life and death. The person speaking in the poem is dead and cannot return to life. Looking at the rural scenes of New England she (?) wants to get out of death, but cannot. It is appropriate that in the scene from life should be the symbol of life, the cucurbit. But the moral of the poem is that reunion will come in any case, not through herself returning

PART ONE: 'PREGNANT GOURDS' AND 'DELIRIOUS PUMPKINS'

to life, but by the fact that everything living will die. Therefore the scene from life is already autumnal (seasonal symbolism) and the pumpkins are being gathered in.

The flippant tone of the sections of the poem that deal with death is well suited to the ambivalence of pumpkin as a symbol and its ridiculous connotations. The poet talks irreverently of her stocking in heaven hanging too high for Santa Clause to reach, thus mixing moods, serious and comic, to reach a better effect. In this mixture the pumpkin is a perfect symbol because it serves both moods, being intrinsically, at the same time, both serious and comic.

In another poem (no. 1407) by Emily Dickinson, the fourth line originally read 'It's Pumpkins to – the Bin', but she changed 'Pumpkins' to 'Triumphs':[193]

> A Field of Stubble, lying sere
> Beneath the second Sun –
> It's Toils to Brindled People thrust –
> It's Triumphs – to the Bin –
> Accosted by a timid Bird
> Irresolute of Alms –
> Is often seen – but seldom felt,
> On our New England Farms –

The substitution was possibly caused by a desire not to undermine the antithesis by anticipating the ambiguity in 'Bin' with another ambiguity ('Pumpkins') in the earlier part of the line.

A passage in one of the apocryphal books of the Bible, Baruch 6:70 (a letter of Jeremiah on the folly of idolatry), also, we think, plays on the ambiguity of the symbol. The text warns against idols and compares them to a scarecrow in a cucumber patch:

> These wooden gods of theirs, plated with gold and silver, give no better protection than a scarecrow in a plot of cucumbers. They are like a thorn-bush in a garden, a perch for every bird, like a corpse cast out in the dark. [NEB]

Though the cucurbits are, on the one hand, valuable and highly positive, and therefore worthy of protection (in the same way that the garden is), they are on the other also absurd, which reinforces the absurdity value of the scarecrow. A scarecrow is trebly absurd if it not only looks absurd and fails absurdly to perform its task, so that it becomes a perch for the very birds it should have scared away, but in addition is set to guard something intrinsically absurd (cf. the jack-o'-lantern; Hawthorne's 'Feathertop'; Lowell, etc.).

PART ONE: 'PREGNANT GOURDS' AND 'DELIRIOUS PUMPKINS'

In the novel *Portnoy's Complaint* by Philip Roth, the Jewish protagonist has a very ambivalent relation to his own nationality or religion. He is obsessed by it, he suffers from self-hatred, and he often vents his love-hate for the Jewish religion and the background of Jewish culture from which he comes. But he cannot escape his identity, and often his upbringing, his loyalty to his people and his prejudices tend to come to the surface after all. His interest in the *shikse* girls around him is partly an interest in forbidden fruit; and his relation to the gentiles is very ambivalent. At one stage he has a *shikse* girlfriend and the relation is on the brink of becoming serious; he even visits her parents. But throughout the episode the theme that dominates the narrative is her non-Jewishness and the non-Jewishness of her home, her parents, etc. At one stage he asks her whether she would convert if they got married. She asks why. Eventually the relationship ends.

The ambivalence of the protagonist in relation to the girl has throughout the episode been well expressed in the epithet he mentally uses for the girl: 'the pumpkin'.[194] On the one hand this is highly positive (cf. Theopompus) and particularly in America, where 'some pumpkins' is a colloquial phrase which expresses something very good; cf. the following example: 'Driving . . . from Piccadilly to Hammersmith, he [H.W. Beecher] quaintly said: "London is some pumkins, I tell you" – a profound Americanism, which is supposed to convey a wholly unutterable approbation and surprise.'[195] 'Pumpkin' also means 'important person'; cf. Bristed (1852): 'A slang expression of young New-York for people of value and consequence'.[196]

'Pumpkin', apart from meaning sexually attractive, valuable and important, also means thick, stupid, fat and absurd. In addition there may be an ethnic dimension in Roth's book. There may be some connection to the fear of an ethnically mixed marriage in the use of the word.

A whole chapter of cucurbitologic analysis could be written on the subject of Negroes and cucurbits. In America white people with racial prejudices use watermelon as a word of abuse for the blacks. Many symbolic undercurrents converge here. In the former aristocratic society of the South agricultural work was usually carried out by black slaves and the prejudice of upper-class whites was expressed in the cucurbitic team, which here has connotations ranging from 'rustic peasant' to 'manual labourer'. In regions where cucurbits grow easily and manual work is despised, cucurbits develop negative class connotations. And anyway there is always, with cucurbits, the possibility of

PART ONE: 'PREGNANT GOURDS' AND 'DELIRIOUS PUMPKINS'

an association with the lower classes: as for example in the following parody written in 1773: 'from his melon-ground the peasant slave/Has rudely rush'd, and levell'd Merlin's Cave'.[197]

One of the reasons for this development is of course also that when cucurbits are cheap they are eaten by the poorer classes, and thus the 'staple-diet abuse' development operates: 'A very favourite dish, especially among the poorer classes of America, is pumpkin pie – pronounced "punkin".'[198] There is also something undignified about the natural way of eating a slice of watermelon (what in modern Greek is known as eating a watermelon 'harmonica-fashion' – the polite way of eating a watermelon is to use knife and fork), and thus some Americans with a cruel talent for ethnic jokes say that the only time a Negro washes is when he eats a watermelon. If no Negroes live in the neighbourhood the same thing can be said about Italians or any ethnic group that the teller of the joke (if it can so be termed) happens to dislike. The aim is to convey the idea of dirtiness, an allegation that is always made when you wish to dehumanize someone; and in accordance with the rule that we have noted – that symbols cluster – the idea of dirty suggests the idea of ablutional liquid – water – and water gives the idea of connecting the target of the prejudice with a negative vegetable that has water associations.

But the sexuality myths of white prejudice are certainly also an element in the term watermelons for Negroes. In a modern absurdistic short film 'Ah, Dem Watermelons' this is clearly one theme.

In serious American literature Negroes are often associated with cucurbits, occasionally in a malicious way, but usually detachedly or often even in a positive sense. The connection can be found in almost any American classic.

In Stephen Crane's masterpiece 'The Monster', the first part of the narrative depicts the enormous vitality and beauty of the Negro Henry Johnson in strong terms in order to create contrast with the latter half of the work, when burning acid, dropping on Henry's face while he is saving his employer's son Jimmie during a fire, has turned him into a monster. Henry's girlfriend, who admires him immensely before the disaster, is almost scared to death by his appearance afterwards. She lives on a street called Watermelon Alley, a name suggesting that Negroes live there. But the name has more significance than a momentary allusion. Watermelon Alley becomes an area that Henry is shut out from after the fire has deformed his face. Cut off from Watermelon Alley, from his fiancée and from family life, he is thus cut off from

PART ONE: 'PREGNANT GOURDS' AND 'DELIRIOUS PUMPKINS'

reproduction and a normal existence. It is appropriate that the symbol of vitality should name the street where his lost life should have been lived.[199]

There is some gradation between the varieties of cucurbits, so that in negative use 'pumpkin' often carries the most negative connotations whereas watermelon or melon is seldom degraded completely.[200] In *The Adventures of Huckleberry Finn* Mark Twain links melons and watermelons to Mississippi life and to humour (particularly in a scene where Jim and Huck haggle with their conscience over which types of fruit they may steal, and reach a compromise, i.e. that they can steal some – the ripe ones – but not others – those that are not in season); but even in this novel, when the characters need a really contemptuous and biting cucurbitic curse they resort to 'punkin-heads'.[201]

One of the nastiest documents ever written on the subject of Negroes and cucurbits was produced by Thomas Carlyle in 1849 in *Frasers Magazine*.[202] Carlyle argues in favour of slavery, saying that the Negroes of the West Indies should be whipped and forcefully put to work to produce sugar and other valuable cash crops instead of being allowed to eat their pumpkins. He argues that might is right, that serfdom is preferable to slavery limited in time; and he draws a picture of the blacks as lazy, brutish, indolent and stupid. He believes that their inferiority is innate.

Carlyle, or his 'persona', says he does not hate the Negro (p. 357), but the pumpkin symbolism of the essay tells us otherwise.[203] Through the whole essay he hammers away at 'pumpkins, pumpkins' in a curious mixture of irrationality and logic. His technique is to mix the two in order to make prejudice seem respectable. He does this by creating a private language and a private world within the essay and bringing logic to bear on that private world so as to make everything he says seem patently true. The error occurs in the premisses, not in the conclusions he draws from them. The private world of his essay starts as a symbol or metaphor and then gradually and imperceptibly becomes accepted truth.

Carlyle thinks than men are born unequal and that the master–servant relationship is a manifestation of divine order. He thus dismisses unemployed seamstresses as being, in reality, runaway serving-girls (p. 366):

> Who has not heard of the Distressed Needlewoman in these days? We have thirty-thousand Distressed Needlewomen, – the most of whom cannot sew a reasonable stitch; for they are, in fact, Mutinous

PART ONE: 'PREGNANT GOURDS' AND 'DELIRIOUS PUMPKINS'

> Serving-maids, who, instead of learning to work and to obey, learned to give warning: 'Then suit yourself, Ma'am!'

Shortly after this he cites a lady he knew who had voiced the same opinion: 'As well call them Distressed Astronomers as Distressed Needlewomen!' (p. 366). After unemployment has been dismissed this way the seamstresses for the rest of the essay appear as 'Distressed Astronomers' (p. 379: 'our thirty-thousand Distressed Astronomers'). The scrupulous logic of the arguments is thus complemented by the unscrupulous manipulation of the materials the arguments are made of – 'distressed Astronomers' is hardly an objective name for the unemployed.

In the same way as he makes the unemployed seamstresses astronomers, Carlyle creates a pumpkin-world for the Negro which allows him to express hatred and contempt, while at the same time seeming logical and rational. The references to pumpkins begin with the idea that Negroes are now well off, which Carlyle sees in terms of sufficient food: 'Our beautiful Black darlings are at last happy; with little labour except to the teeth, *which* surely, in those excellent horse-jaws of theirs, will not fail!' (p. 350). Next, he suggests that pumpkin is the Negro food (p. 350):

> Sitting Yonder with their beautiful muzzles up to the ears in pumpkins, imbibing sweet pulps and juices; the grinder and incisor teeth ready for ever new work, and the pumpkins cheap as grass in those rich climates: while the sugar-crop rot round them uncut, because labour cannot be hired, so cheap are the pumpkins; . . .

also 'and beautiful Blacks sitting there up to the ears in pumpkins' (p. 351). Immediately after this we slip into one of those typical passages where the symbol of Negro life, the pumpkin, is used in a rational-seeming passage, a passage that in reality is highly irrational, because no matter how much West Indian blacks in the mid-nineteenth century may actually have liked cucurbits, the pumpkin remains a metaphor or symbol, and does not turn into an objective fact about Negro diet except for Carlyle's propagandistic purposes (pp. 352-3):

> The West Indies, it appears, are short of labour; as indeed is very conceivable in those circumstances. Where a Black man, by working about half-an-hour a-day (such is the calculation), can supply himself, by aid of sun and soil, with as much pumpkin as will suffice, he is likely to be a little stiff to raise into hard work! Supply and demand, which, science says, should be brought to bear on him, have an uphill task of it with such a man. Strong sun supplies itself

PART ONE: 'PREGNANT GOURDS' AND 'DELIRIOUS PUMPKINS'

> gratis, rich soil in those unpeopled or half-peopled regions almost gratis; these are *his* 'supply'; and half-an-hour a-day, directed upon these, will produce pumpkin, which is his 'demand'. The fortunate Black man, very swiftly does he settle *his* account with supply and demand: – not so swiftly the less fortunate White man of those tropical localities. A bad case, his, just now. He himself cannot work; and his black neighbour, rich in pumpkin, is in no haste to help him. Sunk to the ears in pumpkin, imbibing saccharine juices, and much at his ease in the Creation, he can listen to the less fortunate white man's 'demand,' and take his own time in supplying it. Higher wages, massa; higher, for your cane-crop cannot wait; still higher, – till no conceivable opulence of cane-crop will cover such wages. In Demerara, as I read in the Blue-book of last year, the cane-crop, far and wide, stands rotting; the fortunate black gentlemen, strong in their pumpkins, having all struck till the 'demand' rise a little. Sweet blighted lilies, now getting-up their heads again!

Through the rest of the essay, again and again, pumpkins recur (thirty times altogether after this) as a symbol that dehumanizes the Negroes, making them seem ridiculous, absurd, brutish and lazy. In the same way that he connects pumpkins with Negroes, Carlyle connects the 'noble' (p. 373) cash crops with the Anglo-Saxon British so as to suggest by analogy that the British are as much better than the Negroes as the cash crops are better than pumpkins (p. 373):

> West-India Islands, still full of waste fertility, produce abundant pumpkins: pumpkins, however, you will observe, are not the sole requisite for human well-being. No; for a pig they are the one thing needful: but for a man they are only the first of several things needful. . . . Who it may be has the right to raise pumpkins and other produce on those Islands, perhaps none can, except temporarily, decide. The Islands are good withal for pepper, for sugar, for sago, arrow-root, for coffee, perhaps for cinnamon and precious spices; things far nobler than pumpkins; and leading towards Commerces, Arts, Politics, and Social Developments, which alone are the noble product, where men (and not pigs with pumpkins) are the parties concerned! Well, all this fruit too, fruit spicy and commercial, fruit spiritual and celestial, so far beyond the merely pumpkinish and grossly terrene, lies in the West-India lands: . . .

He then goes on to argue that the Negroes have no right to grow pumpkins in the West Indies because it was the British who cleared the land, and that the Negroes should be made serfs.

Carlyle was too much out of touch with the times in Europe for his ideas to have much significance in Britain, but in the United States where slavery was still very much a live issue the article aroused some

PART ONE: 'PREGNANT GOURDS' AND 'DELIRIOUS PUMPKINS'

indignation. Whittier wrote an answer in which he denounced Carlyle's views as uncivilized, evil and unjust. It is interesting that Whittier apparently found Carlyle's views so shocking that he did not even report them in their original form, but toned them down considerably, particularly on the symbolism of the diet of the Negroes. Whittier sensed that the real contest of opinion was over symbols, names and attitudes, and did not grant Carlyle these false premises from which to build a logical argument.[204]

Since cucurbits are associated with the Negroes, the black authors in America became interested in cucurbitic symbols at the same time as they became interested in themselves. It is natural that when a group of people grow in self-consciousness and self-confidence they wish to explore everything connected with themselves in order to realize their identity. When what you explore is prejudice the process means exploring taboo subjects relentlessly. In Ralph Ellison's *Invisible Man* the drawn-out scene of incest is preceded by explicit melon symbolism. While the poor Negro tells the story of how he committed incest with his daughter, Ellison's uncomfortable protagonist is writhing with shame. How *can* the man bring himself to talk like this when he should know that this is precisely what some white people want to hear!

The incest scene in *Invisible Man* is preceded by a symbolic dream in which watermelons stand for sexual temptation. The incest scene forms an epi-action to the dream:[205]

> It's still comin' at you though. Still comin'. Then you hear it close
> up, like when you up in the second-storey window and look down on
> a wagonful of water-melons, and you see one of them young juicy
> melons split wide open a-layin' all spread out and cool and sweet on
> top of all the striped green ones like it's waitin' just for you, so you
> can see how red and ripe and juicy it is and all the shiny black seeds
> it's got and all.

The chain of events initiated by the melon scene then continues with equally obvious symbolism until finally the dream is mixed with reality.

Melons are no more than incidentally important in the attitude of Ellison's protagonist at this stage, but violent revulsion at the narrative is not only natural but heightened by the Negro aspect of the thing. Later on in the novel the protagonist is liberated from self-hatred and joyfully accepts himself and his black identity. His liberation from self-hatred is epitomized in an act of vegetable symbolism. As long as he was ashamed to be a Negro, the protagonist always made a point of avoiding dishes that he thought were associated with the Negro, above

PART ONE: 'PREGNANT GOURDS' AND 'DELIRIOUS PUMPKINS'

all pork chops and yams. Now when he is liberated from self-hatred he celebrates his new-found identity by going out and buying a roasted yam from a street vendor and eating it with butter, the way he used to back home in the South during his childhood. He expresses his new-found freedom in a vegetable aphorism: 'I yam what I am.'[206]

Cucurbits are used in a very revealing manner in Alex Haley's *Roots*, a work that is openly and professedly a search for an ethnic identity. When Haley's ancestor, Kunta Kinte, is forcibly brought to America as a slave, his enslavement – symbolized by the chains which limit his freedom to decide his own movement – exists only at the most superficial level. Only his body, not his soul, has been enslaved as yet. A far worse form of slavery will have begun as soon as he has become a slave in his own consciousness – as soon as he has learnt to identify with the blacks in America. His slow and reluctant drifting away from his Mandinka heritage and gradual acceptance of the role as a black slave in America is therefore an important theme in the book.

At the end of chapter 45, when Kunta Kinte is trying to puzzle out the strange things around him, he wonders at a new word that is used repeatedly all around him. 'What, he wondered, was a "nigger"?'[207] His question thus concerns the identity of the American black men (who were slaves); and, not surprisingly, cucurbits are mentioned immediately before, and immediately after, this passage. Earlier in the chapter we are told how much the American blacks loved watermelons (p. 207):

> Some days they served foods Kunta knew of from his home,
> such as groundnuts, and kanjo – which was called 'okra' – and so-so,
> which was called 'black-eyed peas'. And he saw how much these
> black ones loved the large fruit that he heard here being called
> 'water-melon'. But he saw that Allah appeared to have denied
> these people the mangoes, the hearts of palm, the breadfruits, and
> so many of the other delicacies that grew almost anywhere one
> cared to look on the vines and trees and bushes in Africa.

In Kunta Kinte's mind at this stage the black slave culture in America is poor – it is associated with fewer varieties of fruit than the African Mandinka culture. The process of Kunta Kinte's mental enslavement naturally includes Kunta's gradual identification of himself with the slave blacks – and thus also the fruit associated with them. The very next chapter opens with Kunta Kinte picking 'punkins' (pp. 209–10):

> With the cutting and piling of the cornstalks at last completed, the
> 'oberseer' began assigning different blacks to a variety of tasks after

PART ONE: 'PREGNANT GOURDS' AND 'DELIRIOUS PUMPKINS'

> the conch horn blew each dawn. One morning Kunta was given the job of snapping loose from their thick vines and piling onto a 'wagon', as he'd learned they called the rolling boxes, a load of large, heavy vegetables the colour of over-ripe mangoes and somewhat resembling the big gourds that women in Juffure dried out and cut in half to make household bowls. The blacks here called them 'punkins'.
>
> Riding with the 'punkins' on the wagon to unload them at a large building called the 'barn', Kunta was able to see that some of the black men were sawing....

Thus Kunta Kinte is soon working with the fruit associated with slave blacks, and in chapter 50 the word 'punkin' is already so familiar in his vocabulary and in his state of mind that he reflects that the bandage on his foot seems as big as a 'punkin' (p. 234). Part of the process of becoming a slave is completed. He has been forced into the chains provided by the white man, into the work provided by him, into the symbolism provided by him, and into the vocabulary.

But the symbolic role of the word 'punkin' in this occurrence is not restricted to the demonstration of Kunta's acceptance of a foreign slave vocabulary. The word is also used very appropriately as regards the entire range of its semiotic aspects.

The wound has been inflicted by the white men, i.e. the enslavers, after his last attempt to run away. The whites have cut off part of his foot with an axe. The mutilation is both physical and symbolic (Kunta is allowed to choose between castration and crippling). Symbolically, the loss of part of his foot, and thus of part of his ability and liberty to move around, finally crushes his spirit as a free man.

He is now a slave; slaves are associated with punkins; therefore the bandage on the wound that makes him a slave seems as big as a 'punkin' to him.

White racists do not have a monopoly on pumpkin symbolism. It serves black racists equally well, at least judging from the poem by Enoch Tindimwebwa which supplied Denis Hills with a title for his book on Uganda, *The White Pumpkin* (pp. 291-2):

> The White Pumpkin
>
> His gun on his shoulder,
> A hat pulled like a basin over his head,
> The white pumpkin came over the hill.
>
> His shorts looked like a woman's skin skirt,
> His gun like a baking stick,
> He resembled and was taken for
> A woman.

PART ONE: 'PREGNANT GOURDS' AND 'DELIRIOUS PUMPKINS'

Crying in terror
The naked children fled,
Followed by their mothers
With babies dangling on their backs.

'An evil white spirit!' men cried,
'A white monster!'
And within the blink of an eye
The village was empty.
Far away they fled
Into the deep forest's breast,
Among mosquitoes and potholes of elephant.

Expecting a roll of drums,
The white pumpkin wondered
To find the village empty and still.

. .

I saw it. I saw it all.
And I saw him wash himself
Behind a grain bin.
I saw his chest
That was hairy as a dog's, and pumpkin white.

The white man is called an 'evil white spirit', 'a white monster'; he is indirectly compared to a dog; and with the aid of the pumpkin symbolism, doubt is cast on his masculinity, as well as on his intellectual and emotional capacity.

The names of the cucurbits are suitable as words of abuse, and if the reason for the application of abusive words is ethnic antagonism it follows that cucurbitic words will acquire ethnic meanings. In southern France 'melons' is a word of abuse for Arabs. E.A. El Maleh seeks a predominantly phonosemic explanation of the word:[208]

> Le vocabulaire raciste survit à la colonisation et trouve dans l'immigration une source de renouvellement. Tahar Ben Jelloun a noté qu'à Nice on pouvait lire sur les murs le slogan suivant: *"Dehors les melons!"* Aucune difficulté pour les habitants de la ville: tous comprenaient de quoi il s'agissait. Le slogan ramasse en une graphie inattendue le *meu* du beuglement et sans doute le museau noté par l'adjectif long. Il y a peut être une autre explication, mais l'intention péjorative ne fait aucun doute et témoigne de l'agressivité raciste.

These observations seem fairly convincing. But probably there are purely semic connotations too. These are likely to be predominantly sexual, since another word of abuse for Arabs is 'tronc de figuier', and

PART ONE: 'PREGNANT GOURDS' AND 'DELIRIOUS PUMPKINS'

the fig is the fruit whose connotations most closely parallel those of the cucurbit in this respect (cf. also El Maleh's comments on 'Amed et Fatima').

Another group that has become more actively self-conscious during the 1960s and 1970s is the feminists, and since cucurbits are part of the female myth, the feminists naturally sooner or later had to explore this aspect. In 1975 the Swiss-born German feminist Verena Stefan published a book, *Häutungen,* in which the narrator decides that she does not have to conform to the current ideal of feminine physical beauty – that she likes her body as it is with its 'kürbisbrüste'. She accepts being a 'kürbisfrau':[209]

> ... im spiegel neigten sich zwei zartbraune weiche kürbisse dem waschbecken zu. in der sonne auf dem land waren weisse härchen zum vorschein gekommen. Cloe lachte laut auf. igelbrüste! murmelte sie. kürbisigel, igelkürbis ... sie dachte an die verbannten ovalen und runden formen. die gebärmutter eine kürbisfrucht. [xxix]

Apart from getting reconciled to her breasts, she also lets her hair grow, another conventional symbol of female sexual abandonment (p. 123):

> ... vor einem jahr hatte sie die haare ganz kurz scheren lassen. sie wollte noch einmal das gefühl ihrer kopf form und ihres blossen geschichtes spüren (und sie hatte gehofft, die strassenbelästigungen dadurch zu vermindern). die haare waren kräftiger und voller geworden. sie waren schnell gewachsen. jetzt konnte sie sie schon wieder aus dem gesicht streichen. sie dachte an die frau, die sie vor einem jahr gewesen war und an die frau an das jahr zuvor und –
>
> Häutungen.
>
> Dies ist das jahr der kürbisfrau! sie erhob sich, und ging in ihr zimmer. nicht mehr der möchte-gern-schmal-sein-frau, der hätte -ich-doch-flache-brüste-frau. . . . [xxx]

The author's calling herself Cloe could be an allusion to the well-known love story by Longus from the third century, *Daphnis and Chloe,* which is set in Lesbos. The connection with Lesbos again is that Verena Stefan has at this point finally decided to give up men and become a lesbian. As Daphis and Chloe gropingly found their way to a consciousness of their love for each other in a heterosexual relationship, so Verena Stefan's Cloe has found her way to a consciousness of her own role in a homosexual relationship. The cucurbit is therefore primarily associated with femininity, and when she becomes a lesbian she accordingly begins to like her gourd-like breasts because they are feminine. In the quotation above she reacts very negatively to the advances of men, the 'strassenbelästigungen'. It is significant that the whole book opens with a male comment on her breasts, a comment that she takes very badly, and in the first chapter she also compares her breasts to gourds. At that point, however, she feels hurt by the negative sense she reads into the cucurbitic symbol; in the last chapter, on the other hand, when she has rejected men, the symbol has been reinterpreted and its positive meaning joyfully and defiantly accepted.

It is a rule of good workmanship for parodists, caricaturists, satirists and authors of mock-heroic works to drag in pumpkins, wherever they can, since these are ridiculous in their own right.[210] We have already mentioned a number of humorous and satiric authors in this study.[211] As an example of a pumpkin episode mocking the traditional genre of traveller's tales, let us finally take Lucian's story of the Pumpkin-pirates, these seafaring savages who use boats made of pumpkin rinds and fight the Nut-sailors who have boats made of nutshells (nuts are also often regarded as funny).[212]

Everything you wish to make ridiculous should be connected with cucurbits.[213] Conversely, everything connected with pumpkins has a latent ridiculous dimension. When Richard Nixon during the 1950s searched for communists in the USA, he once appeared in a newsreel where he showed how a suspected communist had hidden a secret microfilm in a pumpkin. Nixon's opponents returned to this episode with obvious glee again and again during the campaigns of the 1960s. They wished to make Richard Nixon look ridiculous (cf. the film 'Milhouse'), and for their purpose it was a godsend that the secret film had been hidden in a pumpkin. It would not have been half as funny if it had been hidden in, say, a hollow oak – the traditional, dignified place for hiding and finding secret objects.

Anyone with political ambitions should stay away from pumpkins (the present American president and Australian premier may have sufficient problems with their nuts). In the American cartoon series 'Peanuts' with Charlie Brown, Snoopy and all the others, there is one character, Linus, whose highest ambition is to become the president of his classmates at school. His campaign goes well, and everything looks fine, until he gives in to the temptation to start talking about a mysterious, mythical 'Great Pumpkin' that he believes in. Then his campaign collapses and he is unmasked as absurd, ridiculous and potentially mad. In Ben Jonson's *Volpone*, act II, sc. 1 (67–74), there is a character, Sir Politique Would-Bee, who suffers from paranoia and believes that all sorts of secret agents send messages in cabbages,

PART ONE: 'PREGNANT GOURDS' AND 'DELIRIOUS PUMPKINS'

oranges, musk-melons, etc.[214] This character is an early foreshadowing of the anti-Nixon cucurbitic campaign in the 1960s.

It is a dangerous thing to connect oneself with pumpkins (which, incidentally, does not bode well for the critical reception of this study). Mentioning pumpkins produces incredulous and contemptuous smiles as inevitably as the sound of a bell produced saliva in Pavlov's dogs after they had been conditioned. But the human public have not only been conditioned by accumulated cucurbitic tradition; they also have the mental capacity to deduce for ever anew the ridiculous meaning from the anatomy and physiology of the cucurbits. It was a thankless task for Rufinus and St Augustine to defend the 'cucurbita' translation of the Vetus Latina against the 'hedera' of St Jerome's Vulgate, because to argue from a pumpkin platform is difficult.

Even in one of the most beautiful poems ever written on the subject, Andrew Marvell's 'The Garden', melons have a slightly comic role. Marvell depicts the peace of mind that comes over him in the garden. He mentions many plants in his poem. The stanza in which melons occur goes as follows:[215]

> What wond'rous Life in this I lead!
> Ripe Apples drop about my head;
> The Luscious Clusters of the Vine
> Upon my Mouth do crush their Wine;
> The Nectaren, and curious Peach,
> Into my hands themselves do reach;
> Stumbling on Melons, as I pass,
> Insnar'd with Flow'rs, I fall on Grass.

The poet marvels at the beauty of his existence, the happiness that in another stanza annihilates all 'that's made/To a green Thought in a green Shade'. In the quoted stanza the poet is completely passive. He is the object of actions: apples drop about his head, grapes crush their wine upon his mouth, nectaren and peach reach themselves into his hands, melons trip him up. Several of the plants have mildly exaggerated comic tasks, but none as much as the melon on which the poet stumbles. Naturally the size of the melons earmarks them for the job but we notice the predictable associations to abundance, size and comedy.

The first 3,000 to 5,000 years of the history of the cucurbits in human culture are difficult to study because of the scarcity of historical evidence and the ambiguity of the material that has survived (often haphazardly). From about 300 BC to AD 500 there is sufficient material

PART ONE: 'PREGNANT GOURDS' AND 'DELIRIOUS PUMPKINS'

to make out a fairly clear picture both of Greek and Roman use.[216] During the early Middle Ages the material is again poorer, possibly because (as it is believed)[217] cucurbits were not cultivated very extensively, and human culture in general went through enormous changes in Europe (and written texts of importance in this context are scarce). After Walafrid Strabo in the ninth century the material gradually begins to pick up at about 1500, and the tradition after that rapidly becomes so rich that we have restricted our examples mainly to the Anglo-American tradition and to those examples that we needed to illustrate our arguments.[218]

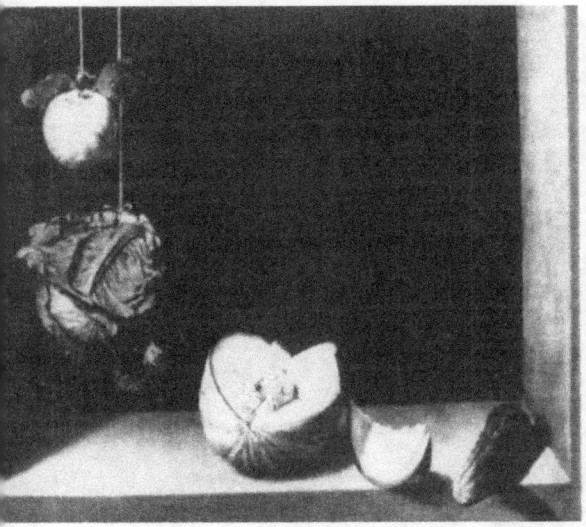
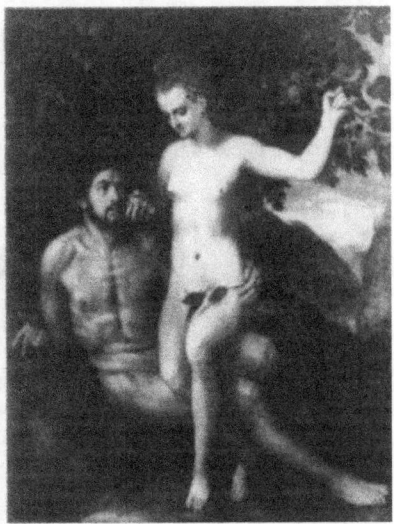

PLATE I
Juan Sánchez Cotán (1561–1627), Still Life, *Quince, Cabbage, Melon and Cucumber*, 1602, collection of the San Diego Museum of Art.

Is there a message in a still life? If so, what is its degree of articulateness, and how can it be 'read'?

One of Cézanne's still lives is called *Nature morte au melon*. See e.g. R. H. Wilenski, *Modern French Painters*, 4th ed., London: Faber & Faber, 1963, p. 133 and plate 48B. That the melon, symbol of life, should be likely to occur in a 'still *life*' is obvious, but it is furthermore also obvious that the artists should try to bring death to mind, since one of the senses of 'still' is 'dead'. Melons in still lives therefore often have slices cut out of them.

PLATE II
Frans Floris (1516–70), *Adam and Eve*. Cognac Museum. After Leo van Puyvelde, *Die Welt von Bosch und Breughel*, München: 1963, picture no. 184.

Through the centuries the Bible has been one of the favourite sources for artists in search of a motif. Of the women in the Bible it is very predictable which ones will occur in connection with cucurbits. The foremost of these is Eve, as in this picture, because Eve and sin go together. At the other end of the scale is the immaculate Maria, whose purity makes it semiotically impossible to have cucurbits in the same picture. To put in cucurbits with the Holy Mother is probably, by the majority of the public, construed as blasphemy.

Carlo Crivelli's *Madonna and Child*, in which a cucurbit does appear together with the Madonna, is classified by Angus Fletcher, in *Allegory: The Theory of a Symbolic Mode* (Ithaca and London: Cornell University Press, 1964), as surrealistic (p. 379; see also p. 372 and *passim*).

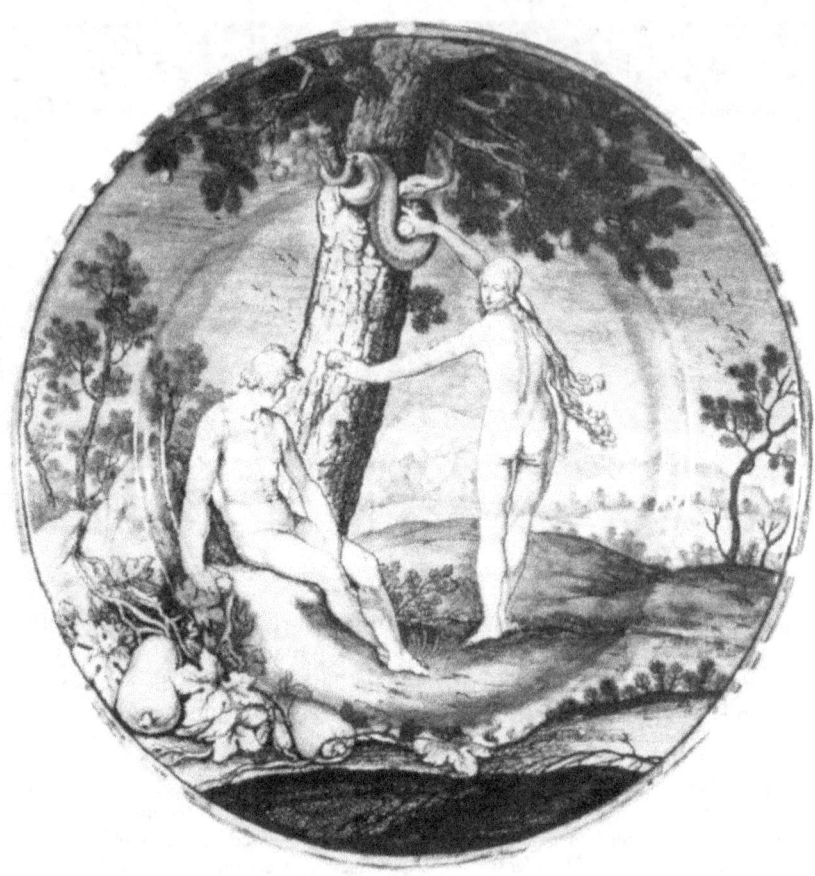

PLATE III
Ferdinando Maria Campani (1702–71), *The Temptation of Adam*. Siena: about 1735. Ashmolean Museum, Oxford, Fortnum Collection.

Here, as in the *Adam and Eve* of Floris, cucurbits have irresistibly crept into the picture because they are semiotically appropriate. The artist sees the temptation as specifically sexual and accordingly brings a sexy fruit into the scene. Cucurbits, in pictures like these, must not be mistaken for incidental ornament or material chosen at random and included in order to balance the composition. They are certainly decorative, but they are semiotically appropriate too, and the way they get into pictures like these is not a random process, no matter whether conscious or unconscious.

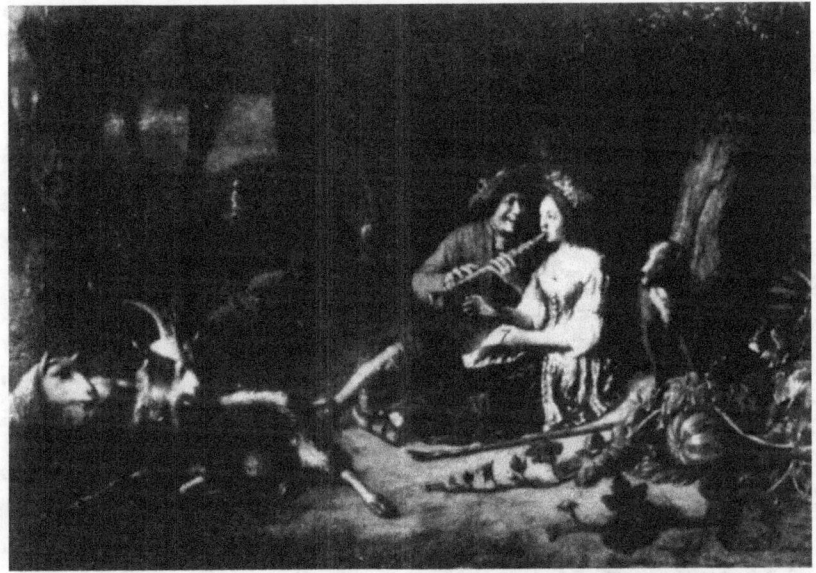

PLATE IV
Lambert Doomer, *Hirtenstück*, Oldenburg (Cat. no. XI).

The tendency for symbols to cluster operates in pictorial art as well as in verbal, and, of course, especially in emblematic representation, where the semioticity of the painting becomes very pronounced – when the various elements quite recognizably stand for something; often functioning as pictorializations of verbal clichés.

In the picture a pair of a shepherd and a shepherdess (or maybe pseudo-shepherd and pseudo-shepherdess) play a flute together. In the background is another loving couple. The cucurbits as symbol of love or sex are reinforced by the he-goat who gives us a sheep's eye. The ambiguity of that glance is reinforced by the symbolic dog who is, probably, a symbol of either fidelity or lack of fidelity (though dogs appear in many of Doomer's paintings).

Wolfgang Schulz, in 'Lambert Doomer als Maler', *Oud Holland*, 92, no. 2 1978, pp. 69–106, points out that the interpretation of the picture must be multi-layered; Doomer has carried on a tradition in a special way (pp. 90–1):

> Mit dem städtisch gekleideten Paar in Sitz-Liege-Haltung auf dem Waldboden klingt ein verbürgerlichtes 'joie de vivre' an. Das symbolträchtige Blasinstrument (Potenzsymbol?) wird durch seinen eigenartigen Gebrauch – der Mann hält die im Mund der Frau steckende Schalmei-Oboe – zum drastischen Hinweis auf die Liebesbeziehungen des Paares. Die Redensart 'Koeri loeri, 't gaet al om het fluiten' gilt nicht zuletzt auch in der Hirtenromantik. Das Paar wird beobachtet vom Hirtenhund, einem positiven oder negativen Treuehinweis. Die auffällig in den Vordergrund gesetzten Kletterpflanzen (Kürbisranken), die kaum als Bildrahmung oder Repoussoir verstanden werden können, sind im Zusammenhang des Bildgeschehens Liebessymbole. Vielleicht muss selbst der Ziegenbock ähnlich interpretiert werden.

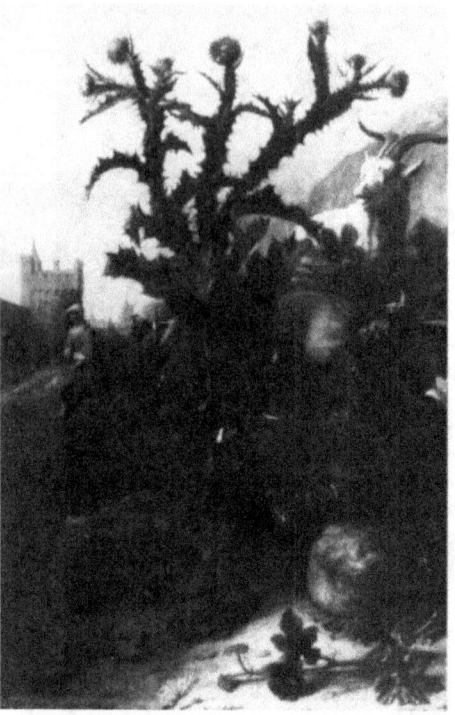
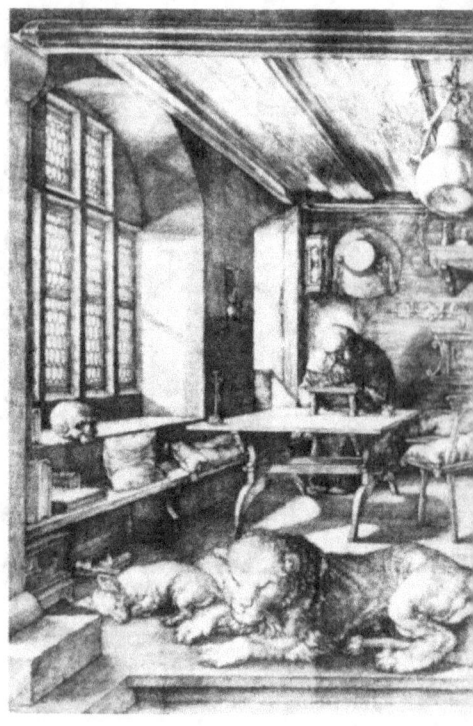

PLATE V
Lambert Doomer, *Distelstaude*, Copenhagen (Cat. no. X), 1675.

This picture illustrates even better than the other painting by Doomer (plate IV) the tendency of symbols to cluster. The thistle in the foreground, according to Schulz, is a sex symbol, said to be known as such even from Pliny. The thistle, says Schulz in 'Lambert Doomer', pp. 91–2, had become

> um 1500 in der Kunst zum Symbol ehelicher Treue mit der Bezeichnung 'Mannentrouw'. Diese Tradition hielt sich im 16. Jahrhundert lebendig und war noch im 17. Jahrhundert breiten Volksschichten bekannt. Durch erneute Zuwendung zu Emblemata und Devisen fand sie ihren ikonographischen Ort in der holländischen Malerei und wurde in ähnlicher Weise wie Weinlaub und Kürbisranken Bedeutungsträger auf Figuraldarstellungen.

But even if the thistle were here taken to stand for 'Mannentrouw' there is still some taste of multi-layeredness in this picture. The thistle is thrown in together with not only a he-goat but with a sex symbol that is also slightly absurd or grotesque – the cucurbit. The thistle is made grotesquely and absurdly big through a trick of perspective.

In any case, in the pastoral scene, where love imagery can be expected, it is in this case tripled: the thistle, the he-goat, the cucurbit.

PLATE VI
Albrecht Dürer's copper-engraving *St Jerome in His Study*, 1514.

That the gourd suspended from the ceiling is an allusion to the Jonah controversy is obvious, but whether there is a specific message (or several specific messages) is difficult to establish. Peter W. Parshall, in 'Albrecht Dürer's *St Jerome in His Study*: A Philological Reference', *The Art Bulletin*, 53, no. 3, September 1971, pp. 303–5, lists a number of possible specific messages. However, we think that one should be wary of jumping to conclusions. It is a very difficult case, and it may be that the gourd is ambiguous, or merely suggestive of the connection between St Jerome and the Jonah–gourd controversy.

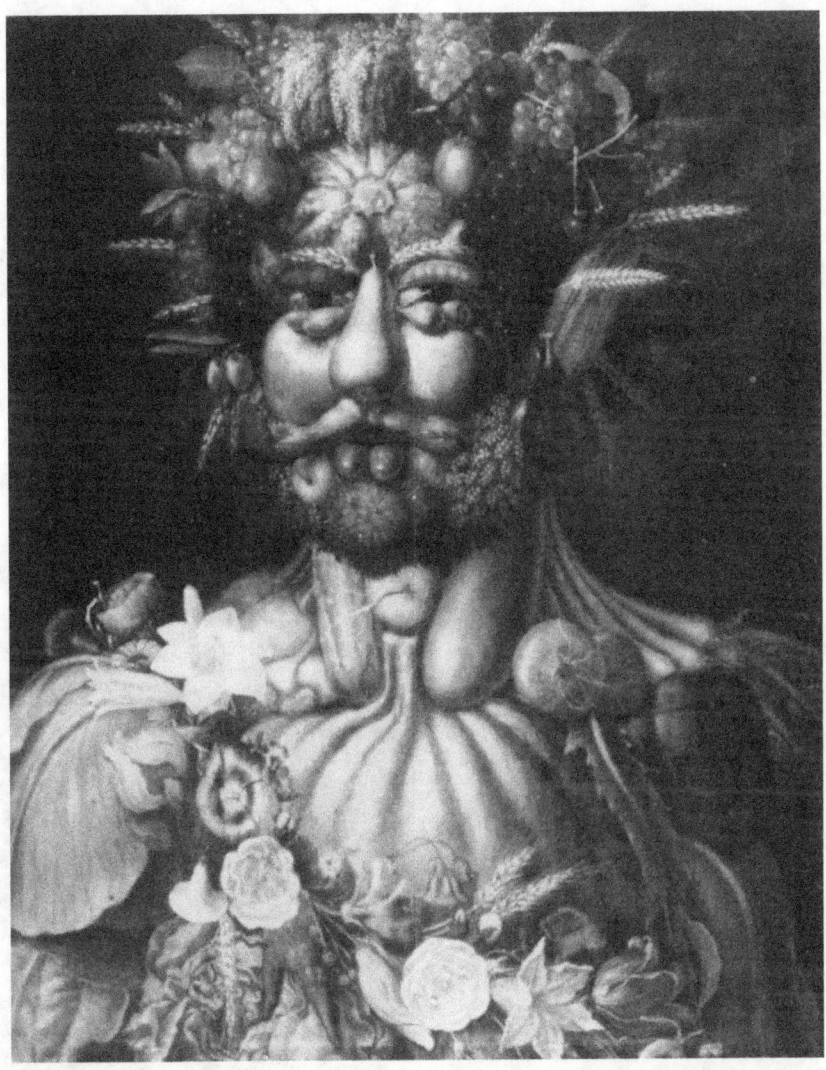

PLATE VII
Giuseppe Arcimboldo,
Vertumnus – Rudolf II, oil, *c.* 1590,
Skokloster.

This picture covers the whole range of connotations, from fertility and abundance to absurdity. For a comment see Sven Alfons, *Symbolister 2 Giuseppe Arcimboldo: En biografisk och ikonografisk studie, Tidskrift för konstvetenskap XXXI*, pub. Ragnar Josephson, Malmö: Allhems förlag, 1957, pp. 134-9 and *passim*; see also Francine Claire Legrand and Félix Sluys, *Giuseppe Arcimboldo et les Arcimboldesques*, Aalter: André de Rache, 1955.

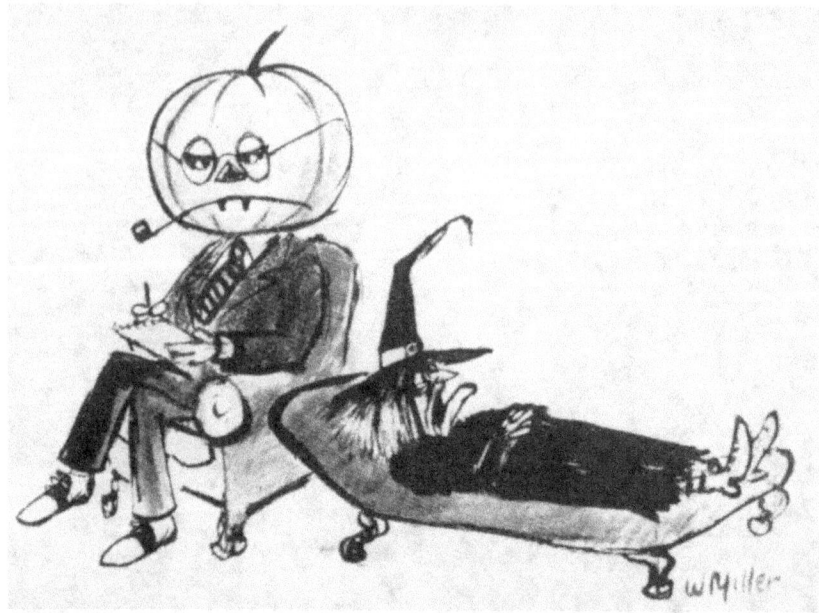

PLATE VIII

Drawing by W. Miller, © 1976, *The New Yorker* Magazine, Inc., 1 November 1976, p. 45. *Pumpkin psychiatrist treats witch lying on couch.*

The drawing was published without a caption. Obviously the artist felt that the message was sufficiently verbal without words – the picture is a typical case of a 'heightened verbal cliché' (or in this case, of two). The artist does not think highly of psychiatrists who are superstitious ('witch-doctors') and stupid ('pumpkin-heads').

PLATE IX

American comic postcard from 1901, J. Stanley Lemons Collection.

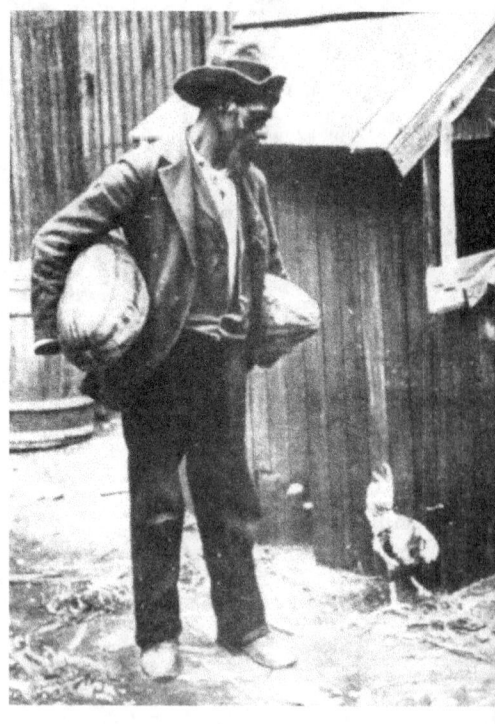

The Negro is made to seem all the more stupid and funny by being put in a situation of an *embarras du choix*, which by its nature makes stupid the person facing the choice – stupid as a 'donkey between two bundles of hay'. In addition the two alternatives that he has to choose between, cucurbits and chicken, are intrinsically negative as well.

Caption: 'Dis Am De Wust Perdickermunt Ob Mah Life'.

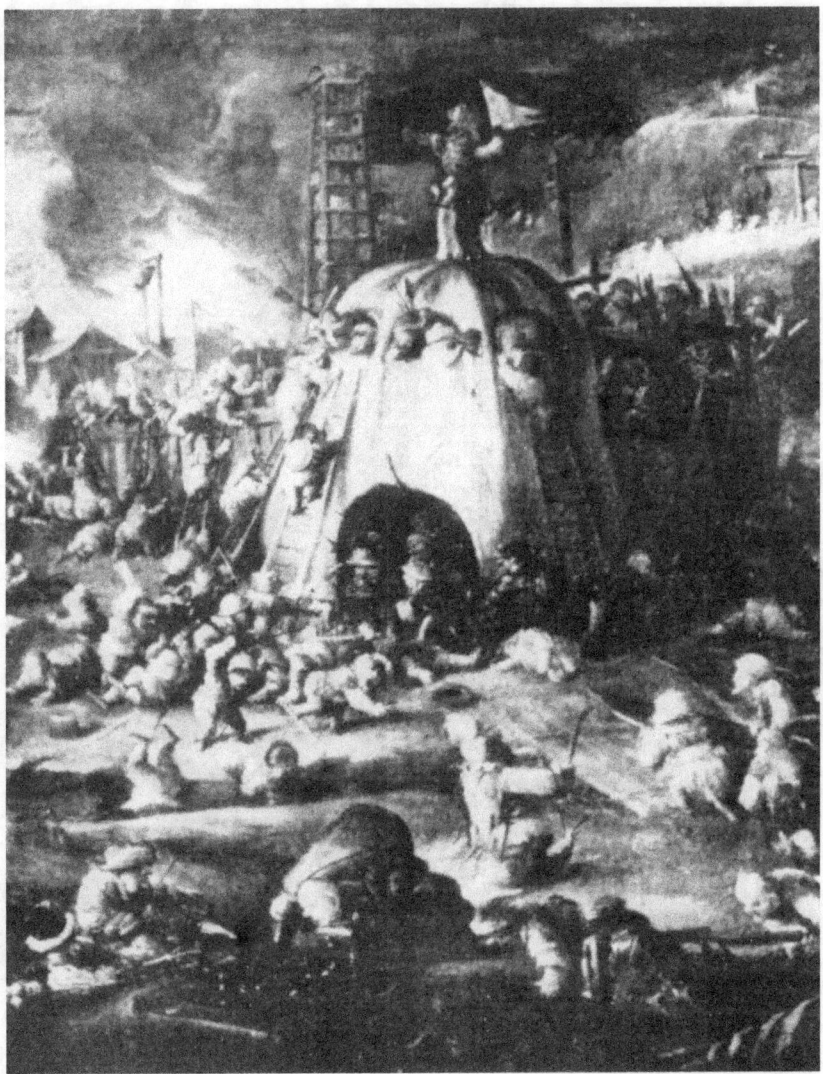

PLATE X
Faustino Bocchi (1659–1742), *Bambocciate*, detail. Painting. Brescia, Galleria (about 1700).

Pumpkins and dwarfs are antithetical as to size, the pumpkin being extremely big and the dwarfs extremely small. They are united by their absurdity; thus we have here extremes on the same absurd continuum. The dwarfs are waging war, some are defending themselves using a pumpkin as a fortress; others are attacking from without.

Is there perhaps a trace of pacifist tendencies and misanthropic realism in some of the black humour of the bamboccianti? If the picture is 'read' verbally with the aid of the juxtaposition of its major concepts (big–small + absurd) maybe the text could be said to be something like this: 'Small absurd men are committing a big absurd mistake'.

On dwarfs see E. Tietze-Courat, *Dwarfs and Jesters in Art*, London: The Phaidon Press, 1957, p. 81 and *passim*.

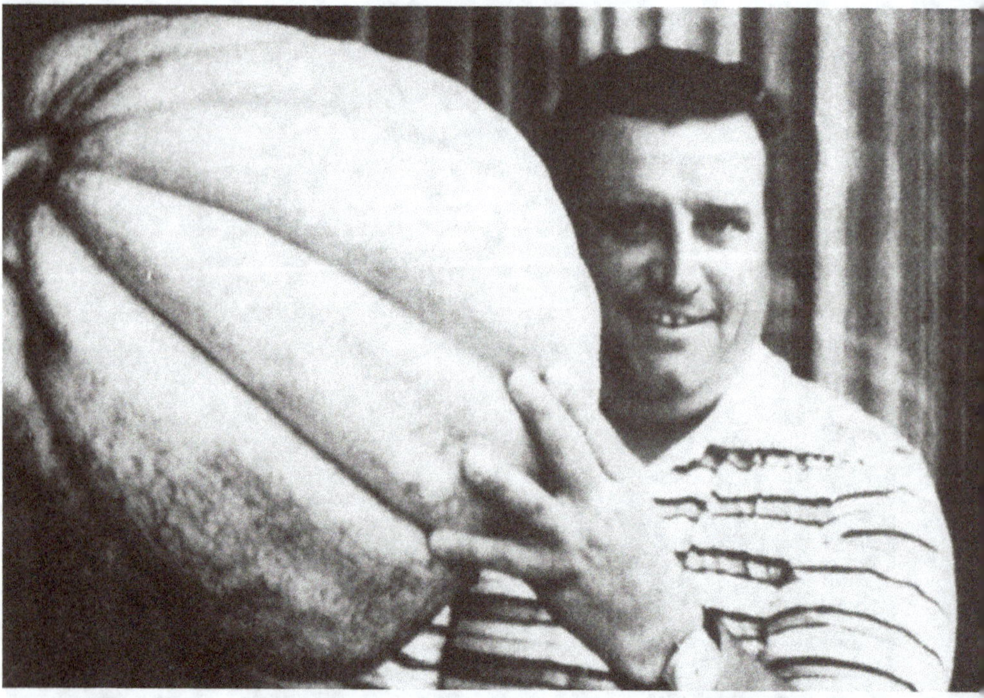

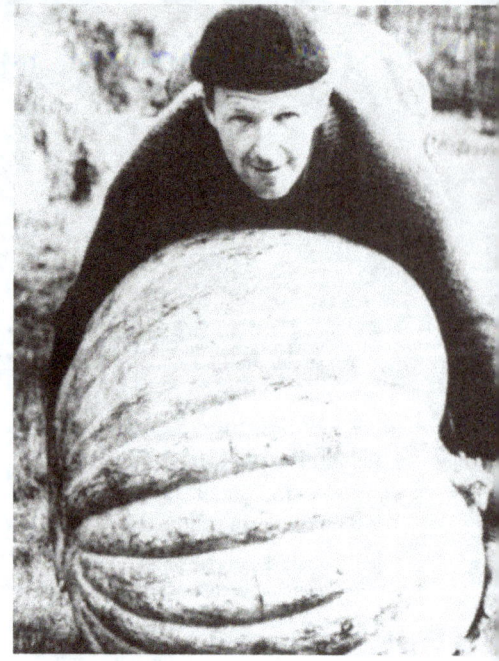

PLATE XI
Above Ed Weeks and his monster watermelon of 197lb (89.3kg), grown in 1975. *Guinness Book of Records*, 25th ed., 1978, p. 54.
Right A pumpkin of 209lb 4oz. (94.913kg) grown by Colin Bowcock in 1976. *Guinness Book of Records*, 25th ed., 1978, p. 55.

The cucurbits are a typical 'record' species in garden produce. Thus they acquire in a heightened form the connotations they pick up, and become the epitome of whatever class of concepts they belong to in one or another dimension of their existence.

Part 2: Implications

τὸ γὰρ εὖ μεταφέρειν
τὸ τὸ ὅμοιον θεωρεῖν ἐστιν.

      Aristotle, *Poetics*

1 Is a literary work written by the author or by the readers?

In addition to 'message', two central concepts of all semiotic theory are 'sender' and 'receiver'. The process of communication is something collective; sender and receiver share the communicative code. If literature is seen as communication one can concentrate on either the role of the sender (the author) or the role of the receiver (the readers). Thus one may ponder the question whether literary works are written by the authors or by the readers; whether the author creates something that he forces upon the readers or whether the author is merely 'borrowed' to formulate something that is essentially created by the readers. In other words, is the author on his own when he writes, or has he merely, after some process of selection, been entrusted with the task of formulating individually what had already been created collectively – the essential part of creation being the establishment in the collective consciousness of readers of a disposition to accept a certain work, and its actual appearance being of secondary importance?

This is one of the perennial questions of literary theory. Recent semiotic literary scholarship, such as French structuralism, has brought about a renewal of interest in the question, but answers to it are as many and contradictory as before. In general, a view of literature as communication tends to weaken the emphasis on the role of the author and to strengthen the emphasis on that of the readers. Communication presupposes a code, and a code is something collective. It is hardly surprising, therefore, that there should be a shift in attention from the individual (the author) to the collective (the readers and the author – an author who is free to create, but only within a code, or codes, that he shares with his readers, or at the most is able to *create for* his readers).

Some structuralists have dissociated themselves from an extremist reader orientation, particularly if such a position implies the recognition of some concept of literary *competence*, because of the alleged authoritarian and restrictive implications of the model. But one branch of structuralist thought on literature has tended in the direction that literature expresses itself in man rather than that man expresses himself in literature.

Language, myths and literature in such structuralist opinion almost have a life of their own. The author is the tool of literature, rather than vice-versa; the author does not borrow literature to express himself – literature borrows the author to express itself. Man does not think in language; language thinks in man. These structuralists quote philosophers who stress the role of the collective language, e.g. Heidegger, who said that 'die Sprache spricht, nicht der Mensch. Der Mensch spricht nur, indem er geschicklich der Sprache entspricht'.[1]

The literary branch of French structuralism is influenced by the anthropological branch, where there has been a similar shift of focus. In his introductory chapter of *Le cru et le cuit* Claude Lévi-Strauss says that he attempts to show not how men think in myths but 'comment les mythes se pensent dans les hommes, et à leur insu'.[2]

But probably the strongest influence has been the linguistic analogy. There has been an attempt to see how far the properties of the metaphorical concept of 'the language of literature' correspond to those of language in the proper sense of the word. What critics have sought is the analogical equivalent in literature of 'languages' – even of languages in the sense of English, German and French.

In natural languages, said Ferdinand de Saussure, signs are arbitrary. The animal that the English call 'dog' is known to the French as 'chien' and to the Germans as 'Hund', and all three arbitrary signs serve equally well. Yet, naturally, the signs are not arbitrary in the sense of being so relative to an individual in a speech situation. In order to make himself understood the speaker has to use 'Hund' in German-speaking areas, 'chien' in French and 'dog' in English.

Analogically, one could argue that in order to be understood the author has to cater to the expectations and stay within the literary 'language' of his audience. He has to accommodate to the opinions, beliefs, prejudices, etc., of his audience – in a word, to *tradition*.

It is at this point that the linguistic analogy breaks down, or at least becomes very flimsy, and certainly very controversial. Anyone can see that there is some truth in the analogy – do we not all recognize that authors pander to their audience? – but not such a neat truth as in language proper. Even in language proper individuals exerting a strong influence may occasionally succeed in changing the code and introducing new words and constructions. This is true to a far higher degree in 'the language of literature', because, first, the codes are not very rigid; second, there always exists a multitude of codes (and a multitude of publics – the population of any country is literarily 'multilingual'); and third, literary codes are often provisional, so that humans not only tolerate but even expect and long for a certain amount of change of the codes. Literary codes are to a large extent the toy of author and reader, and if readers are willing to play a game with signification this increases the creative authority of the writer.

Dogmatic views on the 'author-versus-reader' issue are not very fruitful. It is obvious that there is reciprocity in the process of literary communication. The author has to consider the audience, but the audience is usually also to some extent willing to consider the author. How the respective share of the author and the readers may vary from case to case is more important in the study of individual works than for the construction of general theory.

There is, however, one notable exception, namely naturally motivated signs. The evidence of our cucurbitic material points unambiguously in one direction: *the readers* write these passages. Ultimately this may amount to saying that the passages write themselves – a question that we shall return to in chapter 2. If a sign came into existence because of natural suitability and is then preserved by tradition, it is the readers who write the works. If not only the birth of the sign but also its life is influenced by natural suitability, then the work writes itself.

People sceptical of the notion that the readers write the literary works, or that the works write themselves, may wonder at the technicalities involved in such 'writing'. How, precisely, does a literary work create itself in an author? The answer would seem to be that the natural motivation of the sign is the guiding force that takes an element as far as possible towards a predetermined latent state of perfection.

The best variant of the American story of the 'self-made man' – the underdog who rises from insignificance and obscurity to importance and greatness – is the version in which the hero begins his career as an elevator-boy. It is the best because the elevator is an appropriate symbol. This version also seems to be one of the most popular. It is easy to see its superiority. The hero should not, for instance, start his career as a butler. A butler stays with the same family; he knows his place and so on. The image of a butler reinforces the idea of social stability; what is needed is an image of mobility. Neither should the hero start as a dealer in luxury cars. If he is to start in business at all he must buy and sell something seemingly worthless, such as dirty sacks or empty oil-barrels; otherwise his humble state at the beginning of his career is not sufficiently underlined or sufficiently contrasted with his rise-to-come. He must be associated with something humble, and at the same time associated with mobility.

To start as an elevator-boy is perfect because it includes a symbol of vertical mobility, which prefigures the hero's rise in the world in social and economic terms. It is true that an elevator goes down as well as up – every second time in fact – but this is not the function that takes the primary place in people's consciousness. To the American and to the English mind at least it is the up-going function of this transportational device that is important; at least judging from the names, which both in American ('elevator') and in English ('lift') stress the up-going function – naturally enough, since walking up a stairway is more exhausting than walking down and the lift is given its name from the tiring activity it eliminates.

Assuming that the self-made man starting his career as an elevator-boy is the perfect form of the story, we may imagine several explanatory models for the birth of the perfect version. The first could be called the sieve- or filter-model. This assumes a rich reality, with a rich material from which the story can be created: thousands of poor young boys making it, in thousands of different ways, but finally only the case of the elevator-boy being accepted as material, because of its intrinsic appropriateness. The perfect form of the story should be thought of as latent. When it happens, by chance, to be triggered into materialization, it will be accepted by the public, who have hitherto acted as a sieve or filter, sifting the rich material of reality and rejecting imperfect or less perfect forms.

This idea is analogous to Darwinism: it postulates a rich reality, author-induced chance variation, and a controlling force (the audience) who ensure survival of the fittest version.[3] One could also compare it to American pragmatism, with its two forces of 'tychism' and 'synechism'.

The second explanatory model could be called the 'lie-model'. This involves selection too, but active rather than passive selection, whether conscious or unconscious. The model assumes a greater amount of participation on the part of the author, though not in inventive freedom, but in willingness to cater to the demands of the readers. Of all the boys, and of all the things the boys did, the formulators of the story chose the self-made man who started as an elevator-boy; and of all the things that he did (we may imagine that he did many), they chose to use his work as elevator-boy – all because of intrinsic appropriateness. But above all, even if he did not work as an elevator-boy at all they must still say so – lie – because of the intrinsic appropriateness of the untrue element, which is so true symbolically that it does not matter whether it is true literally as well. 'Fiction', after all, means 'lie'.

The third model seeks the explanation of the birth of the perfect form of the story in life itself. As a boy the self-made man was ambitious; he wanted to rise in the world and therefore, consciously or unconsciously, he sought out as his first job a function that symbolized his social desire.

The idea that a work is written by its public often infuriates people. There is apparently something degrading in the thought of the author as a mere projection of the desire of the public. These violent feelings are obviously connected with the second of the suggested models of literary autogenesis. The public regard the mimetic theory of literature as the only one giving a perfect legitimacy.

The uproar over Alex Haley's *Roots* is an instructive example. The saga of Haley's ancestors is supposed to be based on fact. Fact and fiction are mingled in faction but the readers, anxious to accept the work, want a perfect legitimacy for it, and seek that legitimacy in the belief that Haley is telling the truth. Evidence for this is provided as much by those who attack the factual foundations of the novel as by those who defend them; both appeal to the same authority: the idea of literature as a direct imitation of reality.

Why is Kunta Kinte, Haley's eighteenth-century ancestor, a Muslim in *Roots*? One explanation is that he is a Muslim in the book because he is thought to have been a Muslim in reality in eighteenth-century Gambia in the village of Juffure. Any adducing of further reasons will anger many, since the first is an 'absolute' reason, needing no support, and leaving no choice.

But if there was, somehow, a choice, then it is obvious that Islam was a very good one. The indigenous religions of Africa are of fairly low status in present-day America. These religions are associated with primitivism, barbaric rites and superstitious beliefs. Islam on the other hand was always of fairly high status in the first place, and with the oil money pouring into the Arab world, which is the centre of Islam, the status is steadily rising. The Black Muslims in the United States, a movement that Haley has been in close contact with, try to improve the self-respect of the blacks; and part of this improvement arises out of simply being or becoming a Muslim. Making Kunta Kinte a Muslim in the book gives him a culture that is superior, or at least equal, to that of the white man. Islam brings with it, in *Roots*, literacy, civilization, humanity, refinement.

For the suitability of Islam in *Roots* in relation to a set of values in the minds of prospective readers, it ultimately does not matter whether the real Kunta Kinte was a Muslim or not. *Roots* as we know it was the perfect form of the book for those readers, and Haley came along and spelled it out. If Haley (with his Muslim ancestor Kunta Kinte) had not appeared – on our first explanatory model – the readers would have had to take, and possibly wait for, another author to formulate the work; or – on our second model – it would not matter what Kunta Kinte was in reality; in the book he *must* be Muslim. For the 'fiction' half of faction he must be Muslim; if he happens to have been Muslim in the 'fact' part as well that is all so much to the better.

One cannot argue that the popularity or the sales of a book indicate the degree of reader participation in its creation. There may be books written for (that is, *by*) certain small audiences in which the participation of the audience is great even though the figures of sales are low. Nevertheless, in its tremendous popularity, *Roots* is a phenomenon comparable only to a handful of other American works, such as *Uncle Tom's Cabin* or *Gone With the Wind*, and in terms of complying with something common to the thought of the entire American nation there must be some sort of correlation.

The prominence given to Islamitic culture in the opening section of the book was thus predictable. Even more predictable was the use of cucurbits which we explained in Part 1. *Roots* is an ethnically conscious work. Therefore the symbols that the environment has imposed on the ethnic group, the Negroes, are bound to occur, and to occur in predictable fashion.

In popular white prejudice the Negroes are, or at least were, chicken-stealing watermelon addicts. Typical of this stereotype is the situation depicted in Plate IX, a comic postcard from the turn of the century, showing a black man who has just stolen two watermelons and who stands, one fruit under each arm, outside a shack, looking wistfully at a chicken. The captions reads: 'Dis Am De Wust Perdickermunt Ob Mah Life'.

The stereotype is used to help enslave the black man in white public opinion. In the definition of the Negro's position in the world, with the aid of something from nature, the Negro is coupled with a fruit that has ridiculous and other negative connotations. Against the background of material like this it is natural that Haley in *Roots* should use watermelons and 'punkins' at the crucial stage in the development of Kunta Kinte's identity from free man to slave.

The section devoted to Chicken George in *Roots* may at first seem disproportionately long to people such as Europeans who may not be aware of, or understand, the connection Negro-chicken. But, as Stanley Lemons points out, next to watermelons, chickens are the thing most intimately connected with Negroes in the stereotypes of popular culture at the time of the postcard.[4]

Chickens are stupid (a characteristic feature usually attributed specifically to the female of the species, the hen, because the idea of stupidity can then be reinforced by anti-female sexist prejudice).[5] Chickens are food and the negative effects for the Negro of being coupled with a dish are triple: first, you tend to despise anything that you eat; second, with Negro servants as cooks the act of preparing the food is menial and as despicable as the food itself; and third, there is the staple diet abuse. In the last case, since chickens are not always the cheapest kind of food, a 'moderator factor' – stealing – is brought in to complement the myth so that it can operate in connection with the Negroes. Thus even if it were not true that Negroes eat chicken all the time, that is only because they cannot get it: if they could they would, and given half a chance they will.

An additional boon is that this form of the myth makes the Negroes criminals (thieves), and criminals of a desirable category. Chicken-stealing is a petty crime, ridiculous in the extreme. In stock descriptions of chicken-stealing, when you try to steal a chicken, it slips out of your grip, cackles immoderately, wakes the rest of the roost, wakes the watchdog, and – with the hens cackling and running round in confusion, the dog barking, the owner of the chickens coming out on the porch in his underpants swearing and shouting; all this in a cacophonous symphony – comedy is definitely assured. For the communicative purposes of the postcard it was better for the Negro to be coupled with an insignificant and ridiculous crime than a serious one. A serious one, apart from destroying the humour, which is essential for a feeling of superiority, would also have destroyed that feeling in another way, i.e. by the image of the Negroes growing threatening.[6] (You cannot quite feel superior to someone you feel threatened by.[7]) Therefore the crime should be petty, and chicken-stealing is therefore perfect.

A similar reason determines the fact that the Negro has to choose between two alternatives which are equally good. For the situation of choice to have a stupidifying effect it is necessary that the choice be between two alternatives that are equal; but they could be either equally bad or equally good. To have made the Negro choose between two equally bad alternatives, between 'pest and cholera' as the saying goes, would have made him slightly tragic and a potential object of compassion and other noble feelings; and the humour would have seemed cruel. The choice between two equally good alternatives on the other hand suggests that even the problems of the Negro are somehow a luxury; he has no real problems; he will be all right in either case; it is just his boundless greed that creates problems in his otherwise carefree and idyllic existence.

Chicken, apart from being part of the paradigm mutton, beef, venison, etc., is also part of the paradigm foal, whelp, calf, etc. It is a name for the young, and one persistent type of prejudice against blacks was to regard them as children; that is, human in a sense, certainly, but not worthy of freedom and independence.

Of course Haley had to take up this symbol and destroy it, to re-create it and turn it to use. Chicken George is connected with chickens, but in a sense that destroys all the negative connotations for the blacks. Chicken George is a breeder and trainer of cocks for cock-fighting. 'Chicken' in American means 'coward'. Haley's chapters on Chicken George destroy this meaning because a fighting cock is anything but cowardly. Destroying the sense for the chicken, the chapters naturally also by analogy destroy the sense 'cowardly' in connection with the people associated with chickens, the blacks.

To breed and train fighting cocks demands skill. Cock-fights mean betting, and betting means money, and money means status. The fighting cocks are of no practical use; they are a luxury which leads the Negroes via these cocks to associations with aristocratic idleness, which turns the tables on the laziness issue. Negroes are supposed to be lazy, and blamed for it. The aristocracy is supposed to be idle, and admired for it. The same thing – inactiveness – means a different thing for the poor and the rich. Money makes the difference; and this is why money in the betting sequences of the Chicken George episode is important. The sums of money are huge, the people betting do not deal in 'chicken-feed'.

Cocks are also, like watermelons, associated with sex, and at the time of the postcard this probably worked against the blacks as well. It presumably brought to mind the view that Negroes shop around very freely in matters of love; that there were many black families with only one parent (usually the mother), etc. The aim of the postcard would have been to reinforce indirectly the idea that Negroes were incapable of stable love relationships. The attitudes to sex have changed during this century, and many of the negative connotations have become less negative or even positive; thus Haley did not have to destroy the cock's associations with sexual prowess. In *Roots* Chicken George accordingly has a lot of women and extra-marital love.

All these arguments depend on the assumption that a choice exists, whereas the opposite opinion maintains that in books based on fact there is no choice, because things have to be told as they are, or as they were. But even in autobiography, which is supposed to relate facts, there is an overwhelming amount of choice. Anyone who attempts to write a chapter of his or her autobiography will soon find how little the facts of one's past determine the shape of the narrative. Most is selection, arrangement and manipulation. And even though one may wish to deny it, one still writes for an audience, and the process of accommodation to that audience begins very early.

Naturally, the idea that the audience exerts influence is far from revolutionary. A major consideration with publishers is always whether readers will buy, and a major consideration with authors is always whether publishers will publish. If readers will not buy, then publishers will not publish, and authors will not write. But the audience influences the birth and shape of works in a wide and sophisticated variety of ways.

We have dealt with Haley's *Roots* at such length in order to show both how an author can smash a semantic tradition (particularly if there is an audience waiting to see it smashed) and at the same time, if the tradition is based on naturally motivated signs, how the author is nevertheless forced to accept the basic meaning of the signs. Haley put the cucurbits to his own special use, but he did not touch their basic meaning as signs; indeed he *could* not.

If signs are arbitrary, then teleological arguments are impossible. But if signs are naturally motivated, then the immutability of nature provides the factor of stability that makes such arguments possible. The whole of Chapter 2 will be based on such arguments, but even in this chapter – which is meant to deal with the role of the public – the conclusion should be that the address of a message influences its form and shape to a high degree. What the message will be like is very much determined by its destination.

IS A LITERARY WORK WRITTEN BY THE AUTHOR OR BY THE READERS?

If one stresses the role of the public as a major guiding force in the birth of cucurbitic passages, it follows that one has to believe rather strongly in the existence of a cucurbitic *competence* in readers. There is no doubt in our minds about the existence of a very remarkable cucurbitic *competence*; people master the symbolic grammar of cucurbits very well, whether they are aware of it or not. Anyone who doubts the ability of the public to recognize a cucurbitic epithet as an insult is advised to test a few (and to be prepared for particularly emphatic results of verification during the experiment).

A less hazardous but equally amusing and revealing empirical test is to mention to people that Shakespeare calls only one of his characters 'pumpkin' ('pumpion'). People familiar with Shakespeare's plays will almost always immediately name Falstaff, who is fat (iconic relationship), absurd like a pumpkin, humorous like a pumpkin, a glutton (cucurbits being a glutton's food); who drinks (wateriness connotations), and is at this stage in the *Merry Wives* unsuccessfully trying to seduce a woman (sex connotations).

Before closing the chapter we should comment briefly on the qualitative and evaluative dimensions of the question. In choosing our examples for Part 1 we did not use literary quality as a criterion. We included a few examples illustrating each connotation, whether these examples happened to come from respectable texts or not. Looking back over the material it is not surprising to find that the best use of the cucurbitic symbols, from an artistic point of view, is made by those writers and artists who are even otherwise regarded as the best. But it is striking how their use of the symbols is not only the fullest and richest but at the same time quite unadventurous. The good writers have produced, in a sense, excellent stereotypes. The stereotypes of the bad writers differ from those of the good writers more in their degree of artistic subtlety than in kind.

What is literary genius then? Is it only some subtle form of conventionality? Is literary talent a special sense of what will be acceptable to the mind of the reader or listener, and a special gift for formulating something that will appeal to hitherto-untapped springs of response in the receiver, without disturbing the consistency of the new material with the old?

In the case of naturally motivated signs at least this is so, and indeed has to be. Such is the nature of signs in plant symbolism. Good and bad authors have to use these in the same way; to both the good and bad author the meaning of the plant, in the audience of each, is the same, which in turn is due to the fact that nature is the same. Steel is hard and wax is soft to the good and the bad writer alike. Nature offers her systems for use in metaphors and similes impartially. The good writer and the bad both know what cucurbits are like. It is what the authors make of that knowledge that counts. But the range of variation is limited. The best symbol of wateriness *will be* the most watery fruit. It will be expressive of wateriness-meaning to the degree that it differs from other fruit in wateriness. The choice of sign for wateriness is thereby predetermined, and elegant variation, for instance, can be indulged in only at the cost of expressiveness.

Perhaps it would be fair to say that bad authors often master only the paradigm and rely too much on the 'signalling value' of inherently funny elements and thus produce clichés. They expect that by the mere dragging in of pumpkins humour will be engendered and laughter generated. The good authors, in contrast, work on the context, making it funny, and then, for a slot in the syntagm, where the textual neighbourhood is already very funny, they choose an element (cucurbits) which in addition is inherently funny; success thus being ensured by a combination of maximal effect in the syntagmatic and the paradigmatic dimensions. The good author puts humour in the one and humour in the other (if humour is what he aims for), and the mark of his genius is his perfect knowledge and mastery of both.

The author's mastery of the material is at the same time, however, the material's mastery of the author. The romantic view of literature stresses the individual, independent, creative and inventive genius of the author. Classicist periods believe less in invention than in craftsmanship. But one area of literature is special, and that area is literature which makes use of naturally motivated signs. In this area of literature writing has always been, is, and will forever remain 'classicist', and the best the artist can aim for will inevitably be 'what oft was thought, but ne'er so well express'd'.

2 Does a literary work write itself?

In plant symbolism, in addition to the role of the sender and the receiver, the message itself plays a very important part. Cucurbitic passages often formulate themselves, as it were, because their perfect, their given, form is latently in existence, only waiting for the sifting or filtering processes of human thought to bring it forth into materialization. In Chapter 1 we argued that the author is free to create only within certain limits, and that those limits are largely determined by the ability of his audience to decode the message. Actually, however, it often seems as if the restrictions were not even imposed by the public but by the material itself. Certain elements of the works have, in a sense, latently a given form which forces its way into speech or print. Passages involving plant or animal symbolism are such elements.

In this chapter we shall exemplify four ways in which cucurbitic passages 'write themselves'.

Maximal appropriateness

The cucurbits are in many respects somewhat extreme – they are a typical 'record' species in garden produce, as a perusal of the *Guinness Book of Records* will confirm. Thus they acquire in a heightened form the connotations of the place they grow in; they become the epitome of whatever class of concepts they belong to in one or another dimension of their existence. They are the prime produce of a garden; thus they acquire the connotations of gardens in a heightened form, whether this be the scorn of the city-slicker, or the enthusiasm of the back-to-nature romantic. They are usually delicious, and thus acquire the symbolic role of the dainty *par excellence*; very suitable for gluttons.

'Suitability' is the key word.

DOES A LITERARY WORK WRITE ITSELF?

The principle involved could be called simply 'maximal appropriateness', and the way the selection works is of course quite obvious; when you choose something from nature to illustrate an idea, you choose something suitable. If you want an image of hardness, for instance, you take iron rather than wax.

As we pointed out in Part 1, cucurbits, particularly the melon, are delicious. Gluttons and gourmands are fond of delicious food; therefore a good story of a gourmand or glutton should ideally depict him as eating cucurbits. Investigating this, we find that cucurbits are a stock item in stories of gourmands and gluttons. The Roman emperor Clodius Albinus, a glutton on the throne, is said to have eaten 'melones Ostienses decem' during one single meal, in addition to a fair amount of peaches, grapes, figs and oysters.[1] Of Carinus it is said that he 'inter poma et melones natavit'.[2] And in stories of divine retribution, when his lack of moderation becomes the bane of the glutton, the instrument is often cucurbits, as in the case of the Chinese emperor who was so immoderately fond of musk-melons that he died of overeating them.

The rule that cucurbits occur in connection with gluttons holds irrespective of genre or stylistic level. It is equally to be expected in a children's book (for example, one by Richard Scarry) as in the *Historia Augusta*. A perfect story of a glutton should have cucurbits as an element, and through some process of selection such stories often seem to acquire them.

An observer unfamiliar with the thought that literary passages could write themselves might object that the *Historia Augusta* states that Clodius ate ten melons from Ostia not because this is semiotically appropriate at this point, but because the emperor really did so. But the mimetic element in literature does not work in such a crude and simple way. The emperor eating the melons from Ostia may be a necessary but not a sufficient requirement for the action to be included in the *Historia Augusta*. Life is immeasurably rich in detail. Therefore literature cannot be indiscriminate imitation; instead it inevitably turns into selection, manipulation and arrangement of the selected material. Literature imitates not life but a refined image of it.[3]

From the numerous things that the emperor can be expected to have done that day, the author of the *Historia Augusta* selects one, his eating ten melons from Ostia, which distils the essence of the emperor's gluttonous nature as the author saw it. The story creates, syntagmatically, a convincing picture of a glutton: Clodius eats, and he eats a lot. In the choice of a dish for his zenith of gluttony (eating ten of something) the author chooses melons, a fruit that is inherently associated with gluttons. Thereby the author displays his mastery of the paradigm as well as the syntagm. The well wrought context fits perfectly the well chosen element he puts in it.

To explain how the cucurbit found its way into the *Historia Augusta* let us return to the three models we suggested in Chapter 1. Adopting the first model, we may imagine that of all the things the emperor did the author chose the characteristic one; or else the passage, in order to come into existence, had to 'wait' for the emperor to do the characteristic thing. According to the second model, we may assume that, no matter what the emperor did in reality, in the *Historia Augusta* he has to eat ten melons, because this is symbolically so true that it does not matter whether or not it is literally true as well. The third model, again, would base the argument on life itself – being a glutton, the emperor did eat ten melons and thus provided the symbol of his gluttony, i.e. lived up to his image.

These are all thinkable, but the role of the third should not be exaggerated. In the distribution of emphasis to either art or life, many arguments that may at first seem to favour a shift towards life will prove, on closer inspection, to be false. It might have been argued, for instance, that when the assassin in the book and film *Day of the Jackal* (see Part 1) uses a watermelon as target in his shooting practice it is not an artistic choice (semiotics of art) but a choice in the reality depicted (semiotics of life).

In order to scrutinize this argument let us consider a parallel. In the Australian film *Walkabout* by Nicolas Roeg there are two suicides, both of them connected with heavy fruit symbolism. At the end of the film the aborigine male hero, having become disillusioned with the white heroine, hangs himself from a mango tree. With his body dangling among the ripe and over-ripe mangoes (which, like melons, are a symbol of life) the parallel with the human life, ripe for death, is obvious.

The other fruit symbolism occurs at the beginning of the film. A father takes his daughter and son for a picnic in the desert. Before they leave their home in Sydney, the girl takes several varieties of melons from the refrigerator and puts them into the picnic basket. The alerted watcher realizes that since the symbol of life has figured so prominently there will soon be death; and once out in the obligatorily melon-antithetical desert (see section below on 'Antithesis') the father promptly tries to shoot the children and then succeeds in shooting himself. Some of the bullets hit the picnic food spread out on a blanket.

DOES A LITERARY WORK WRITE ITSELF?

The scene ends with a photographic shot of flies swarming over the slaughtered melons, i.e. two symbols of *Vergänglichkeit* or ephemeral life.

This film illustrates yet another argument about why the choice of melons belongs to art rather than life. As an artistic choice it makes sense – over-abundant sense. An argument to the effect that bringing the melons was a choice in life, on the other hand, must totally ignore their symbolic value, since the plot is such that the daughter is not supposed to have known what was going to happen. The artist–creator who wrote the script knew what was going to happen; the character (the heroine) did not. It is a strong argument in favour of regarding choices such as these as belonging entirely to art and not to life that many elements acquire their symbolic meaning only in retrospect.

Death was primary, and once it was a given it brought the melons in with it. The melons cannot be primary; and the choice of them, if it is symbolic, cannot be a choice in life rather than art, because in that case anybody bringing melons to a picnic would be stopped by the police for his manifest intention of killing himself and others. If the cucurbitic element has symbolic meaning, it is art, not life, that gives it that meaning.

In Chapter 1 we tried to argue the probability or even inevitability of the occurrence of cucurbits under certain conditions, seeking the explanation in the symbolic status of the cucurbits in the minds of the public. But actually we may go a step further, and argue the probability or even inevitability of the existence and structure of that status too, and root the explanation in the physiology of the plant. The physiology determines the symbolic status of the cucurbit in the minds of readers and therefore its status when used by authors in symbolic passages.

Since the cucurbits are record species in so many respects, the probability or inevitability of their occurrence is assured when an author wants to epitomize, through the use of a symbol, one of the connotations of the cucurbits. We saw in Part 1 how again and again cucurbits have been used to epitomize something connected with one of their chief connotations. They were used to symbolize the sexiest, the most absurd, the extremely bathetic, the quickest-growing, the fastest-dying, etc.; and since they somehow excel in all these departments in reality, their being picked to stand as a sign for it in literature is not surprising.

To show the best of earthly splendour, Eve in Milton's *Paradise Lost* goes to pick the 'juiciest Gourd' (see Part 1). The cucurbit in Tennyson

DOES A LITERARY WORK WRITE ITSELF?

(see Part 1) was second only to grapes, just as it tends to occur in a prominent position in any hierarchy of fruit. Walafrid Strabo's 'altipetax', the *cucurbita*, overshadows its competitors in his garden both literally and symbolically (see Part 1).

Examples abound, and it is easy to find instances where the role of a cucurbitic element as the epitome of something is not only implied but is spelled out. As a final example, to illustrate this let us take a passage where the cucurbit epitomizes sexiness. The symbol involves a Negress, and as we pointed out in Part 1 there is a well attested connection between cucurbits and Negroes. With the sex connotations of the cucurbits, and the sex myths about the Negroes, a triangular relationship Negro–sex–cucurbit has come into existence.

In John Updike's novel *Rabbit Redux* the protagonist, Rabbit, has to imagine some character in order to be sexually aroused. The most prominent imaginary character is a fat and slightly absurd Negro woman:[4]

> He always has to imagine somebody, masturbating. As he gets older real people aren't exciting enough. . . . He takes to conjuring up a hefty coarse Negress, fat but not sloppy fat, muscular and masculine, with a trace of a mustache and a chipped front tooth. Usually she is astraddle him like a smiling Buddha, slowly rolling her ass on his thighs, sometimes coming forward so her big cocoa-colored breasts swing into his face like boxing gloves with sensitive tips. He and this massive whore have just shared a joke, in his fantasy; she is laughing and good humor is rippling through his chest; and the room they are in is no ordinary room but a kind of high attic, perhaps a barn, with distant round windows admitting dusty light and rafters from which ropes hang, almost a gallows.

Later on, at the very end of the novel, when Rabbit's lack of sexual energy grows worse and worse, his incapacity is antithetically contrasted with the epitome of sexuality: 'Lately he has lost the ability to masturbate; nothing brings him up, not even the image of a Negress with nipples like dowel-ends and a Hallowe'en pumpkin instead of a head' (p. 403). The cluster of symbols is now complete: rabbit (with connotations not only of running but also of sex)–Negress–cucurbit. Since the image was already slightly absurdistic in the earlier passage, the cucurbit carrying on the tradition is a pumpkin (the most absurd of the cucurbits), and a jack-o'-lantern to boot. The absurd and comic undertones of the passage are, however, of secondary importance; its primary importance – as testimony of the semiotic role of cucurbits – lies in the use of a cucurbit in an image of the sexiest thing that the author and his protagonist can imagine; an image that is furthermore set up in contrast to impotence.

In the use of cucurbits as the epitome of something the weight of the paradigmatic and syntagmatic dimension respectively may vary. The textual chain may be so strong horizontally (syntagmatically) that it could well stand on its own without paradigmatic props. In some genres (realistic novels, for instance) the use of paradigmatically over-obvious elements is frowned upon and given the name of cliché. In other genres again (allegory, satire, fable) the primary strength of an element may lie in the vertical (paradigmatic) dimension and paradigmatically strong elements are desired and given names such as topoi, archetypes, 'flat characters', etc.

But naturally the most interesting case is when these two meet, and paradigmatic and syntagmatic suitability reciprocally reinforce one another. When paradigmatic appropriateness is matched with syntagmatic, even if the former is only ancillary, some sort of 'semiotic economy' seems to be in operation – the text is made to bear as much meaning as it can.

A typical example of this in Part 1 is Hawthorne's story 'Feathertop: A Moralized Legend'. As we pointed out, the story is kin to the Hans Christian Andersen tale of the emperor's new clothes. In Hawthorne's story a witch makes a scarecrow with a pumpkin for a head, infuses life into it and sends it into polite society where it is much admired for its wit and intelligence, and takes everyone in (except children, just as in Andersen's story). Hawthorne is making fun of people who are fooled by illusions and appearances and cannot see through to reality; who deludedly think the scarecrow intelligent when in fact he is a pumpkin. It is absurd not to see through to reality, and very absurd if the reality is an intrinsically absurd pumpkin. In Andersen's tale the corresponding element was nakedness. People did not wish to admit that the emperor was naked because it would have been a sign of stupidity, or proof that they were unfit for their office – so the swindlers had explained. Instead, people pretended to admire the emperor's new clothes. The mistake – preferring a fiction to reality – was shameful, as shameful as nakedness.

Hawthorne's tale could probably be classified as allegory, and Andersen's story as something similar, with a strong element of the didacticism of the fable. For a final example of a passage of satire to illustrate the principle of 'auxiliary symbolism' working in this fashion, let us turn to one of the masters of satire, Jonathan Swift.

In *Gulliver's Travels,* in the book on the voyage to Laputa, Swift's satire is directed against scientists wasting their time on useless speculation and abortive projects. The Laputans are habitually so deeply immersed in thought that they have to be stirred into life by a *Flapper* carrying an inflated bladder containing peas or pebbles (cf. Plato and his colleagues, Part 1). When the narrator visits the Academy of Lagado he finds that the scientists are all madmen pursuing crazy ideas and impossible projects. The first scientist is trying to extract sunshine from cucumbers:[5]

> *The* first Man I saw was of a meagre Aspect, with sooty Hands and Face, his Hair and Beard long, ragged and singed in several Places. His Clothes, Shirt, and Skin were all of the same Colour. He had been Eight Years upon a Project for extracting Sun-Beams out of Cucumbers, which were to be put into Vials hermetically sealed, and let out to warm the Air in raw inclement Summers. He told me, he did not doubt in Eight Years more, that he should be able to supply the Governors Gardens with Sun-shine at a reasonable Rate; but he complained that his Stock was low, and intreated me to give him something as an Encouragement to Ingenuity, especially since this had been a very dear Season for Cucumbers. I made him a small Present, for my Lord had furnished me with Money on purpose, because he knew their Practice of begging from all who go to see them.

The next scientist is trying to produce food from human excrement. In the light of Swift's scatological vision in general (and perhaps an Irish literary tradition starting as early as *The Tain*), this was of course predictable. It was also predictable that two such elements as excretion and cucurbits should occur together to reinforce the idea that the scientists connected with such things are ridiculous and mad.[6]

The satire is effective because there is precisely that element of reason in the madness that makes it psychologically convincing. To try to extract sunshine from cucumbers is very reasonable in mad logic, because, as we have seen in Part 1 (Karlfeldt, Tennyson, etc.), there is a persistent connection between cucurbits and sunshine. But Swift uses another symbolic dimension of the cucurbits – their absurdity – as 'auxiliary symbolism' in his devastating attack on the scientists.

In Part 1, commenting on the word 'pumpkin-head' for Puritan, we stated our scepticism as to the explanation of the origin of the word given in S. Peter's *A General History of Connecticut*. Peter thought the word originated from the Blue Laws, which enjoined every male to have his hair cut round by a cap, and that when caps could not be had a pumpkin-shell was substituted. We maintain that no shortage of caps is necessary; the tool should be changed from cap to pumpkin-shell in accordance with the principle of 'auxiliary symbolism' to achieve semiotic economy. In this case, and in similar cases, it should be changed, and studying world literature, we find that usually such elements have been changed. In order to delve deeper into the question, let us contemplate for a while that swarm of cucurbitic symbols clustering around the subject of *sex*.

A quick review of these shows how thickly they cluster around the kernel, and how well all possible directions are covered. We have cucurbits in connection with a desirable woman (Theopompus; Ruxton's *Life in the Far West*); in connection with music and cucurbit-shaped musical instruments (John Updike's *Couples*); melons and love (Alemán's *The Rogue*); melons and wife or marriage (Lear; Whittier's 'The Pumpkin'; Perrault's *Cinderella*); sex myths about Negroes ('Ah Dem Watermelons'); moon and menstruation (Columella; *Maison Rustique*); sterilization (Penelope Mortimer's *The Pumpkin Eater*); 'forbidden fruit', such as girl of another ethnic group in a culture favouring endogamy (Philip Roth's *Portnoy's Complaint*); sexual perversion (Juvenal's *Satires*); effeminate male (Seneca?); Eve and sin (Floris and Campani); incest (Ralph Ellison's *Invisible Man*); castration (Alex Hayley's *Roots*); feminism and lesbianism (Verena Stefan's *Häutungen*); we have cucurbits reinforced with other sex symbols, such as thistle and he-goat (Doomer); infidelity (DuCange's 'cucurbitare'; 'Peter, Peter Pumpkin-Eater'; Penelope Mortimer's *The Pumpkin Eater*); pumpkin and rabbit (John Updike's *Rabbit Redux*); cucurbits to restrain sexual appetite (Boorde's *Dietary*); prostitution (James Joyce's *Ulysses* – see below); sexual intercourse (anonymous parody of James Whitcomb Riley's 'When the Frost is on the Punkin'; John Updike's *Couples*); masturbation (John Updike's *Rabbit Redux*); sexual taunt (Tove Jansson's *Pappan och havet* – see below); sin (Tennyson's 'The Vision of Sin'); *droit du seigneur* and defloration (Fletcher and Massinger [?], *The Custom of the Country*); lechery (Shakespeare's *Merry Wives*); pregnancy (Joyce's *Ulysses* – see below; Pliny; Virgil's *Georgics*); nymphomania (Procopius); chastity (*Vitae Patrum*).

Having come even this far in the list the state of affairs is obvious. Take any connection with sex; the cucurbits have it. Anything connected with sex magnetically attracts cucurbits. In the making of devices and contraptions connected with sex (contraceptives, etc.) the cucurbits are accordingly seen by authors as the proper material. It is of course also inevitable that the terminology for those parts of the body that are relevant to sex will cucurbitize in literature. 'Cucumis' for the male organ occurred in Plautus' *Casina*, and it is easy to find such expressions as Mod. Gk. ἀγγούρι. Though cucurbitic words (usually 'cucumber') for the male organ are frequent and widespread, it seems that cucurbits in connection with parts of the body of woman are even more frequent. For watermelon split open, see the quote from Ralph Ellison's *Invisible Man*. For cucurbits and breasts, see Verena Stefan's 'kürbisbrüste'.

In a work by the Danish author Jørgen Nash, breasts are likewise named 'pyntegraeskar' (ornamental gourds). This novel also provides a splendid example of a link between cucurbits and *numse* ('melons grown together'). In Nash's book, as so often when cucurbits are used symbolically in connection with women, the cucurbits are meant to suggest a sound animalic or vegetabilic closeness to nature – including a frank acceptance of nature in the sense in which the word could be used during the nineteenth century to mean sexual instinct. Nash's narrator uses a set of vegetables, and particularly cucurbits, to characterize a girl called Lis Nemesis Jensen:[7]

> Husk på, jeg kom fra en rå og tung bondeverden med landlige teorier om dit og dat, der slet ikke svarede til storbymenneskets kultur. Hun oplevede gaderne som brede havegange, og husraekkerne var drivhuse.
> – Hver aften går jeg ned og vander brostenenes blomster, sagde hun, og det var tydeligt, at når hun snakkede, levede hun fuldkomment med i det. Men denne fremmede indfølingsmåde drillede unaegtelig min hårde realitetssans. Nu bagefter kan jeg godt se det latterlige i mine indvendinger, for selvfølgelig var det i pagt med sandheden, når hun haevdede, at hendes arme var slangeagurker, munden en tomat, øjnene mirabeller og i visse tilfaelde stikkelsbaer. Min kaereste hjemme i Jylland ville aldrig finde på at sige, at hendes numse var to sammenvoksede meloner. Da jeg spurgte Lis Nemesis Jensen, hvad hendes bryster så var, knappede hun snydeblusen op og sagde:
> – De er kvindens pyntegraeskar.
> Jeg kom pludselig i tanke om, at jeg selv nyligen i et brev til min kaereste havde skrevet, at hendes bryster var to turtelduer. [xxxi]

Lis, whose arms are cucumbers and who says that her breasts are a woman's ornamental gourds ('pyntegraeskar') is contrasted with the narrator's former fiancée in Jutland who would never have said that her behind was 'two melons grown together'. But the narrator too is changed by this new vegetabilic sensuality and he suddenly recalls that he had recently written to his fiancée that her breasts were two doves.

DOES A LITERARY WORK WRITE ITSELF?

Throughout the rest of the chapter, breasts, mouth and other parts of the body are referred to by their new vegetabilic names so that the love-making is related in a suitably sensual medium. Significantly when Lis at first puts up some resistance to the narrator's amorous advances, her breasts are referred to by the chaste synonym 'turtelduer' (p. 24), but when she gives in the terminology again cucurbitizes: 'slangeagurker' for arms, 'melons grown together' for *numse* (p. 24) etc.

An even more extreme example is that of Sven Holm's *Jomfrutur*.[8] In Holm's novel, which is a love story between two high school pupils, the girl's father is a gardener. The entire love affair is related in vegetables, cucurbits playing a prominent part, and the youth declares his love in vegetables (pp. 7-9). The book is overrun with vegetables; vegetables determine the lives of the characters and even their vocabulary has been vegetabilized. Of their various experiences and acts love is insistently throughout expressed in cucurbits. To catch the girl's attention the young man in particular brings melons, marrows and gourds to school (p. 8), and in conversation the connection between gourds and breasts is again made: 'Du blev naturligvis bestyrtet ved det blotte syn [of the cucurbits] og undersøgte instinktivt om det var bh'stroppen der var sprunget. Men det var ikke dig der havde mistet grøntsagerne.' (p. 8) [xxxii] For the first time the girl really notices him, and the narrator wonders that she prefers him and not one of the other 'idioter, der både var flottere og fastere i kødet' (p. 8).

The division of labour between different types of vegetables in the cited works of Nash and Holm eloquently testifies to the connection cucurbits-sex.

Denis Hills also connects breasts and cucurbits: 'The breasts of the older women had shrunk to flaps like dried seed pods, and they were honoured for them; for these flaps, when full and large as pumpkins, had suckled sons'.[9]

Nash's narrator saw Lis's *numse* as two melons grown together. Philip Roth also comments abundantly on the posterior anatomy of the big-bottomed Kay-Kay, 'the Pumpkin' (see Part 1). The best passage illustrating this, however, must surely be the following from James Joyce's *Ulysses* (p. 719):

> In what final satisfaction did these antagonistic sentiments and reflections, reduced to their simplest forms, converge?
>
> Satisfaction at the ubiquity in eastern and western terrestrial hemispheres, in all habitable lands and islands explored or unexplored (the land of the midnight sun, the islands of the blessed, the isles of Greece,

> the land of promise) of adipose posterior female hemispheres, redolent of milk and honey and of excretory sanguine and seminal warmth, reminiscent of secular families of curves of amplitude, insusceptible of moods of impression or of contrarieties of expression, expressive of mute immutable mature animality.
>
> The visible signs of antesatisfaction?
>
> An approximate erection: a solicitous adversion: a gradual elevation: a tentative revelation: a silent contemplation.
>
> Then?
>
> He kissed the plump mellow yellow smellow melons of her rump, on each plump melonous hemisphere, in their mellow yellow furrow, with obscure prolonged provocative melonsmellonous osculation.

Thus the relevant zones of the body are well represented in cucurbitic symbolism. Even in *Sut Lovingood*, when Sut calls the waist of the girl 'the huggin place' and George fails to understand the reference, Sut's language immediately cucurbitizes when he goes on to abuse George, calling him an 'oninishiated gourd'.

Against this background it is easy to understand the semiotic appropriateness of the substitute element in those passages in literature in which artificial sexual body characteristics made of cucurbits are mentioned. The perfect form of such stories prefers the material to be cucurbits. For an example of artificial breasts made of gourds, see the following passage from another Sut Lovingood yarn:[10]

> Ketch me rockin' cradles, or totin meal home for a palpitytator toter, or buyin' stockin's for a par ove bran bags, or givin' an 'oman a legal right tu bite me, with teeth made out ove delf. *No sir,* I'd marry the figgerhead ove a steamboat first. I jis' can't sit still, an' think 'bout thar menyfold shams an' traps an' gewolly-tockery, speshuly the palpititytators. Why don't you believe, that even Ratsnes' hes got her a par, a homemade par.
>
> 'Who the dickens is Ratsnest, Sut?'
>
> Why sister Sall, an' be durnd to you, she saw'd a round dry gourd in two, a gourd as big as my head, an' then made a hole in the middil ove each half, an' stuff'd in white oak acorns, butt first, an' dad shave me if she dident hist the whole contrapshun intu her buzzum. I wish I may be dam if you cudent see the bulge ove the acorns across a field. Then she went on a rale turky gobbler strut to church, a leanin' back from 'em like a littil boy totin a big drum. She looked like a dairy, by geminy. I sware I jist wanted tu kill the damfool, that's what ail'd me.

We have dwelt unduly long upon the sex connotations in order to prepare the ground for yet another discussion of the interrelationship between fact and fiction. The relationship between the two is often far from easy to sort out. On the one hand we argue that the symbolic roles of the cucurbits are determined by the physiology of the plant, i.e. by a fact; but the role of fact in explanations of the genesis of cucurbitic lore should be kept strictly in perspective. Isolated, unsystematized fact usually does not help interpretation very much.

Consider the role of cucurbits in folk-medicine. Pumpkin seeds are eaten for virility, for example, in Greece and Roumania. Cucurbits were used in pregnancy tests in ancient Egypt (see also Hippocrates). Young girls being recommended to use slices of cucumber, or the juice of cucumber, to improve their complexion is common in folk-beliefs. We have come across examples from Scotland, Ireland, New Zealand, Greece (ἀγγουρόνερο),[11] Finland,[12] and England.[13] Against the background of the overwhelmingly rich evidence of the ubiquitous connection cucurbits–sex, the connection cucurbits–(female) beauty falls neatly into place as a natural sub-category. We amassed the examples of the connection cucurbits–sex in order to demonstrate this and soften the impact of a question that has to be asked at this point, even though one may feel embarrassed in spelling it out. The question is *whether such beliefs and practices as cucurbits for beauty work or not*, and the interest of the question is of course in the general theoretical aspect, not in the specific of any one example.

Probably these passages, beliefs, practices, etc., find their form more or less regardless of such fact. If cucumber juice works as a skin beautifier then so much the better; then the fact that it works will surely cement its role and stabilize the custom. If, on the other hand, it works as little as anything else, then it will nevertheless acquire its role; because, in comparison with the other quackery, at least it is *symbolically right*.

At any rate, we are convinced that interpretations should be of systems, not of scattered and isolated instances. An anthropologist studying, say, folk-customs in the Igbo areas of west Africa will find that in some Igbo villages a pregnant woman is advised to eat plenty of pumpkin from five months on. It would be ridiculous for the anthropologist to look merely for a factualistic explanation of this, and to see whether pumpkins *are* good for a woman during the later stages of pregnancy; instead, the anthropologist should persevere and see if there does not exist a symbolic grammar of this fruit and plant in Igbo culture. If he does, he will find that in marriage ceremonies in some Igbo areas it is a custom that old women who come to congratulate the bride wish her to 'multiply like a melon'. A successful person is called a 'fruitful calabash'; and thus, in general, the symbolic role of the cucurbits is the same in Igbo as elsewhere.[14] The question whether pumpkins are wholesome food for a pregnant woman is really not relevant.

The value of scattered factualistic explanations as a tool in hermeneutics has been greatly over-estimated. Much of nineteenth-century and early twentieth-century *Realphilologie* scholarship suffers from this weakness. Unless factualistic explanations are organized into a coherent system, an exaggerated belief in such explanations may lead to a kind of naive positivistic outlook which gives free rein to one's tendency to believe in facts merely because they are facts.

The explanatory appeal of *the fact* is enormous: *how* enormous is realized fully only by those who have begun to question it. A case in point is the debate over the dietary rules of Leviticus 11 and Deuteronomy 5 preceding and following Mary Douglas's analyses.[15] Her interpretations are a brilliant example of an attempt to get inside a system of thought. What is so typical about the history of the previous attempts to explain the dietary rules, particularly the ban on pork, is the enormous appeal of explanations such as that which proposes that pigs were declared unclean because they may carry parasites. In the face of a hard, solid, isolated fact like this – taken, moreover, from the most prestigious of sciences, medicine – marginal things fade: it does not matter to the factualist that the ban on pork is only one of several rules; rules that, moreover, occur together in the same contexts and might thus be expected to form a system; it does not matter that parasites are not given as a reason in the text; it does not matter that another reason *is* given (cloven feet but no chewing of the cud); it does not matter if the parasite-explanation does not tally with the rules on other animals – for the ban on them another factualistic and isolated but neat explanation must be found.[16]

It is easier to believe in a fact than to adjust one's whole vision to see the patterns in a system. Mary Douglas began her analyses by considering the explanation that was there under everyone's nose all the time. The text makes no secret of the reason why the swine is unclean; it is unclean because, though it does have cloven feet it does not chew the cud. If the factualist believes more in parasites than in the desirability of cloven feet and cud-chewing that is not necessarily a sufficient reason for the ancient Hebrew to do the same.

In studying the cucurbits one must not make scattered piecemeal interpretations of isolated phenomena, but rather must try to see cucurbitic lore as a system and understand its structure. Even though it is true that gourd has meant 'dice-box' during some periods of history, it is still a daring speculation, in our opinion, to pick on this isolated fact and explain the *Apocolocynthosis* as an allusion to the Emperor's putative predilection for gambling.[17] Instead, an explanation should be sought through an understanding of the whole semiotic matrix of cucurbits at that time in history. Likewise we think that the explanation 'cucurbitae caput non habemus' as an allusion to baldness is farfetched, despite the *fact* that cucurbits *can* associate with baldness, and actually do, in the same period, and even in the same author.[18] There should be some consistency and order; details should be explained as parts of a coherent system.

The principle of 'maximal appropriateness' can operate with one or several elements. The examples we have given so far have usually entailed the auxiliary use of one element. For an example of a use of two, let us return to the comic postcard from 1901 (see Plate IX).

The communicative aim of the sender (the designer of the postcard) seems to have been to ridicule the Negro(es). To achieve this goal he constructed an optimal economy in the message. The situation is one of choice and it does not take much reflection on the position of the 'situation of choice' as an element in life and literature to realize its significance in this case.

To have to face situations of choice is one of the less pleasant experiences in life, because choices are often very important, and you may be given only one chance to choose. Therefore authors find the use of images like that of crossroads such a potent symbol (see, for instance, Robert Frost's poem 'The Road Not Taken', from the volume *Mountain Interval*). Faced with the ambiguities and ambivalences of life in a situation of choice, man may well wish that there were someone he could turn to for guidance; that there were, say, an oracle at Delphi whither he could repair and ask for advice. The semiotic significance of the stories about the oracle, however, is that help is not to be had – insecurity in the face of a situation of choice is the human lot. The oracle returns the ball to the askers by giving answers that are so amphibolous or ambiguous that to decide between the two (or several) alternatives of interpretation puts the asker in front of a choice that is just as difficult as his original one.

The situation of choice is thus a special one, and men have special attitudes to it. But these attitudes may vary from compassion to scorn, depending on whether, for example, a friend or an enemy is involved.

One important part of the anatomy of the 'situation of choice' is its paralysing and stupidifying effect. People walking into a street, out in front of an approaching car, are paralysed by their choice of either continuing or jumping back, and often they remain frozen to the spot looking extremely stupid. 'Situation-of-choice'-induced stupidity is so well observed by man that it has got into several standard phrases in language. We talk about an 'embarras de choix' or 'embarras de richesse'. Even more revealing is the expression 'as a donkey between two bundles of hay', the donkey being a stupid animal and the rustic bundles of hay also scoring low on a status scale.

By putting the Negro in a situation of choice the designer of the postcard was able to make him seem stupid and funny. To make the message perfect for his purposes through the use of auxiliary symbolism, he then picked, for the two alternatives that the Negro was to choose between, two things, chicken and watermelons, that not only are in every aspect in perfect agreement with each other, but also are both in agreement with the semiotic relevance of the situation.

Antithesis

Another principle that leads to literary passages determining their own shape is antithetical juxtaposition, which, of course, is closely related to the principle of maximal appropriateness. Dualistic structuring of reality, one of man's simplest intellectual models, also seems to be one of his dearest. Antonymic or antithetic structuring naturally makes the other half of the oppositional pair predictable once the first is given. The contrasting element must be different, and as different as possible.

As examples of antithetical structuring we shall take passages where the cucurbit symbolizes life, particularly when this is connected with the wateriness of the fruit. Cucumbers and melons consist chiefly of water (95–99 per cent), and wateriness fits in well with associations with life – water is a life-giving and life-sustaining factor.

The cucurbit as a symbol of life is frequent and widespread through the ages. Explicit testimony of its role can be found in those occurrences where the juxtaposition of opposites is expressly signalled by an adversity-marker such as 'either–or', and the semiotic significance of its partner is known. As we pointed out in Part 1, the lily for the Greeks was the flower of death. In the pair 'ἢ κολοκύντη ἢ κρίνον' it is obvious that, since the lily stands for death, the antonymic symbol, the pumpkin, must stand for life. Recall also the antithetic juxtaposition of lily and cucurbit in Tennyson's 'The Princess' (Part 1). The lily has some natural suitability for its role such as its pallor but let us here consider another partner for the cucurbit; a partner whose pure intrinsic appropriateness is perfect.

Deserts and cucurbits, as semiotic elements, are perfect natural antitheses. Deserts are sterile, dry, deathly; cucurbits are fertile, watery, life-giving. When authors think antithetically in extremes, the perfect opposite of desert is cucurbit and the perfect opposite of cucurbit is desert. The perfect opposition is so obviously neat that it leads to different literary practice in different modes and genres. In those genres where stereotype is cultivated and desired, such as caricature or allegory, the juxtaposition of deserts and cucurbits predictably occurs, whereas realism tries to avoid such perfectly neat constellations and structures. It is therefore only in artistically poor realist works that one finds the perfect antithetic structuring deserts–cucurbits.

One such work is Henry Rider Haggard's novel *King Solomon's Mines* (1885). In this work there is hardly any cliché that the reader need wait for in vain. At one stage when the expedition is trekking through an African desert they are in very bad shape: at the limit of thirst and exhaustion. The hot merciless sun beats down on the party, who fear that the end is close at hand. They can see no escape from the hostile desert which is sterile, dry and deathly. Since, in a work of this nature, effect is sought by maximization of the function of the device used (in this case contrast), and since the extreme opposite of the desert is the cucurbit – which is fertile, watery and life-giving – the inevitable happens: they discover a patch of melons![19]

> So we sat down under the rocks and groaned, and for one I wished heartily that we had never started on this fool's errand. As we were sitting there I saw Umbopa get up and hobble towards the patch of green, and a few minutes afterwards, to my great astonishment, I perceived that usually very dignified individual dancing and shouting like a maniac, and waving something green. Off we all scrambled towards him as fast as our wearied limbs would carry us, hoping that he had found water.
> 'What is it, Umbopa, son of a fool?' I shouted in Zulu.
> 'It is food and water, Macumazahn,' and again he waved the green thing.
> Then I saw what he had found. It was a melon. We had hit upon a patch of wild melons, thousands of them, and dead ripe.
> 'Melons! ' I yelled to Good, who was next me; and another minute his false teeth were fixed in one of them.

After this they kill a bird and by and by get out of the desert. Things improve gradually, whereas before the melon passage they had been growing gradually worse. At the point of juxtaposition (the structural node), the two intrinsically antithetical elements, desert and cucurbit, were employed to heighten the dramatic change in fortune.

What we are again trying to stress here is the high probability of the choice of cucurbits. To supersede and be maximally contrasted with the least watery thing imaginable (desert) there is one suitably watery thing: a melon. The only improvement on this passage would have been for the party to discover water itself, but this possibility was discarded by the author for several reasons. Melons, at this stage, which is the climax of the desert episode, appeal more to the imagination. In the escalation of the thirst theme, which reappears cyclically, 'finding water' is an appropriate element at the beginning, but it cannot be repeated; that would blunt the effect. Each new episode must be an escalation in relation to the preceding, and to find water now would be an anticlimax. Part of the way the picture of the plight of the party has been created has been the tacit assumption that they will not find water. Finding water would damage the maximal appropriateness of desert as the driest thing imaginable – a place could hardly be said to be dry if you find water in it! As it is they find water; yet do not find water.

There was the same juxtaposition of wilderness and cucurbit in the story of the Christian hermit who hung a tempting cucumber in front of himself (see Part 1). We also saw in Part 1 how two watery species of cucurbits were introduced into Numbers 11 in one of those grumbling passages that recur as a *leitmotif* at regular intervals through the whole of that book in the Bible. The Jews, we recall, were displeased with the diet (manna), and being in the sterile Sinai their thoughts antithetically went to the fertile Goshen [NEB]:

> Will no one give us meat? Think of it! In Egypt we had fish for the asking, cucumbers and water-melons, leeks and onions and garlic. Now our throats are parched; there is nothing wherever we look except this manna.

It is next to irrelevant here to inquire into the plants actually grown in Goshen at the time the Jews were there. What is relevant is the state of the Jews at that moment in the narrative – hungry, thirsty and bored – and the semiotic position, in the lexicon, of the things they mention, which in each case is antithetical: hungry (meat and fish), thirsty (cucumbers and watermelons), bored (leeks, onions and garlic). In addition there is the juxtaposition cucurbit–desert (i.e. life–death), expressing the ominousness of their present situation and its difference from their memory of Goshen.

Doubtless one of the reasons for the appeal of the κολοκύντη/cucurbita reading in the debate over the translation of Jonah 4:6 is man's propensity to make deserts and cucurbits antithetical in literature (since they seem to him antithetical in life). Jonah is in the desert, in a bad mood, the sun torturing him; it is obvious that a cucurbit would be very fitting as an antithetic element.

As an antithetical partner of deserts, melons slip into texts with particular ease if the logic of the text is dependent on 'free association'. If the mind is free to have its pick – as it is supposed to be in dreams, or under the influence of opium – then the place of melons as a contrasting companion of deserts is assured, as in the following example from Christina Rossetti:[20]

> While with sunk eyes and fading mouth
> She dreamed of melons, as a traveller sees
> False waves in desert drouth
> With shade of leaf-crowned trees,
> And burns the thirstier in the sandful breeze.

These examples, we hope, have sufficiently illustrated the element of predictability in the way certain literary passages involving antitheses find their own shape. Indubitably, the author played *some* part – let us assume that it was Haggard's decision to put his group of characters in a desert. Once he had made that decision, however, everything else more or less followed. Melons are antithetical to deserts, and, going through material like ours, one becomes aware of the extent to which antithesis is one of the intellectual models in which man habitually thinks. Antithesis is actually often a link as good as any between two elements. Some periods, such as the baroque, seem to have been particularly fond of antithesis, as well as some authors. Use of oppositional structuring is, however, all-pervasive and extensive. This explains why there are such curious seeming inconsistencies and dualistic contradictions in cucurbitic symbolism, as when, for instance, cucurbits are thought either to induce or to restrain sexual appetite.

On the continuum of any symbolic role there seems to be a pull towards the extremes. That pull is basically the same as in maximal appropriateness except that now there are two elements maximally appropriate, and in contrasting ways. An ambiguous symbol like the cucurbits, which appeals so strongly to the imagination, will be taken up and each possible aspect of its complexly ambiguous nature exaggerated, cultivated, isolated and purified until it can stand as a strong unambiguous sign even though it stands unambiguously for the opposite in a different (also unambiguous) text. There is a kind of centrifugal force which catapults the sense towards the extreme periphery.

In Part 1 the cucurbit figured in many antithetical structures where the pattern varied and the position of the cucurbit varied. Sometimes it symbolized the elevated or sublime, sometimes the bathetic; it was high or low, desirable or undesirable. The authors who were technically most adroit made use of the fact that it is a latently ambiguous symbol when used in one of its specialized roles, and they often manipulated the context so as to activate one or two potential secondary meanings and thus enrich the effect. How they were able to do this would be explained if we assume that every specific meaning that exists in the open in one cucurbitic occurrence exists latently in every other occurrence in which the specific open meaning is something else.

Symbols cluster

Another principle, which like the preceding is also closely related to 'maximal appropriateness', is the tendency of symbols to cluster and interrelate, and seek companions that are not only in keeping with the general semiotic drift of the passage in which they occur but also paradigmatically congenial.

The principle is one of *amount*, simply that more is better than less, and the simplest cases are those where an author doubles (or trebles, etc.) his symbolism for good measure.

The cucurbit grows very quickly. It is therefore often combined with mushrooms when authors wish to double the symbolism of fast growth. The cucurbits also die easily (none can tolerate frost). Dying as quickly as it grows the plant has accordingly become the image of short-livedness (an aspect significant in the Jonah translation controversy).

The life of some insects is also proverbially short in many languages (Sw. 'dagslända' or Eng. 'ephemeron'), which explains why gourd in the following example should be mentioned with a fly:[21]

> we should have been but as an Ephemeron, Man should have lived the life of a Fly, or a Gourd, the morning should have seen his birth, his life have been the term of a day, and the evening must have provided him of a shroud.

An author wishing to double his symbolism and wanting to use the cucurbit in its role as a symbol of stupidity can for instance couple it with a stupid animal, such as the sheep, as in our example from Jerome K. Jerome's *Novel Notes* (1893) in Part 1: 'Surely as to a matter of this kind, I, a professed business man, must be able to form a sounder judgment than this poor pumpkin-headed lamb' (p. 24).

In these examples two signs were involved. The principle of 'symbols cluster' is related to 'maximal appropriateness' in that the symbols in this case too, as in the examples from 'maximal appropriateness' (which may be hierarchically superior – an inclusive concept), have to suit, as to their paradigmatic nature, the slot in the syntagm that they are chosen for. Their additional, specific feature in 'symbols cluster' is that they are paradigmatically related to each other as symbols. This is fairly simple if the symbols are two and their task is to convey one significance (the same). It becomes much more intricate when you increase the number of items and the number of connotations – then the number of relations increases geometrically.

There is a certain numskull story which according to folklorists is spread over large parts of Asia, Europe and the southern part of the United States. The numskull thinks that a pumpkin is an ass's egg. He throws it into a bush. A rabbit that has been hiding in the bush is frightened and jumps out. The numskull thinks the egg has broken and the rabbit is the ass's colt.[22] In this story practically all the imaginable streams of symbolism converge. The subject is sex; what the numskull is ignorant of are the facts of reproduction. Thus not only is the pumpkin appropriate, with its sex connotations, but the rabbit is also – rabbits are proverbially fertile. But not only in the sex aspect is the connection from pumpkin both ways – to the subject and to the animals – appropriate. The man is stupid; pumpkins symbolize stupidity, and so do asses. The interlacement of relationships in the story is such that every element fits every other. Because of the nature of the case, with two basic ideas involved, sex and stupidity, and three elements of narrative – man, mother-animal and egg/baby-animal – and the simple mathematics following from this, there exists latently a perfect form of the story, which tends to force its way into existence. In cases like these man does not think in literature but literature in man.

In orally transmitted literature of this kind there is ample scope for changes towards perfection; for imperfect forms to be discarded; and for a transmitter, who may be more clever than the last teller of the story (and master the semiotic matrix of the elements more fully), to touch into life the element that was waiting for him to take it into the story, where it will strive to remain if it improves the story. Perfect semiotic economy may be one factor influencing the stabilization and canonization of a certain version of an orally transmitted work.

In addition to the tendency of symbols to cluster, there is another closely related principle at work in literature. Not only symbols but connotations too have a tendency to flock together. If a sign has been used in a passage because of one of its connotations, it tends to be used because of another in the immediate vicinity in the text, and often to run the whole gamut of connotations. For reasons of presentation our explications in Part 1 usually ignored this tendency; we had to make use primarily of the chief connotation in each case in order to illustrate each point as clearly as possible. But often several or even all of a cucurbit's connotations are brought into play in literary passages, and sometimes with extraordinarily neat predictability.

In one of the adventures of Asterix the Gaul, by Goscinny and Uderzo, Asterix and his companion Obelix visit Britain. Among all the curiosities and idiosyncrasies they encounter is an anachronistic rugby match.[23] The game is played 'avec une calebasse et trente Bretons, partagés en deux équipes de XV' (p. 36). To make the sides play with 'une calebasse' for a rugby ball gently mocks the Britons, since people fighting over something worthless seem stupid.

This is the main symbolic use of 'calebasse' and it is quite straightforward. But during the game one of the players, refreshed with magic potion which gives him superhuman strength, kicks the ball (the *calebasse*) so hard that it temporarily vanishes into the sky. It redescends a little later, now far away at sea, hitting the Negro pirate of a pirate ship on the head, knocking him down from the mast where he was supposed to keep watch. The pirate captain asks: 'Corne de bouc garçon! Qui t'a permis d'abandonner ton poste de vigie?' The Negro answers: 'J'ai 'eçu une calebasse su' le c'âne!' (p. 40) – which is funny, since it should be so patently improbable, yet in this case is not. In this episode, once the 'calebasse' had been introduced and first used for its primary connotation of ridiculous absurdity, a little later, because of the tendency of more connotations of the same element to be brought in if one has been, the two further specific connections with head and Negro were made. Of all the places the *calebasse* could have landed, it landed on the only Negro in the story, and on his head.[24]

Even when it serves no specific purpose to bring in secondary connotations, authors nevertheless often weave them into the same episode

DOES A LITERARY WORK WRITE ITSELF?

in which they use a meaningful primary connotation. In the final episode of William Styron's *Lie Down in Darkness* the watermelon rind that drops from La Ruth's hand is primarily a symbol of destroyed life (Peyton's death); and the fact that La Ruth is black, and Peyton's unhappiness was connected with her lack of success in love, should be incidental. But on some level of logic subtler than the main layer of story it pleased the author to create a pattern in which not only the main connotation of cucurbit (life) is used, but two others are thrown in as well.

Similar yet different

If the principle of 'maximal appropriateness' was hierarchically superior; and if the first sub-category, 'antithesis', meant the addition of an abstract relation 'difference' plus the introduction of a numbering of the items (two); and if the second sub-category, 'symbols cluster', depended on the abstract relation 'similarity' (two or more items; one or more connotations), it is to be expected that there should also be a category combining the abstract relations of sub-categories 1 and 2. Let us call this case simply 'similar yet different'.

This, of course, is usually thought of as the basic chart of the metaphor. In 'the man is a lion' the man is similar to the lion in his courage, yet different from the lion in that he is not really a lion but a man.

In Part 1 we had the slang expression 'punkins' meaning 'people of value and consequence' quoted from C. Astor Bristed's *The Upper Ten Thousand* (1852). It is interesting to note that the expression occurs in a passage abundant in other vegetable symbolism; symbolism that illustrates very strikingly the principle of 'similar yet different'.

'Cabbages' are of extremely low semiotic status. Their low value is sometimes rivalled by that of the cucurbits, but cucurbits are a potentially ambiguous symbol, whereas cabbages are purely negative. The other fruit or vegetable that occurs in the passage, 'pea-nuts', is also very negative (pp. 216–17):

> Mrs R. had been trying to poke fun at us, behind our backs of course, on the subject of cabbages and pea-nuts. Well, not long after she gave a big ball, and we, being punkins, were of course among the invited. So I went to a clever working jeweller that I knew, and gave him an order to be filled up in all haste from a design of my own, ear-rings imitating pea-nuts in dead gold, and shirt buttons in green enamel, to be the counterfeit presentment of two cabbages; and Clara and I wore our

> ornaments at the ball (where they were much admired for their originality), and made a point of bringing them under Mrs Robinson's notice.

In the discussion preceding the story, an Englishman has found it strange that his American friend confesses his regrets at not having become a wine merchant. The American is militantly self-confident and does not want to give up his identity or be above his origin – his ancestors have made their fortune in peanuts and cabbages. So he creates a paradox, a representation of vegetables of the lowest possible value (peanuts and cabbages) in material of the highest possible value (gold and enamel). The nineteenth-century American attempt to reconcile the ideas of democracy and social hierarchy was paradoxical. The paradox involved in uniting the two ideas demanded an equally paradoxical symbol, in this case involving a link through similarity in colour: nuts–yellow–gold and cabbages–green–enamel. With the aid of the paradoxical symbol the American is signalling to Mrs R. a message about his similarity and difference: 'I may be rich like you, but I am different, and proud of it'; or maybe: 'You may think I am different from you, and so I am, but at least I am as rich as you'.

To illustrate the role of the principle 'similar yet different' in the autogenesis of literary passages, let us return to the role of the cucurbit as a symbol of life.

Since the cucurbit symbolizes life, the act of cutting a cucurbit sets the human imagination in motion. Thus a number of related symbolic patterns have come into existence. One finds for instance that an eclectic, slightly hedonistic attitude to life and its pleasures (especially love) can be likened to the arbitrary knife of the melon-vendor, as in the passage from Alemán's *Guzman de Alfarache* which we quoted in Part 1 from Mabbe's 1622 translation. The original goes as follows:[25]

> No falta en Roma bueno, y mas bueno, a menos peligro, y costa, cõ mas gustos, y me nos embaraços: no sè si lo haze, q̃ nuc̃a yo quiero por querer, síno por salpicar, como los de mi tierra: soy cuchillo de melonero, ando picando cantillos, mudando hitos; oy aqui, mañana en Francia; de cosa no me concoxo, ni en alguna permanezco; a mis horas como, y duermo, no suspiro en ausencia, en presencia bozeço, y con esto las muelo.

Or else, in a case where the tension of the co-present principles similarity–difference is already felt, if the body of a man is cut the way a cucurbit would be, one feels there should have been a difference, but alas there is not. We already had a good example of this in Part 1, from

DOES A LITERARY WORK WRITE ITSELF?

Stephen Crane's short story, 'The Blue Hotel'. The knife cuts the body of the Swede as it would have a melon (p. 505):

> There was a great tumult, and then was seen a long blade in the hand of the gambler. It shot forward, and a human body, this citadel of virtue, wisdom, power was pierced as easily as if it had been a melon. The Swede fell with a cry of supreme astonishment.

Two prominent examples of life, melon and man, are different in that the melon is insensitive. But where, alas, was the difference! What seems similar but should nevertheless be different turned out to be similar after all.

The difference between cutting human flesh and cutting a melon, i.e. the material of two varieties of life, one sensitive and the other insensitive, is a cliché that is utilized particularly in connection with ideas of callousness or cruelty.[26] In a thriller by Edgar Wallace there is a female character who is supposed to be the epitome of cruelty. One of her acts is to slash the hand of an admirer to teach him that his attentions are not welcome. The idea of the following quotation is that to normal people there is a difference between cutting a melon and cutting human flesh, but that to this cruel woman it is all the same.[27]

> 'She is wonderful, really, Mrs Meredith, wonderful! I find myself thinking about her at odd moments, and the more I think the more I am amazed. Lucretia Borgia was a child in arms compared with Jean – poor old Lucretia has been malignated, anyway. There was a woman in the sixteenth century rather like her, and another girl in the early days of New England, who used to denounce witches for the pleasure of seeing them burn, but I can't think of an exact parallel, because Jean gets no pleasure out of hurting people any more than you will get out of cutting that cantaloup. It has just got to be cut, and the fact that you are finally destroying the life of the melon doesn't worry you.'
> 'Have cantaloups life?' She paused, knife in hand, eyeing the fruit with a frown. 'No, I don't think I want it. So Jean is a murderess at heart?'

Consider, for a moment, this quotation and its implications for the idea that art imitates reality! 'The realist myth', with which we sometimes delude ourselves, would claim that art imitates real life. However, it simply is not a fact of real life that one's partner in a conversation happens always miraculously to have a cantaloup in her hand any time one needs to make a point about cruelty! Neither is it true in life that people make points about cruelty only when their interlocutresses happen to be cutting cantaloups – though this is much more likely.

117

DOES A LITERARY WORK WRITE ITSELF?

It is well known that art imitates not so much life as other art. A sonnet imitates not only life but above all other sonnets. But, as the Edgar Wallace example demonstrates, even when art does imitate life it is not life in its raw, unordered state, but life as she should have been lived ideally.

A special mutation of the idea of co-present similarity and difference is a pattern that we would like to call 'chiastic inversion', which is related to the pattern of 'similar yet different'. The mechanism of this pattern is that '*a* is not what it *should* be; but *is* what it *should not* be, i.e. the same as *b*' and '*b* is not what it *should* be, but *is* what it *should not* be, i.e. the same as *a*'. This variation of the well-known formula of 'appearance and reality' is a stock-in-trade with many authors, both good and bad.

One of the artistically most pleasing executions of the theme is Guy de Maupassant's short story 'Boule de suif' (1880). In this story, of half a dozen people leaving Paris in a stagecoach, because of the German invasion, the character from whom the story derives its title, a prostitute, is contrasted with the rest of the passengers, who are assorted Parisians: some characters from the *bourgeoisie* or the lesser nobility, two nuns and a revolutionary.

At the beginning of the story the low social position and humility of the prostitute is contrasted with the status of the rest of the company who all have some claim to excellence in one way or another: the upper class (refinement), the *bourgeoisie* (wealth), the nuns (holiness, chastity), the revolutionary (political vision, social conscience). When the journey begins the other passengers have left in such haste that they have had no time to bring any food, but the prostitute has brought an overflowing basket of various delicacies (she is slightly corpulent, which explains both her nickname and her popularity among customers). The prostitute generously shares her provisions with the other passengers. This scene contrasts with a similar scene at the end of the story when it is the others who have brought food and the girl who has not; then the others do not share their meal with her.

Thus they are outdone by her in generosity. During the course of the story the author gently and unostentatiously shows how she surpasses them in every virtue. At an inn a German officer stops them and refuses to let them continue their journey until the girl has slept with him. At first she refuses – a sign of her patriotism – and the others support her. But by and by, as time passes, the others change their mind and talk her into it in order that the journey may continue.

In the abstract pattern of the story the prostitute *is* whatever the others could have been supposed to be but are not. The nuns could have been expected to be charitable but they are not; whereas the prostitute is. They could have been expected to have firm opinions, but they bend their doctrines to suit the occasion and use their influence to talk the girl into sleeping with the German officer by quoting as parallel cases similarly self-sacrificing holy women from the scriptures and church tradition; whereas the girl is unwilling and has simple but stable views. The revolutionary could have been expected to feel compassion and comradeship with a fellow-citizen, but he joins the others when his own plot of sleeping with the girl falls through; whereas the girl is always compassionate and loyal. The upper-class members of the party could have been expected to behave in a civilized fashion, but while the girl is sleeping with the German officer they have an orgy of vulgar behaviour; whereas the girl always behaves correctly; and so on and so forth.

In the primary half of the inversion the girl *is* everything that the others *should be* but are not. The reciprocal inversion is of course that the others *are* everything that the girl *should be* but is not. Taken to its logical conclusion this means that *they* are the real prostitutes, and that as she surpasses them in everything else she surpasses them, paradoxically, even in chastity: *she* sells only her body.

This, then, is one of the ways in which the 'chiastic inversion' pattern was used by a literary master. Another master who was extraordinarily fond of this pattern – as he tended to be fond of abstract patterns in general (maybe as a result of his admiration for the French 'well-made play') – was Henry James. He was fond of the 'appearance and reality' formula, and fond of 'the irony of destiny'; and the combination of the two, often, in his works, leads to endless mutations of multiple 'turning-of-the-tables' tricks, involving ironic inversions according to a complicated (sometimes slightly mechanical) pattern. In a story such as, for instance, 'Lord Beaupré' (1893), the girl who is supposed to guard the young Lord Beaupré against scheming mothers who are eager to marry off their daughters suddenly finds that she herself has a scheming mother who is eager to marry off her daughter (herself); and having taken on the job to ward off other girls because she was not herself supposed to be in love with his lordship, she by and by realizes that she is; and is prevented from acting on her realization by her scruples, which are created by her compromising situation, and so on. James was particularly fond of ending the inversion half-way, so as to leave the chiastic switch as an ambiguous suggestion. Thus in *The Turn of the Screw* (1898) it is gradually suggested that the two ghosts, who are at first supposed to be a threat to two children, may actually be rather harmless, whereas the governess, who was supposed to guard the children, may in fact be more of a threat.[28] In 'The Liar' (1889) Colonel Capadose, who is supposedly the liar, is by and by revealed as a harmless Baron von Münchhausen character, whereas the narrator (whose name 'Lyon' is partly homophonous with 'lie' in an alternative pronunciation) is shown to lie 'with intent'.

But there is no need for more examples merely to illustrate the principle; we must proceed to cucurbitic examples of chiastic inversion; and Henry James is one of the authors in whose works the reader is least likely to come across cucurbits – which actually is a literary statement characterizing James and his *oeuvre* as well as any.

Several of the authors we have dealt with in Part 1 play with various incomplete forms of 'chiastic inversion' in connection with 'appearance and reality' themes or 'turning-of-the-tables' irony. Traces of the pattern can be found in Hawthorne's 'Feathertop' (where particularly the 'appearance and reality' is worked out) or in Browning's 'The Melon-Seller' (where particularly the 'turning-of-the-tables' irony is worked out).

The inherent ambiguity of the pumpkin makes it very suitable for the patterns of chiastic inversion, and authors like Tompson probably make use of this (see Part 1). It is probably also made use of in Seneca's *Apocolocynthosis* (from where, of course, Tompson may have got his idea).

According to some theories[29] an initial confusion and an ultimate renewed clarification of borders between classes or groups is an important element in certain literary genres such as comedy. Chiastic inversion, either in its complete form or partially, is a useful tool in the final process of re-establishing order and dealing with anomalies. The new class status of the anomalous individual(s) is legitimized historically with the aid of chiastic inversion; of a character rising in status it can be explained that although he seemed to be lower-class he actually was not, and that although he did not seem upper-class in actual fact he was – hence all the paraphernalia of foundlings, etc. Chiastic inversion is probably an element in *Cinderella*, and the use of the pumpkin therefore more sophisticated than it seems at first. Cinderella is seemingly lower-class but really, as will later appear, is upper-class, and fit for marriage to the Prince. Her two rivals are chiastically contrasted with her in a see-saw pattern: above her at the beginning of the story, beneath her at the end of it. It is a well documented wish, among large groups of women, to marry men who can give them a socially and financially secure position. In popular fiction, for instance, the social position of the heroes is often well above that of the readers. A literary mechanism like the 'chiastic inversion' pattern and a symbol, the pumpkin, that could facilitate such upward mobility has a great potential appeal. The Cinderella story is found all over the world, but it seems to have reached a high degree of perfection in Perrault's version.

As this is a paradigmatic study our explications usually explain little about any work as a whole, although we hope that they will explain as well as possible the single element that we deal with. But for a final example of 'chiastic inversion' let us choose a work where cucurbits are the dominant metaphor and an understanding of the key metaphor could be expected to bring with it an understanding of the whole work.

In Richard Brautigan's book *In Watermelon Sugar*, first published in 1968, all events are enacted in the sugar of watermelons, and watermelons colour the lives of the characters, both metaphorically and literally – watermelons and sunshine change colour with the day of the week. The book begins with a proclamation:[30]

> *In watermelon sugar* the deeds were done and done again as my life is done in watermelon sugar. I'll tell you about it because I am here and you are distant.
> Wherever you are, we must do the best we can. It is so far to travel, and we have nothing here to travel, except watermelon sugar. I hope this works out.

Watermelons and watermelon sugar are thus, apart from everything else they turn out to be in this book, also the vehicle for communication between the implied author and the implied reader. This vehicle is worth a more thorough scrutiny, but first let us make a rapid survey of the multiple role of watermelons and particularly watermelon sugar in the book.

The shack in which the narrator lives at iDEATH is 'small but pleasing and comfortable as my life and made from pine, watermelon sugar and stones as just about everything here is' (p. 1). The narrator has a 'lantern that burns watermelontrout oil at night' (p. 1). In iDEATH there are bridges 'made of watermelon sugar' (p. 2); there are the Watermelon Works where the sugar is made from watermelons (*passim*), watermelonseed ink (p. 8), a dress made from watermelon sugar (p. 17), statues of vegetables in watermelon sugar (pp. 25–6

121

and *passim* – the statues are of vegetables of fairly low semiotic status like bean, artichoke, carrot, head of lettuce, bunch of onions, potato), a bed with watermelon covers (p. 37), beams of watermelon sugar in the ceiling of a shack (p. 60), bells hanging by small watermelon chains (p. 84), trays and ponds in a hatchery made from watermelon sugar (p. 92), lumps of watermelon sugar to put in your coffee (p. 108), golden planks of watermelon sugar made at the Watermelon Works (p. 113), blue watermelon shingles to nail down on a roof (p. 117), a sauce made from watermelon sugar and spices (p. 123), watermelon bricks made from black, soundless sugar (p. 126) and death robes made from watermelon sugar (p. 132).

More important than these details, however, are the passages where watermelons and watermelon sugar express the entire existence at iDEATH. After a bad moment in the narrative the narrator wakes up feeling refreshed and stares at his watermelon ceiling (how nice it looks) before getting out of bed (p. 105). In this passage the watermelon (ceiling) has a soothing effect. In a similar passage the narrator says that he likes his bridge 'because it is made of all things: wood and the distant stones and gentle planks of watermelon sugar' (p. 12). Watermelon sugar is often used metaphorically or semi-metaphorically in passages which express a positive feeling: 'Old Chuck's voice slowed down. His body kept relaxing until it seemed as if he had always been in that chair, his arms gently resting on watermelon sugar' (p. 20). The narrator's girl is naturally associated with watermelon sugar: '*Pauline's shack* is made entirely of watermelon sugar' (p. 28), even the windows.

The community at iDEATH live entirely in watermelon sugar: 'There are about 375 of us here in watermelon sugar' (p. 25), and the narrator says frankly about his 'life lived in watermelon sugar' that 'There must be worse lives' (p. 9).

The symbol of watermelon and watermelon sugar is thus clearly used on the one hand in a way to make much of the positive connotations, particularly those combining cucurbits and life or vitality. On the other hand there is inevitably also the absurd or the fantastic dimension to watermelons. In the chapter 'The Watermelon Sun' (pp. 38–9) we learn how the watermelons change colour during the week; there is a colour for every day of the week and the black watermelons of Thursdays are soundless, and clocks are made from black soundless melons (p. 39). These fantastic details are included partly because a life in watermelon sugar should be to some extent fantastic, but even these details further the picture of iDEATH. The soundless clocks do not keep time any more; time is unimportant.

At the beginning of the book the narrator states (p. 2):

> We make a great many things out of watermelon sugar here – I'll tell you about it – including this book being written near iDEATH.
> All this will be gone into, travelled in watermelon sugar.

What, then, is the watermelon message of this watermelon book? If we are not wrong in reading too much allegorical meaning into it, the use of watermelons would suggest that the author has picked on them because they are an ambiguous symbol. The watermelons stand for life and everything associated with life on the one hand; and on the other they stand for fantastic absurdity. The message would thus appear to be, in chiastic inversion, that the seemingly fantastic or absurd may in actual fact be the most life-affirmative and vital, and the watermelon symbol is thus an essential part of the author's apologia for a life of the sort that the community at iDEATH live.

The people at iDEATH, who tend to play down hysterical or violent emotions, are contrasted with the inBOIL gang, who drink, intoxicate themselves on forgotten things (books? history?) and re-discover violence. The apollonian culture at iDEATH have the idea; the dionysic culture of inBOIL have death. Brautigan intends to turn the tables on the absurdity issue and show, in reciprocal inversion, that the inBOIL people are more absurd than the people at iDEATH, who should have been absurd because of the watermelons, but who are not.[31]

The creation of a literary work, or a literary passage, is a joint affair in which the author, the readers and the work itself all participate. The share of each may vary. In Chapter 1 we tried to argue that in the case of plant symbolism the role of the readers may be more than usually important. In this chapter we have suggested four ways in which the work itself, too, may be more than usually important.

3 Sign and signification

When is a rose a rose, and when is a cucurbit merely a cucurbit?

Invoking the linguistic analogy again, one could imagine in 'the language of literature' a distinction similar to that between phonology and phonetics. All differences of speech sounds are not relevant for meaning: there is some free variation. Phonetics studies all sounds, but phonology only those differences and similarities that are relevant for the meaning. Whether features of pronunciation affect the meaning or not varies from code to code (dialect to dialect, or language to language). Analogically, in the varying codes of literature what is meaningless in one code may be meaningful in another. The hero going into a pub and ordering a whisky is probably not a very important narrative element in a detective story, but in a story in a teetotaller pamphlet it is outstandingly important.

There are naturally passages in literature where the cucurbits are merely cucurbits as when an author lists the wares in a fruiterer's shop. Nevertheless the cucurbit very easily becomes a symbol.[1] On a borderline case in pictorial art is the debate over the semioticity of still lifes (in which cucurbits often occur; see Plate I). Is there a message in a still life? If so what is its degree of articulateness, and how can it be 'read'?

We may imagine a three-part classification of cucurbitic meaning. First, the cucurbit sometimes functions merely as a cucurbit. Second, it often functions almost purely as a symbol. Third, there is an area of overlap between these, when, although it is merely a pumpkin on one level of interpretation, yet it is also a symbol on another. An example of the last case would be Washington Irving's 'The Legend of Sleepy Hollow'. The pumpkin that Brom Bones throws after the frightened Ichabod Crane should of course be thought of as a real pumpkin in one sense, but also, in a variety of senses, as a symbolic pumpkin. Other examples from Part 1 could be Hawthorne's 'Feathertop', or *The Scarlet Letter* - it is the essential nature of allegory that it lends itself to interpretation at several levels. The use of pumpkins in Carlyle's essay in *Frasers Magazine* is also multi-layered; his ubiquitous pumpkins are both real pumpkins and symbolic pumpkins used for a propagandistic purpose.

When cucurbits are used both as cucurbits *per se* and as symbolic cucurbits, the respective share of each role may vary - there may be just a barely perceptible tinge of symbolism in a cucurbitic passage; or the symbolism may almost totally crowd out the literal meaning. Most of our examples in this study are cases when the cucurbits occur in a pronounced symbolic role. That they are used thus is often well known to both speaker and listener, or author and reader. Elegant testimony of this is the fact that in their use as symbols the cucurbits may obey, e.g., the grammatical rules of inflection according to gender, in languages where this applies.

For an illustration let us turn to a Greek work from the late nineteenth century: *He Ligere* by A. Karkavitsas.[2] The book is usually thought of as an ethographia, describing various local village customs; but it is in many respects highly sophisticated, particularly in reporting language. The local witch, who is also the local match-maker, wants to marry a certain girl to a very promising merchant boy, who has lots of money, has risen from nothing, and is doing well. The witch tries to persuade the slim beauty of the village to marry the boy; but the girl feels nauseated at the thought of marrying him, whom she thinks of as ugly and pimply, with large soft palms (- hands to count money with). The witch tries to bring the girl around and asks her: 'Why are you disgusted, young daughter, don't you like the big cucumber?' (In Greek: 'Γιατί, θυγατέρα; δὲ σ' ἀρέσει ὁ ἄγγουρος;') It is interesting to note that the symbolic use of cucumber is so pronounced that it even determines the gender of the word. 'Cucumber' in modern Greek is neuter: τὸ ἀγγούρι. Here, however, the witch uses a masculine form: ὁ ἄγγουρος.

In addition one would have expected the accent to fall on the penultimate syllable; the witch, however, puts the accent on the initial (the antepenultimate) syllable. She is really playing with the word, going against the expectations that the rules would create. She lengthens the word phonetically, which by analogy makes it seem as if there were that much more of the boy, as it were.

The concept of ambiguity is relevant to the study of cucurbitic symbolism in several respects. In those cases of overlap, when a cucurbit functions both as itself and at the same time as a symbol, some sort of formal ambiguity could be said to exist. This, however, is usually not problematic and not very interesting. But there is more to cucurbitic ambiguity than this.

In order to clarify the discussion we must first make some classifications. One may distinguish between *potential* and *actual* ambiguity. Many signs – most words in the natural languages for instance – are potentially ambiguous, as a quick glance at any page in a dictionary shows. Yet when these signs are actually used there is usually no uncertainty as to which of several senses is intended, because the context determines one *Meinung* within the word's *Bedeutung*. It is not likely, if someone is told to 'take the money to the bank', that he will take it to a river bank.

But sometimes an author, intentionally or unintentionally, structures the context in such a way as to activate one or several latent alternative meaning(s), and *actual* as opposed to *potential* ambiguity results. There are thus several possibilities. A sign may be inherently unambiguous; it may be inherently ambiguous, but unambiguous in the particular instance you are concerned with; it may be inherently ambiguous, and ambiguous in the particular instance you are concerned with.

There are some inherently ambiguous signs that have a propensity to slip into the last category even though users intend them for the penultimate; in other words, signs whose latent alternative meanings will always tend to come to the fore; ambiguous signs that simply cannot be used unambiguously.

If it is important for the sender that only one meaning of a potentially ambiguous sign be activated, he will hate this class of signs and try to avoid them. Consequently many such signs disappear from languages in the course of their development. It is often also an avowed goal of normative grammarians and purists to weed out ambiguity. Whereas some linguists regard ambiguity as one of the normal characteristics of language, these people take ambiguity as a symptom of a pathological state of language.

The role of this class of symbols (whose ambiguity tends to be activated always) varies with the genre of the text and with the subject. Connotations or secondary meanings of words are not equally important to all speech occasions. Waiting for instructions about where to take the money, nobody is likely to stop and reflect very intensely over the various meanings of 'bank'. The interest is in denotations rather than connotations, and the word is used for the sole purpose of communication.

SIGN AND SIGNIFICATION

But communication is not the only function of language. In some circumstances, for instance in political or religious texts, words do not exist merely for communicating a meaning; they have a value of their own. Words that are favourites with one party may be anathema to another, and often a war over words is going on. If connotations are important to the friends of a word they will be equally important to its enemies, and the importance of secondary meanings is hereby further increased. The enemies may wilfully seize on alternative latent meanings which the friends of a word had not intended to activate – thus it might be best not to use the potentially ambiguous word at all. Linguistic taboos begin to operate in connection with ambiguous signs.

Politics is not the only delicate area. Traditional taboo subjects, such as sex, influence usage so that potentially ambiguous words are avoided. The animal which in England is known as 'ass', or 'donkey' is in America preferably called 'donkey', because 'ass' and 'arse' are roughly homophonous in American pronunciation. A few decades ago the animal could be known as 'ass' in the English version of a book published in parallel issues on both sides of the Atlantic, and as 'donkey' in the American.

The cucurbits often tend to belong to this category of signs whose latent secondary meaning(s) will always be activated. Even though the cucurbit in many instances functions unambiguously as a sign of purely positive meaning, still the threat of unintended secondary negative meanings is so strong that the cucurbit is not normally found, for example, in pictures of the Madonna. It is usually reserved for other biblical women such as Eve (see Plates II and III).

For an example from political usage let us turn to the debate on euthanasia. In this debate, in England and the USA, 'vegetable' is a word of abuse that the supporters of euthanasia use for the people they think should be left to die. 'Vegetable' is the general negative term, but specific names are also used. This is almost invariably 'cabbage'. Of all vegetables pumpkin has the most negative connotations, but it is closely followed by cabbage, which is prosaic, cheap, low-class, smells when cooked, and often, like the pumpkin, has a shape similar to a head ('pumpkin-head' has a parallel 'cabbage-head' in several languages, e.g. Italian 'testa di cavolo'). After cabbage comes a group of vegetables like turnips, potatoes and artichokes which are vaguely negative.

Obviously the supporters of euthanasia wanted to choose the most negative vegetable. Nevertheless, they stayed clear of pumpkin; because, as we have seen, the pumpkin is an ambiguous symbol. It can be both the most positive and the most negative. Cabbage on the other hand is purely negative. In addition, the comic connotations of pumpkin may have influenced the choice. To use pumpkin, and thus give the public reason to suspect that the supporters of euthanasia find the subject funny, would be a grave tactical error – almost as grave as to use the symbol of vitality for someone you argue should be killed.[3]

Doctors, however, and certainly humorists, need not have the same scruples as politicians, and a passage from a comic short story by the humorous American writer James Thurber confirms our suspicion that the semiotically most appropriate word is really a cucurbitic term, and that cabbage is only a substitute which is used because the vitality connotation and the ridiculousness connotation of cucurbitic words rule out their use in political discourse on the subject:[4]

> Minturn got up and began to pace. The brandy had run out. He sat down and lighted a cigarette.
> 'Of course, the people that doctors refer to as squashes,' pursued Fletcher, 'the invertebrates, you might say, just lie there like vegetables. It is the high-strung cases that manifest the interesting – manifestations. As you just said, Nancy, you think you're so darn smart. I mean, hospitalization moves the mind toward a false simplification. A man gets the idea that he can hold processes in his hand, the way I'm holding this glass. He lies there, you might say, pulling the easy little meanings out of life as simply as if they were daisy petals.'
> 'Daisy petals,' said Minturn. 'Where's brandy? Why isn't there any more brandy?'

Neither is there sufficient reason for a writer of fiction describing 'vegetation' from the point of view of the human vegetable itself to refrain from the use of a cucurbitic word, the way Suzanne Prou uses 'coloquinte' in *Méchamment les oiseaux*. The narrator of the novel is suffering from mental illness and is repeatedly visited by a psychiatrist called Antoine, who is at first euphemistically described as a workman who has come to redecorate the room. The important events of the narrator's past are unearthed one after the other until finally the terrible secret of the birds is revealed. The narrator's illness is a combined illness of body and soul, and he compares his existence to that of a plant:[5]

> Je ne me réjouis ni ne m'attriste. Je vis à peine. Je végète, allongé tout le long du jour, pareil à une plante rampante. Parfois, pour

parfaire la ressemblance, il me semble que des feuilles me poussent, ici et là, que j'atteins objets qui m'environnent avec des vrilles plutôt qu'avec mes mains. Ma tête enfle comme une coloquinte: je réfléchis; j'étudie le présent et le passé. [xxxiii]

Recall in this context also the cases reported in Part 1 where someone through a lack of caution and prudence in the use of the ambiguous symbol of cucurbit (which he intended to be unambiguously positively understood) gave his enemies a chance to seize upon a secondary, negative, meaning and turn the situation to their advantage. Such cases were, for instance, Richard Nixon; the character Linus in 'Peanuts'; St Augustine, Rufinus and the other advocates of the κολοκύντη/cucurbita translation of קיקיון, and James Whitcomb Riley. They all became an easy butt for ridicule, and were given names such as 'pumpkin-lovers', φιλοκολόκυνθοι. The two sides in the conflict between Puritan roundheads (pumpkin-heads) and Cavalier ('rattle-heads'); the emperor Hadrian, the woman character Terry in Updike's *Couples*, etc. – all invited ridicule, and got it.[6]

The victims of cucurbitic prejudice cannot win by avoiding cucurbits because insistent avoidance of the things they have been maliciously associated with would be as meaningful and revealing as habitual non-avoidance. For the tactics of a counter-attack such people usually try not to avoid the symbol but to reinterpret it to their advantage (e.g. Ralph Ellison's 'yam-aphorism', Part 1).

Sometimes, though someone whom an author wants to ridicule has not actually used cucurbits, the author nevertheless imputes or hypothetically attributes such a use, as when Irenaeus makes fun of Valentinus' strange beliefs (see Part 1). Having done this the author then goes on to apply the cucurbitic word of abuse, 'pepo', which Valentinus had not *directly* done anything to deserve.

We wish to deal with two more aspects of ambiguity in this chapter. The first of these is potential ambiguity as it emerges from our material, and the second the question of the extent to which this potential ambiguity has existed or exists in the cucurbitic semiotic matrix of one particular writer, at one particular time, writing for one particular audience.

One major potential ambiguity in our material is the split between positive and negative meaning. Both these meanings are subject to that pull towards the extremes that we already commented upon, and this makes the ambiguity more dramatic in the same degree as the opposite meanings get further and further away from each other. At varying levels of specificity we also have minor ambiguities such as femininity-masculinity; cucurbits used in folk-medicine to either induce or restrain sexual appetite, etc.

At first sight the variety of meanings, and the mutually contradictory nature of some of them, may seem bewildering. It may also at first seem to lend support to a view that arbitrariness of signs exists in areas where we have suggested it does not. How is it that the collective mind of mankind has adopted such widely differing and even contradictory symbolic uses of the plant?

In answering this we must first of all eliminate the source of error inherent in the shortcomings of our own perception and our inability to adjust to different ways of thinking. Otherwise there is a danger that we will project ambiguities on to a material where they do not really exist; that is, on to a material that is not thought of as ambiguous by the people using it. A typical 'translation' bogus ambiguity is caused by differences in the level of specificity. In the classification of hierarchical items, where a is the inclusive concept for subcategories b and c, it often happens that two languages differ from each other so that one has only the inclusive concept whereas the other has only the two sub-categories.[7] English normally uses 'grandmother' for both maternal and paternal grandmother. Some other European languages use specific terms for each of the two sub-categories and do not have an inclusive concept. For the speakers of these continental European languages to imagine that the English are using an 'ambiguous' word ('grandmother') would be a misconception. The English are not aware of using an ambiguous word: their language merely happens to structure reality this way.

This is trivial and self-evident, yet in studying ambiguity one constantly has to guard against the mistakes that arise from the habit of measuring ambiguity with the usage of one's own code as a yardstick. Two conventional examples in this context are the words 'sacer' and 'altus'. Much of what has been written about the alleged ambiguity of such words is beside the point. Certainly they can both express ambiguity (in the case of 'sacer' particularly to Christians). Yet it is only in a culture that divides the gods into good and bad that 'sacer' becomes even potentially ambiguous, the two alternatives of interpretation being 'holy' and 'accursed'. If you do not distinguish between good gods and bad, 'sacer' means simply 'supernatural'. Similarly with 'altus'; it is only if your thought structures reality with the aid of the two specific categories, 'high' and 'low', and you have no hierarchically

SIGN AND SIGNIFICATION

higher word for both of these, that 'altus' is ambiguous. To some other people there exists a word to express the concept of 'high-or-low' and that word is precisely, for instance, 'altus'.

We cannot know for sure that we are not merely prisoners of our limited perception if we find the use of pumpkin-seeds eaten for virility *or femininity* so heavily contradictory. Maybe in the culture where such an apparently self-contradictory state of affairs exists one does not regard femininity and masculinity as such absolute opposites. It is conceivable that to the people using the drug it means roughly 'something that makes you more true to your sex' and the two specific facts – masculinity and femininity – are only surface manifestations brought about by a purely mechanical rule – as when you use the word for the highest official of a school you are thinking primarily of the professional role of that person, and the fact that the word comes out as either 'head-*master*' or 'head-*mistress*', depending on sex, is a fact of little importance.

Because of the way our own perception structures reality some of the ambiguities that we believe ourselves to be noticing are only illusions. Nevertheless, in some sense it is doubtless true that at a level of great specificity the cucurbits have become signs proper and are as such arbitrary. Yet they usually preserve a link with their origin and whether or not one chooses to be surprised by such variations as cucurbits eaten either to increase or to check fertility depends on the type of rationality one brings to the task of observation. Our rationality is result-orientated and our attention concentrated at a level of great specificity. We classify 'sterility-drugs' into two groups: those that cure it and those that induce it. It is different if the effect of medicines is mainly psychological. Then thought moves at a level of lesser specificity. If the matter concerns sex, a fruit with sex connotations is appropriate whatever the complaint.

It is a common experience for folklorists to find the same cultural element interpreted in diametrically opposite ways in different localities. In one village you find the belief that on a certain day you must do a certain thing, whereas in the next village you find the belief that on the day in question you must *not* do this same thing. Thus the kernel of material stays the same but interpretations vary, and often they vary dualistically (must not–must; good–bad; sign of good luck–sign of bad luck; etc.).

Whether we like it or not, this is the way the collective 'rationality' of man works in the case of cucurbitic lore. Such is the psychological

SIGN AND SIGNIFICATION

mechanism at work that it is precisely on the most specific level that variations occur, however strange this seems when it involves diametrical oppositions and inconsistencies. Though cucurbits have both bad and good semiotic value the basis stays the same, so that, even when they are denounced as the devil's plants in some texts, the author recognizes the sex symbolism; it is just the attitude of the writer that varies. If we discount the purely personal element in the varying attitudes to cucurbits, much apparent ambiguity disappears.

We may again take an example from the sex connotations of the cucurbits, this time from the connection cucurbits-courtship. Because of the woman-life-sex-reproduction-loveliness connotations of the melons, finding a wife and picking a melon are perceived as related activities in literature, and in the perfect form of a story of courtship they should be intermixed. We have already quoted the Spanish proverb 'El melon y el casamiento ha de ser acertamiento'. We also found cucurbits and courtship intermixed, for instance, in Sven Holm's *Jomfrutur*, in *Cinderella*, etc.

For an example in a positive tone of voice let us take Ken Kesey's *Sometimes a Great Notion* in which one of the chief male characters, Hank, gets his wife from Rocky Ford, a city in Colorado known as 'The Watermelon Capitol of the World'. Hank passes through the town during the Annual Watermelon Fair ('All the Melon a Man can eat . . . FREE!!!!') and meets his future wife, whose job is to weigh and sell watermelons. Her skill in estimating the weight (and thus the price or worth) of a watermelon is meant to suggest her skill in matters of love. Her name is Viv, with associations both with 'living' and 'wife', both of which tie in perfectly with the main themes of the novel.[8]

If we contrast Kesey's use of cucurbits with a passage from Tolstoy the difference is at first sight very striking. The passage occurs at the beginning of Chapter 7 of Leo Tolstoy's *The Kreutzer Sonata*, or *Spent Passion*, as it is variously called in English (1889). The protagonist, the uxoricide Pózdnyshev, is recounting in his monologue how he met his future wife at a ball; how unprepared he was to resist female arts and schemes; what an easy prey he was for girls in search of a husband and mothers in search of a son-in-law. He was easily taken in by the fineries, by the festive atmosphere and in general by all the little arts that he was totally unprepared for. He was the perfect victim: he had, he says at the beginning of the chapter, grown up in a milieu that produced enamoured young men as cucumbers are forced in intensive cultivation in a hothouse atmosphere:[9]

— Да, так вот меня эти джерси, и локоны, и нашлепки поймали. поймать же меня легко было, потому что я воспитан был в тех условиях, при которых, как огурцы на парах, выгоняются влюбляющиеся молодые люди. [xxxiv]

The use of the cucurbits in connection with courtship in Tolstoy certainly seems very different from the use in Kesey. But is this evidence of a multiple semiotic role of the cucurbits (the two authors making use each of a different one), or is it merely two different authorial attitudes to the same thing (and the semiotics of cucurbits consistent after all)?

Count Tolstoy was not only a pacifist, an egalitarian and an experimenter in new educational ideas: among his many beliefs there was also room for a strong admiration of chastity and even of celibacy. *The Kreutzer Sonata* is prefaced with two mottoes (Matt. 5:28 and 9:10-11):

> *But I say unto you, that every one that looketh on a woman to lust after her hath committed adultery with her already in his heart.*
>
> *The disciples say unto him, If the case of the man is so with his wife, it is not expedient to marry. But he said unto them, All men cannot receive this saying, but they to whom it is given.*

In *The Kreutzer Sonata* Pózdnyshev's monologue is one long inventory of all the unhappy consequences of the wrong attitude to love, and the best attitude to love would actually be no attitude at all. Celibacy would be best; castrati are happy. Pózdnyshev listens to no objections and his ruthless logic stops at nothing. If human beings abstained from love-making, would not the human race die out? So what? answers Pózdnyshev and, at least to some extent, Tolstoy, since Pózdnyshev is undoubtedly a dramatization of one dimension of the author's own self. The themes and views of *The Kreutzer Sonata*, no matter how exaggerated they may appear, were intensely important to Tolstoy and there is a strong autobiographical element in the book.

Naturally the use of the cucurbits in *The Kreutzer Sonata* had to be precisely what it is, with the negative connotations very prominent, considering the general view of the author, and particularly its appearance in a pure and exaggerated form in this book.

But stripped of that part of the context which is determined by personal attitude, the cucurbitic usage in Tolstoy and Kesey is really the same. Cucurbits are associated with courtship; that is the basic truth about the sign, and whether there is ambiguity or not is a matter of definition.

SIGN AND SIGNIFICATION

For exemplification of the two halves of an ambivalent attitude to sex, and specifically to cucurbits as symbols of courtship, we do not actually need two different authors. During those periods of history that have been characterized by an ambivalent attitude to sex, or in authors whose personal attitude is ambivalent, the cucurbits are negative or ambiguous even when their use very clearly indicates that the author recognizes their significance. The Victorian period in England is famous for its prudery. It has been observed that the prude resembles the libertine in that sex is intensely important to both of them. Thus the negative attitude does not in any way impair the prude's ability to recognize cucurbitic meaning. Let us take a Victorian example to illustrate how the appropriateness of cucurbits as a symbol of courtship is endorsed despite a negative attitude.

In Dickens's *Nicholas Nickleby* the protagonist Nicholas and his sister Kate are extremely prudish, priggish and proper. Their mother, the widow Mrs Nickleby, on the other hand, is very silly, and one manifestation of her silliness is her readiness to be flattered by the attention of admirers, real or imagined.

Nicholas and Kate are horrified at the mere thought of their mother being susceptible to this kind of influence, and apparently the author to some extent shares their view. Partly because Mrs Nickleby is not supposed to remarry, and partly because she is so silly anyway, Dickens makes the scenes in which 'the gentleman in small-clothes' declares his passion for Mrs Nickleby grotesquely absurd. The cucurbits involved are the low-status cucumber and vegetable marrow (both highly absurd), and the way they are employed is equally undignified: the suitor throws them over the garden wall.[10]

> 'You may well be surprised, Nicholas, my dear,' she said, 'I am sure I was. It came upon me like a flash of fire, and almost froze my blood. The bottom of his garden joins the bottom of ours, and of course I had several times seen him sitting among the scarlet-beans in his little arbour, or working at his little hot-beds. I used to think he stared rather, but I didn't take any particular notice of that, as we were new-comers, and he might be curious to see what we were like. But when he began to throw his cucumbers over our wall –'
>
> 'To throw his cucumbers over our wall!' repeated Nicholas, in great astonishment.
>
> 'Yes, Nicholas, my dear,' replied Mrs Nickleby, in a very serious tone; 'his cucumbers over our wall. And vegetable-marrows likewise.'
>
> 'Confound his impudence!' said Nicholas, firing immediately. 'What does he mean by that?'

> 'I don't think he means it impertinently at all,' replied Mrs Nickleby.
> 'What!' said Nicholas, 'cucumbers and vegetable-marrows flying at the heads of the family as they walk in their own garden and not mean impertinently! Why, mother –'

The prudish Nicholas immediately understands the meaning of the sign, i.e. interprets the throwing of cucumbers as a gesture of courtship, and he protests violently, exactly the way Kate does later on.

There is no doubt that Mrs Nickleby too has got the message, since the cucumber-throwing immediately puts her in mind of her late husband's courtship of her (p. 568):

> 'He must be a very weak, and foolish, and inconsiderate man,' said Mrs Nickleby; 'blameable indeed – at least I suppose other people would consider him so; of course I can't be expected to express any opinion on that point, especially after always defending your poor dear papa when other people blamed him for making proposals to me; and to be sure there can be no doubt that he has taken a very singular way of showing it. Still at the same time, his attentions are – that is, as far as it goes, and to a certain extent of course – a flattering sort of thing; and although I should never dream of marrying again with a dear girl like Kate still unsettled in life –'
> 'Surely, mother, such an idea never entered your brain for an instant?' said Nicholas.

Later on, when the cucumber-throwing is repeated in Chapter 41, Mrs Nickleby again associates the cucurbitic attentions of the gentleman in small-clothes with Mr Nickleby's courtship (p. 616).

In Chapter 37, when he first hears about the attentions of the gentleman next door, Nicholas is very shocked and says: 'You know, there is no language of vegetables which converts a cucumber into a formal declaration of attachment' (p. 569). As we know, this statement is multiply and repeatedly belied by the reactions of the characters in the novel. The gentleman next door knows what the throwing of cucumbers and vegetable marrows means; so does Mrs Nickleby; so do Nicholas and Kate; so do the readers and so did Dickens. And Dickens created both the prudishly horrified Nicholas (and Kate) and the foolishly susceptible Mrs Nickleby, thereby dramatizing two mutually contradictory attitudes of his own mind and of that of his contemporaries towards the cucurbits, which were by both parties recognized as a symbol of courtship.

At the end of Chapter 37 the matter is clarified. Mrs Nickleby reveals that the suitor has proposed 'marriage and an elopement' (p. 569). The horror of Nicholas is now so great that he pronounces the gentleman mad (pp. 569-70):

> 'There are a thousand ways in which you can show your dislike of these preposterous and doting attentions. If you act as decidedly as you ought, and they are still continued, and to your annoyance, I can speedily put a stop to them. But I should not interfere in a matter so ridiculous, and attach importance to it, until you have vindicated yourself. Most women can do that, but especially one of your age and condition in circumstances like these, which are unworthy of a serious thought. I would not shame you by seeming to take them to heart, or treat them earnestly for an instant. Absurd old idiot!'

Though Dickens makes the final exclamation referentially ambiguous so that it applies to both the suitor and to Mrs Nickleby, it primarily means the suitor. Later on we learn that the man is in fact mad. Nicholas's and Kate's, and partly Dickens's, Victorian revulsion at the thought of Mrs Nickleby remarrying, is thus so strong that sexual desire at Mrs Nickleby's age is equated with madness, and the madness is not only imputed by Nicholas and Kate; its existence is also confirmed by the author – the gentleman in small-clothes is actually mad.

The imagery expressing revulsion reaches extraordinary heights of pathological horror. Some of the images connected with the sex symbolism are incredibly unpleasant. In the sort of haphazardly created chain of free association that Mrs Nickleby habitually indulges in, it is natural that the courtship of the gentleman next door puts her in mind of sex and the begetting of children, and this leads her to a passage of reminiscences in which babies are likened to roast pig (pp. 616-17):

> 'Kate, my dear,' said Mrs Nickleby; 'I don't know how it is, but a fine warm summer day like this, with the birds singing in every direction, always puts me in mind of roast pig, with sage and onion sauce and made gravy.'
> 'That's a curious association of ideas, is it not, mama?'
> 'Upon my word, my dear, I don't know,' replied Mrs Nickleby. 'Roast pig – let me see. On the day five weeks after you were christened, we had a roast – no that couldn't have been a pig, either, because I recollect there were a pair of them to carve, and your poor papa and I could never have thought of sitting down to two pigs – they must have been partridges. Roast pig! I hardly think we ever could have had one, now I come to remember, for your papa could never bear the sight of them in the shops, and used to say that they always put him in mind of very little babies, only the pigs had

much fairer complexion, and he had a horror of little babies, too, because he couldn't very well afford any increase to his family, and had a natural dislike to the subject. It's very odd now, what can put that in my head! I recollect dining once at Mrs Bevan's, in that broad street, round the corner by the coachmaker's, where the tipsy man fell through the cellar-flap of an empty house nearly a week before quarter-day, and wasn't found till the new tenant went in – and we had roast pig there.'

One would have thought the unpleasantness of likening babies to roast pig sufficient, but Dickens actually improves on it by introducing the nice touch of a body that was not found until new tenants moved in.

In Chapter 49, when Mrs Nickleby says 'I would rather, I declare, have been a pig-faced lady' (p. 741), the allusion again equates pigs and babies because it refers to the folklore monster which was a baby but had a pig's face.[11]

At the very beginning of the cucumber-throwing episode, even before the cucumbers have been mentioned, the suitor is already associated with physical abnormality (p. 567):

'There can be no doubt,' said Mrs Nickleby, 'that he *is* a gentleman, and has the manners of a gentleman, and the appearance of a gentleman, although he does wear smalls and grey worsted stockings. That may be eccentricity, or he may be proud of his legs. I don't see why he shouldn't be. The Prince Regent was proud of his legs, and so was Daniel Lambert, who was also a fat man; *he* was proud of his legs. So was Miss Biffin: she was – no,' added Mrs Nickleby, correcting herself, 'I think she had only toes, but the principle is the same.'

Daniel Lambert was the fattest man in the world; Miss Biffin had neither arms nor legs and never grew more than 37 inches tall.

Dickens was able to express horror at the thought of Mrs Nickleby's temptation by playing on the ambiguity of the cucurbit as a symbol. As we have seen in Part 1, cucurbits can easily be associated with bodily deformity and with obesity. In Chapter 41 Dickens includes a bodily defect that is specifically connected with cucurbits: we learn (p. 622) that the gentleman next door has a 'perfectly bald head'.[12]

But despite the strong revulsion expressed in images and associations as unpleasant as these, nobody construes the throwing of cucumbers as anything but a declaration of passion. Dickens insistently associates the cucumber-throwing scenes with other more conventional cases of courtship in the story. One parallel is Smike's love for Kate; he puts all the gravel on her side of the garden (p. 618), and all the roots of flowers.

Mrs Nickleby thinks this is attention to herself (p.618). Kate asks her mother whether she had many suitors before she was married (pp.618-19), and Mrs Nickleby enumerates them. In the midst of this comes another orgy of cucumber-throwing (p. 620):

> Kate looked very much perplexed, and was apparently about to ask for further explanation, when a shouting and scuffling noise, as of an elderly gentleman whooping, and kicking up his legs on loose gravel with great violence, was heard to proceed from the same direction as the former sounds; and, before they had subsided, a large cucumber was seen to shoot up in the air with the velocity of a sky-rocket, whence it descended, tumbling over and over, until it fell at Mrs Nickleby's feet.
>
> This remarkable appearance was succeeded by another of a precisely similar description; then a fine vegetable marrow, of unusually large dimensions, was seen to whirl aloft, and come toppling down; then several cucumbers shot up together; and, finally, the air was darkened by a shower of onions, turnip-radishes, and other small vegetables, which fell rolling and scattering and bumping about in all directions.

Dickens further associates the cucumber-throwing with legitimate cases of courtship at the beginning of Chapter 42, in which John Browdie and Matilda reappear as a newly married couple. He also deals with the relation between Fanny Squeers and Nicholas which had once mistakenly been thought to be an engagement. Finally, in Chapter 49, in which the gentleman in small-clothes makes his last appearance, there is a veritable riot of parallels: the love of the gentleman in small-clothes for Mrs Nickleby is parallelled by Smike's love for Kate, by Frank Cheeryble's love for Kate (which Mrs Nickleby again thinks is his polite 'attention' to herself), by the rumour of Frank's love for a German lady, by Tim Linkinwater's 'flirtation' (p.737) with Miss La Creevy, by Mrs Nickleby's renewed remembrance not only of her late husband's love for herself, but also of the young gentleman 'who used almost every Sunday to cut my name in large letters in the front of his pew while the sermon was going on' (p.741), and finally, at the end of the chapter, by the cucumber-gentleman transferring his attentions from Mrs Nickleby to Miss La Creevy (p.743).

The gentleman in small-clothes is mad; but, as Mrs Nickleby says at the end of Chapter 41, 'there's a great deal too much method in *his* madness' (p.629). There is also a great deal of method in Dickens's employment of cucurbitic symbolism. Dickens's use of cucumbers in connection with courtship shows that basically the meaning of the symbol is stable, and that the variation in usage is caused by differences in people's subjective attitude. In Dickens the widely differing attitudes on Kesey and Tolstoy coexist in the same work.

If it is obligatory to have the connection courtship–cucurbit the logical solution for an author who wants to make discriminations between one courtship and another is to make use of the differences between one cucurbit and another. Doubtless this is why Kesey favoured the watermelon, which is fairly positive, whereas Tolstoy and Dickens chose cucumbers and marrows, which are less so.

The narrator in Alemán's *Guzman de Alfarache* knows that courtship of a woman is always a tricky business. Women are all basically the same; yet how very different they may turn out to be! 'Piensa, que los casamientos, què son sino acertamientos, como el que compra vn melon, que si vno es fino, le salen ciento pepinos, ò calabaças?'[13] [xxxv] You think you have got a melon but she turns out to be a gourd or a pumpkin; all three are cucurbits, but how very different they are from one another. Alemán's narrator manages to introduce the idea of distinction by seizing on the differences between the various cucurbitic species, even though he preserves the obligatory connection courtship–cucurbit. The quotation comes from a chapter in which the narrator, having recounted the sad story of how his wife turned against him when their money ran out, shoots off into a long digression on the hazards of courtship and marriage.

In addition to the subjectivity of the sender there is also that of the receiver to be considered, when the receiver is not only the reader but another character in the work; that is, when the message exists not only as communication between author and reader but also as communication between characters in the work. In the use of a cucurbitic term of abuse as a taunt it is not only what the sender has in mind that matters; the role of the victim's imagination is also important. Ambiguity or vagueness in the taunt may be an asset because, realizing the user's intention to hurt, the listener will interpret the expression in whatever way is worst for his own idea of himself.

An example of a vague cucurbitic nickname used tauntingly can be taken from one of the Moomin stories by the Finlandswedish author Tove Jansson. To take an example from a work written by her is of additional interest because, as readers and critics know, her works are symbolic or allegorical at a very subtle level. It is usually impossible to explain that a certain element in one of her texts 'means' a certain thing in a one-to-one relationship, because she habitually stays clear of clichés and worn-out devices.

SIGN AND SIGNIFICATION

In *Pappan och havet* the Moomin family have migrated to a lone and distant island and the isolation of their new life triggers some sort of personality crisis for most members of the family. For the protagonist, the Moomin troll, this is adolescence, and the awakening need to abandon his family and start thinking of girls.

The girls come in the form of seahorses. The Moomin troll finds a horseshoe and gives it to his mother. The seahorses look alike and Moomin does not know which one is his (pp. 144–5 and *passim*) – a common enough experience for adolescent males looking at girls. The seahorses taunt him, calling him 'sea-cucumber' ('sjögurka') (pp. 145-6):

> Sjöhästarna simmade fram och steg upp på sjöns tröskel, vattnet nådde dem till knäna.
> Det är jag! Det är jag! svarade båda två och fnittrade sig halvt fördärvade.
> Ska du inte rädda mig? frågade den ena. Lilla, lilla tjocka sjögurka, tittar du på mitt porträtt varenda dag? Tittar du?
> Han är inte en sjögurka, sa den andra förebrående. Han är en liten, liten äggsvamp som har lovat rädda mig om det börjar blåsa. Han är en liten äggsvamp som söker snäckor åt sin mamma.
> Är det inte förtjusande! Förtjusande!
> Mumintrollet blev het i ögonen. [xxxvi]

The seahorses make fun of his dreams of performing some heroic deed (saving them), and they make fun of his emotional attachment to his mother. 'Tjock' ('fat') naturally links the fact that the Moomin troll *is* rather corpulent with the obesity connotations of the cucurbit. But since 'tjock' is, paradoxically, in the immediate vicinity of the repeated 'lilla' (small), and cucumbers as a matter of fact are rather slim and not *tjock* at all, the smallness element of the passage ('lilla, lilla') must be diffused through generalization to the whole passage and interpreted as a taunt which is somehow in keeping with the rest of the passage.[14]

In this maze of uncertainty one thing is clear. The Moomin troll feels hurt and takes the episode hard. He has great difficulties rationalizing it and it takes a long time before he can look back at the episode dispassionately. Far from being a drawback to the symbol, the ambiguity of 'lilla, lilla tjocka sjögurka' is an asset. The ambiguity that is achieved not only with the aid of the ambiguous symbol cucumber, but also with the aid of the rhetorical figure of oxymoron, is instrumental. The Moomin troll is more hurt by his adolescent inability to make out what things mean than he would have been by abuse that he could have understood clearly at once. It is important that in this section of the book everything is a kind of projection of the Moomin troll's own self.

SIGN AND SIGNIFICATION

The Moomin troll was ripe to be hurt, and the cucurbitic nickname hurts him, and therefore functions unambiguously despite its ambiguity.

We are dealing with strange kinds of logic in this chapter. But then the types of 'rationality' at work, e.g. in the development of cucurbitic usage, really are very strange, and they demand to be dealt with on their own terms. It is necessary to abandon certain intellectual habits and acquire certain others in order to understand how these mechanisms work.

In particular, one must let go of any notion that links at deeper levels between elements should always be signalled by a corresponding connection in the surface logic of the text. In this material there exist all sorts of connections without any corresponding surface manifestations. Surface logic must therefore be abandoned and patterns traced that depend on another kind of logic at a different level of consciousness. If one looks closely at the examples in this book some extraordinary ramifications and patterns emerge. It is not only a question of the predictability with which you bump into pumpkins in humorous works; or, conversely, the predictability with which you may conclude that the rest of the work is humorous if you find a pumpkin in the first random passage you happen to come upon. The intricacies of some patterns are astounding. Very striking is the regularity with which one finds things symbolically related to cucurbits in the immediate vicinity of a cucurbitic occurrence, even in the absence of any logical relation-marker in the surface text. Time and again we find authors who, having used a cucurbit in a passage, then go on to something closely related to the cluster of symbolic associations that cucurbits have.

Particularly intriguing also are the patterns of sound symbolism, or phonosemic correlations. There are a number of phonetic features in the names of the cucurbits that can be suspected of carrying such symbolism. Heavily under suspicion are the labial consonants *b, p* and *m* (*pump*kin, cucu*mb*er, *p*e*p*o, *m*arrow, *m*elon, *m*usk*m*elon, etc.), since labiality in general is probably suspect. Similarly with velarity, which throws suspicion on 'squ*a*sh'. Further candidates for the list would be, e.g., the '-urk-' of Ger. 'G*urk*e', Norw. 'ag*urk*', Sw. 'g*urk*a', Fi. 'k*urkk*u'; the '-nt-' of 'ca*nt*aloup', etc. Reduplication, which is widespread in the names of the cucurbits, may also, we think, carry some semic significance.

A problem is that if phonosemic correlations exist, one does not know how far they extend geographically. Are they restricted to one language? Are they restricted to a family of languages? The role of the labial consonants, for instance, seems to be quite different in Africa from what it is in Europe. But relative to whatever unit is relevant there did seem to be phonosemic symbolism. We asked a small number of people, speaking different languages, what the names of the cucurbits in their own language 'sounded like', and there seemed to be a tendency for them to 'sound funny' or to coincide with phonetic features found in words from some other areas such as slang terminology for delicate subjects.

The labial consonants *m*, *b* and *p* seem to be used in words denoting, e.g., massive roundedness; but also, in the combination *mp* for instance, movements that come to an abrupt halt. Above all they seem to be used in words denoting phenomena that the user approaches with strong feelings of love, shame, fear, contempt or hatred.

Again and again we met the labial consonants hand in hand with the cucurbits. Recall the quote from *Hermit in London* (Part 1), and the labial consonants of 'qui*mp*e', '*b*u*mp*', occurring not very far from a cucurbit ('her melon-formed head') which was symbolic of corpulence. 'Lu*mp*' did not occur only in Hawthorne's *The Scarlet Letter*, but was a regular companion of cucurbits. So was '*plump*', and not only in the phonetically extraordinarily lush voluptuousness of Joyce's *Ulysses*, where '*plump*' is a neighbour of 'ru*mp*' and cucurbit: 'He kissed the plump mellow yellow smellow melons of her rump, on each plump melonous hemisphere, in their mellow yellow furrow, with obscure prolonged provocative melonsmellonous osculation' (p.719).

When the cucurbitic name occurring in a text was one of those that do not have the combination of double labial consonants ('cucu*mb*er', 'pu*mp*kin') this desirable sound combination, carried by some other word, would often try to sneak into the immediate neighbourhood, preferably into the same sentence or the same line. Thus in Keats's poem 'To Autumn' the cucurbit used is gourd, but since the verb used about the gourd is 'swell' the poet puts in the word '*plump*' in order to get the desired combination of labial consonants even though he attributes 'plump' to the nut: 'To swell the gourd, and plump the hazel shells/With a sweet kernel; . . .'[15] Or take a case of the inverse order from Christina Rossetti's poem 'Goblin Market' where, in her enumeration of various kinds of fruit, having mentioned '*plump* unpecked cherries', her imagination is then presumably unconsciously alerted by the '-*mp*-' so that she puts 'melons' into the next line: 'Plump unpecked cherries,/Melons and raspberries.'[16] Sylvia Plath, thinking of melons, longs so yearningly for the '-*mp*-' sound that she even coins new words in order to get the desired labial consonants into her poem 'Fiesta Melons'. She coins such words as 'thumpable', 'bump-rinded', etc.[17]

In dealing with this kind of material it is very difficult to keep strictly to reasonable observation and avoid solipsistically 'creating' one's findings. It is, of course, inevitable that some labial consonants will happen to be in the neighbourhood of cucurbits by chance. Nevertheless it was our impression that there were more of them than would have been warranted by pure chance.

In this context we wish to add a few words about the whole question of cucurbits and sound symbolism. The study of phonosemic correlations is very difficult and highly controversial. Investigation has to rely mainly on subjective impressions. None of the prestigious methods of measuring the success of a theory can be employed; to use sophisticated statistics is out of the question, since one does not know what to count or what to compare with what. All words are not equally important. Verbs and adjectives, and nouns of certain categories (such as words of abuse, endearment, etc.), are more important than, for instance, pronouns or conjunctions. Above all some stylistic levels of speech and writing are more relevant than others. Slang, and informal language in general, and language needed to deal with delicate subjects, provide the most rewarding material.

So many things have to be dealt with at once – subject matter, stylistic level, parts of speech, etymology, degree of lexical stability, etc. – that simple mechanical methods are ruled out. Moreover, if counter-examples are regarded as refutation there is no point in studying phonosemic correlations at all, since counter-examples can always be found. If sound symbolism *is* to be studied, it will have to be on the basis of a recognition of the fact that phonosemic correspondences do not operate with the same regularity as the 'laws' of, e.g. natural science, and that counter-examples cannot in this case constitute absolute disproof in the same way as they are often thought to elsewhere.

We have not looked into the question of cucurbits and sound symbolism very thoroughly, but we suggest that it might be interesting to consider the following hypotheses:

1. that, given a possibility, e.g. through accidental similarity between the name of a cucurbit and another word connected with one of their chief connotations, the name of the cucurbit

will become mixed up with the other word and the predetermined semantic role hence enhanced;

2   that, if a sound change is optional, the names of the cucurbits will have it if this makes the sound of the word phonosemically more appropriate, or will not have it if the opposite is the case; i.e., the names of the cucurbits will acquire as many as possible of the sounds that are intrinsically funny or otherwise suitable for their role, in a language;

3   that given a chance the names of the cucurbits will acquire suitably expressive morphological elements (such as the '-kin' in 'pumpkin');

4   that, if foreign names of cucurbits are accepted as loan words, they will be more easily borrowed if their sound is intrinsically suited to the symbolic role of the plant in the receptor language;

5   that, if, of two biologically similar species of cucurbits, one happens to have a name phonetically more expressive, that species will be used symbolically more often than the other.

To move to safer ground and yet continue our attempts to trace the strange ways of peculiar logic at work in the material, let us turn to those genres where the logic at work is openly admitted to be different from everyday rational surface logic. The interpretation of dreams, or in general the literature of dreams, is a typical genre where a different sort of logic is acknowledged to be at work. It is satisfying to find that in this genre the cucurbits behave precisely as we would expect them to.

Recall how in that passage from Christina Rossetti's poem 'Goblin Market' that we quoted in Chapter 2 there was no direct link between melons and desert in strict surface logic. But in dream logic (or pseudo-dream logic) they were analogous and suitable to appear together.

Another genre where a 'logic of association' is taken for granted is stream-of-consciousness prose. To illustrate this let us take a case where, in addition, it is combined with a dream – Joyce's *Ulysses* (pp. 47–8):

> 'After he woke me up last night same dream or was it? Wait. Open hallway. Street of harlots. Remember. Haroun al Raschid. I am almosting it. That man led me, spoke. I was not afraid. The melon he had held against my face. Smiled: creamfruit smell. That was the rule, said. In. Come. Red carpet spread. You will see who.'

The cucurbit being connected with 'harlots' is entirely in keeping with what one may expect. The narrative element reappears later in the work: 'Last night I flew. Easily flew. Men wondered. Street harlots after. A creamfruit melon he held to me. In. You will see' (p.215).

And still later on, predictably, in the brothel scene (p. 556):

> The whores
> [*Laughing.*] Encore! Encore!
>   Stephen
> Mark me. I dreamt of a watermelon.
>   Zoe
> Go abroad and love a foreign lady.
>   Lynch
> Across the world for a wife.

Note in the following final example from *Ulysses* how, although the chief connotation of the cucurbitic passage itself (its own sentence) is stupidity or big-headedness, yet the expression occurs in the neighbourhood of references to childbearing (pregnancy and corpulence) and the sentence 'People knocking them up at all hours', which may be meant ambiguously (p. 159):

> Funny sight two of them together, their bellies out. Molly and Mrs Moisel. Mothers' meeting. Phthisis retires for the time being, then returns. How flat they look after all of a sudden! Peaceful eyes. Weight off their minds. Old Mrs Thornton was a jolly old soul. All my babies, she said. The spoon of pap in her mouth before she fed them. O, that's nyumyum. Got her hand crushed by old Tom Wall's son. His first bow to the public. Head like a prize pumpkin. Snuffy Dr Murren. People knocking them up at all hours. For God's sake doctor. Wife in her throes. Then keep them waiting for their fee. To attendance on your wife. No gratitude in people. Humane doctors, most of them.

Readers are used to looking for connections not announced in surface logic in such texts as Joyce. Though surface logic is present in other authors this does not mean that the type of logic that stream-of-consciousness prose relies on is absent. It certainly is not in the case of cucurbits.

A genre rather similar to the literature of dreams is writings on etymologies during earlier periods. The foundations of the discipline of etymology have often been so shaky in the past that with many authors one can again take their statements primarily as evidence of their own opinions, and again disregard 'fact', i.e. the question of whether they are right or wrong.

Some of the varieties of peculiar logic can help explain how an underlying link, at a level of lesser specificity, may be more important and real than a spectacular discrepancy at a level of greater specificity. If a logic of this kind operates there is, despite some inconsistencies which at first seem striking, a definite order and system in the material, and the cucurbit passes from the state of a non-arbitrary sign to that of a sign proper only at a level of great specificity.

Before closing the chapter with a brief note on the relation between our panchronic method and ambiguity, let us finally say a few words about a special type of apparent ambiguity; a false impression created by our organization in Part 1.

As we already stated in the Introduction, the problem with too much order and organization in Part 1 is that it distorts the picture of the semiotic role of the cucurbits. One ought ideally to say everything at once, and deal with all aspects simultaneously. Since this is impossible, we had to simplify (and thereby distort) the presentation by concentrating on only one aspect at a time of the semiotic role of the cucurbits. This created a false impression of diversity; an image of the cucurbits existing as signs at a level of great specificity with highly specialized, clear-cut roles, often mutually contradictory.

Much of this impression is false. We could not return to every example again and again to deal with aspects we had intentionally neglected the first time we brought forth the example, because repetitiveness would have fragmented our arguments; and we thought that readers can analyse each example more fully on their own retrospectively when the whole semiotic matrix has been dealt with.

Much apparent ambiguity and seeming specialization appears in a different light if looked at in the entirety of its own context. We have used the account of the emperors Carinus and Clodius Albinus from the *Historia Augusta* as evidence of the cucurbits used as a sign in a story of gluttons. But this is not the only function they have in this text. In the passages on Clodius and Carinus the cucurbits fit the context in many respects.

Though the writer in dealing with Clodius attributes much of his information to hearsay or to others, and even if he exonerates Clodius of some malpractices (the emperor is for instance reported to have been 'innocent of unnatural lusts'), yet the general drift of the narrative is clear, and for instance, in connection with the last-mentioned element, even if Clodius was 'innocent of unnatural lusts', nevertheless he was at least a noted womanizer, 'mulierarius inter primos amatores'.

The case of the account of Carinus in the *Historia Augusta* is quite clear. One can hardly find a more negative or hostile portrait in the whole series. Carinus was, says the *Historia Augusta*, the most polluted of men, an adulterer and a constant corrupter of youth. He even 'ipse quoque male usus genio sexus sui' (Carus, Carinus, Numerianus XVI.2, *Historia Augusta*). The list of his malpractices is long and detailed.

In the middle of the list comes the account of his gluttony, which shows him exceeding the limits of all moderation, 'swimming among apples and melons'. Naturally the melon fits in not only with the gluttony but also with the promiscuity, etc., in this passage, the ultimate reason being that gluttony and promiscuity themselves combine well in the view of the *Historia Augusta*. Inability to control one's appetite and one's lust are seen as parallel vices. The gluttony and the promiscuity are both signs, signalling the unfitness of the emperor for his office, as the *Historia Augusta* sees it. How could someone who was unable to govern his lust, or govern his appetite, be expected to be able to govern an empire?

The passages could be much more fully explicated. But we could not deal with all passages even to this extent, because our primary interest was to present the semiotic matrix of cucurbits and this was best done by concentrating in each passage on that aspect or connotation whose role was most pronounced. This means that if the full context of all occurrences is examined much seeming ambiguity and apparent specialization disappears.

An objection that could finally be brought against our panchronic method is that we have created, like Dr Frankenstein, a phenomenological monster, with calabash-legs from Borneo, cucumber-arms from Lapland and a Cyclops's eye from Patagonia in the middle of its pumpkin-head – in other words, that the semiotic matrix of the cucurbits such as it emerges from our material is only a construct which has never existed, at least not in its entirety, for a particular author, writing for a particular audience, during a particular period.

But if the physiology of the cucurbit determines its semiotic role, the semiotic matrix is inevitable in the form it takes. On this question hinges our whole view of the case, and if we are right the objection against the monster is invalid. Then it is to be presumed that somehow, at some level of consciousness, most, or even all, of the connotations that exist for one author or reader are always at least potentially available to other authors or readers as well. The corollary of this is that our study is no more than an explicit writing out of the implicit or unconscious reactions of every author or reader.

Ferdinand de Saussure thought that linguistics should be 'le patron général' of all semiology because in the natural languages signs are arbitrary. Moving away from linguistics to literature or social codes, semiotic studies usually stress the extent to which the signs are arbitrary in these systems as well. It is usual to try to convince the readers that there is more arbitrariness than the author expects the readers to have thought. In the case of cucurbitic symbolism, however, there rather seems to be less arbitrariness than one might have thought. Plant and animal symbols are 'symbols' in the sense in which Saussure used the term, i.e. naturally motivated signs.

4 Independent creation versus tradition

One obvious dualistic way to structure an inquiry about our material is to ask the question that anyone studying similarities in works of art from different periods and different locations always has to ask: how much is borrowing and tradition, and how much is independent creation?

If the similarities in the use of cucurbits as a sign in different authors from different periods and countries are explained as borrowing and tradition, it would suggest that man is an extraordinarily imitative creature and that a worldwide network of communication, of astounding proportions and complexity, has existed and exists.

If, on the other hand, the similarities in usage are explained as having arisen spontaneously and independently in different localities and periods, without borrowing or tradition, this would suggest an incredible sameness in the workings of human thought, through the ages, in various places, unless one assumes that some role is also played by the element itself, so that the development of the imagery can be explained teleologically. Our argument is that the physiology of the plant provides the necessary basis for a view that the development of cucurbitic imagery is predetermined.

The study of literary influence, borrowing and tradition is notoriously difficult. The two types of evidence that a source hunter usually has to rely on are either explicit comment (or some other kind of external corroboration), or arguments based on alleged similarity between the imitating and the imitated work.

Ideally the first type of evidence proves the case beyond any doubt. If the author mentions his source that usually clinches the matter. But often much less definite types of external corroboration have to be relied upon. Finding the works of the imitated author in the private library of the alleged imitator is sometimes taken as an indication of literary indebtedness. But such arguments may be over-simplifications. The division between an author's subjectiveness and objectiveness, between his creative self and his receptive self, need not be so clear cut that his own works constitute his subjective activeness and his reading his objective receptiveness. There may be much subjectivity and much activeness in his reading too. What he reads may be just as much a projection of his own self as his writing and the argument for borrowing weakens. It becomes as convincing to argue that since he was already interested in something, and had written on it, he read a work that was similar, as to argue that he read something, became interested and wrote on it.

The argument from similarity is also beset with difficulties. The basic idea is that similarity may indicate imitation. But some similarities are trivial and some the result of chance. In addition there are several curious features of the methodology of similarity-reasoning. It is well known that authors usually do not like to be caught thieving, and most of them, if they borrow, try to hide it. Hiding means making the borrowed element dissimilar, and suddenly, hocus-pocus, we have a situation where everything could be imitation, because if it is similar, then it is imitation, and if it is dissimilar, then the author is furiously trying to hide his imitation. Contributing further to the dangers are the mechanisms of literary allusion. An allusion to another literary work should preferably be veiled; it is aesthetically most pleasing for the reader if the elements signalling the allusion are minimized. In the same way as irony signals should be minimized, so should those of allusion, since it gives the audience a pleasurable feeling of belonging to an 'in-group' if they can catch a veiled and casual allusion, rather than an allusion that vulgarly insists on drawing attention to itself by irritating verbal nudges and obnoxiously pointed stylistic fingers, in a self-conscious poke which insults the reader by underestimating him. Allusions are kin to cryptography.

This contributes even more to a situation that might be a heaven for paranoiacs but turns into a nightmare for anyone else. Now, if two passages are dissimilar, one can not only conclude that the author of the later passage is borrowing, despite the dissimilarity; one can also praise him for his mastery in covering up. The pitfalls become especially dangerous if one's starting point is a high opinion of an author and a conviction that he had cryptographic leanings. It is then easy to produce whatever results one wants, since both ways of reading the evidence can produce the same meaning.

INDEPENDENT CREATION VERSUS TRADITION

Nevertheless, having said all this, we think that even to the very cautious observer it is obvious that cucurbitic traditions of extraordinary complexity have existed and exist. In particular, the two traditions of Jonah and Seneca have developed into quite recognizable super-codes living a life of their own through the centuries in the Christian and Western worlds. With these two one can easily imagine that the cucurbit has passed into a sign which is used by people who do not reflect over the origin of the sign, i.e. its coming into existence because of the biology of the plant. It was therefore capable of spreading north to countries where, because of the climate, the cucurbits are scarce, such as the Scandinavian countries. A rich Jonah tradition existed for some time in the folk-painting of the Swedish province Dalarna. The artists knew the sign even though they had never seen a cucurbit – judging from the form of the plant in their paintings, it does not seem as if they had. We are moving into pure metalanguage here – they were able to use the cucurbitic sign as a man can talk about 'nectar' as 'the drink of the gods' even if he has never tasted or seen nectar and is an atheist. Of course one cannot claim that the use of a cucurbit as a sign is *directly* influenced by the physiology of the plant in the case of users in climates where there are no cucurbits.

But it can be observed that the cucurbit as a sign exists in such localities only if it is introduced with the aid of very strong traditions such as those of Christianity or classical learning. In Finnish and Norwegian literature there are hardly any symbolic uses of cucurbits at all before the nineteenth century apart from those in the classical or biblical tradition, presumably because the cucurbits were introduced to Scandinavia late. It thus seems to be part of the nature of plant symbolism that there should be a possibility for the user of the sign to refresh his sense of the semiotic role of the sign by occasionally deducing it again from the anatomy of the plant – this of course goes for the author as well as the public. Even the tradition is dependent on periodic revitalization.

If we wanted to explain cucurbitic imagery in our material as being primarily borrowing and tradition we could occasionally take such an argument quite far. Often, during our research, when we had found a use such as Tompson's comparison of 'pompeon' to a 'saint' in his New England poem, it was first obvious to us, phenomenologically, that here was yet another instance of that frequent type of occurrence in which the cucurbit is likened to some person high in a social hierarchy (kings, emperors, etc.), and one explanation would then be that because the cucurbits are a record species of garden produce, the most prominent plant of the garden had again been likened to a socially prominent person in a symbolic passage. The same combination of ingredients had once again, independently and spontaneously, with the pleasing regularity of a well-known chemical process, produced the same result.

But then, of course, thinking twice about Tompson and his classical learning, it became obvious that there may have been a catalyst too – that Tompson may have been influenced by Seneca's *Apocolocynthosis* – and we were back to where we started: it is possible to explain the cucurbit in Tompson either as a case of literary influence (Seneca) or as an independent creation of a similar usage as that of Seneca, the similarity being brought about by the inherent nature of the literary element.

The attractiveness of the borrowing theory grows spectacularly if one argues that much borrowing takes place unconsciously. In music unconscious imitation is a well recognized danger (the criteria of borrowing are also very clear – copyright conventions specify a number of bars). Even literary critics are afraid of unconsciously plagiarizing. It seems natural to assume that literary authors imitate earlier texts unconsciously, directly or indirectly. It may be that to Rider Haggard's generation Christianity and the Bible were so familiar that he could not help having Numbers at least unconsciously at the back of his mind when he wrote the desert episode in *King Solomon's Mines*. Then the killing of the bird could be an unconscious parallel to Numbers.

The evidence is usually inconclusive. We think that even if the tradition is undoubtedly strong in some cases, such as Seneca and Jonah, what is usually important is nevertheless not borrowing but the predetermined nature of the cucurbitic passages. What does it matter whether or not an author knew an earlier work which he could imitate if he could have created his own (similar) passage independently anyway?

If a passage in an author can be explained equally well as imitation or independent creation, should imitation be regarded as primary? Authors do not imitate everything they know, only what they think worth imitating; thus there is an element of subjective creativity even in imitation, and it could be argued that authors often imitate what they would have created independently anyway. In a hierarchization of explanations it is sensible to put borrowing higher than independent creation if the character of the element could vary arbitrarily, because then imitation is competing only with pure chance. And even if we know that sometimes pure chance must be at work, we also prefer to explain all such cases as imitation if possible because the explanation is so much more substantial and satisfying.

It is different if the character of the element does not vary arbitrarily. Many national anthems resemble each other. This does not mean that the authors of these imitated each other directly. The likelihood is that national anthems will resemble each other in form since they all resemble each other in content: they are all about the beauty of the native country, its glorious past and its bright future, the love that its citizens bear for it, etc. The authors imitate each others' patriotism rather than each others' poems.

The passages in which authors from different periods and different places have used cucurbits symbolically resemble each other because the cucurbits of different periods and places resemble each other, and because the communicative needs of users of signs in different places and periods all resemble each other.

5 On the nature of signs used in cucurbitic metaphors

When Ferdinand de Saussure presented the principle of the *arbitraire du signe* in his course of general linguistics, he seems to have thought of the sign primarily in a fairly limited sense. In Part 1, 'General Principles', Chapter 1, where he deals specifically with the nature of the linguistic sign, he gives as the first of his two important principles the arbitrariness of the sign, and begins his exemplification by stating that there is no link of an inner relationship between the idea of 'sister' and the succession of sounds s-ö-r which serves as its signifier in French. According to the notes of most students he then further pointed out that the arbitrariness of linguistic signs is exemplified by the very existence of different languages: 'ox' is b-ö-f on one side of the border and o-k-s on the other.[1]

At the end of his treatment of the principle of arbitrariness, before proceeding to his second principle (linearity), he anticipates hostile criticism by dealing with two phenomena that might seem to contradict the idea of arbitrariness. Significantly these are onomatopoeia and interjections; thus his concern is again with sounds.

But between the 'ox' example and his remarks on onomatopoeia came some reflections that have already caused much confusion among followers and will doubtless cause much more. In Bally's and Sechehaye's reconstruction Saussure's ideas are reported as follows (Mauro, pp. 100-1):

> Une remarque en passant: quand la sémiologie sera organisée, elle devra se demander si les modes d'expression qui reposent sur les signes entièrement naturels – comme la pantomime – lui reviennent de droit. En supposant qu'elle les accueille, son principal objet n'en sera pas moins l'ensemble des systèmes fondés sur l'arbitraire du signe.
> En effet tout moyen d'expression reçu dans une société repose en principe sur une habitude collective ou, ce qui revient au même, sur la convention. Les signes de politesse, par example, doués souvent

d'une certaine expressivité natu[r]elle (qu'on pense au Chinois qui
salue son empereur en se prosternant neuf fois jusqu'à terre), n'en
sont pas moins fixés par règle; c'est cette règle qui oblige à les
employer, non leur valeur intrinsèque. On peut donc dire que les
signes entièrement arbitraires réalisent mieux que les autres l'idéal
du procédé sémiologique; c'est pourquoi la langue, le plus complexe
et le plus répandu des systèmes d'expression, est aussi le plus
caractéristique de tous; en ce sens la linguistique peut devenie le
patron général de toute sémiologie, bien que la langue ne soit
qu'un système particulier.

On s'est servi du mot *symbole* pour désigner le signe linguistic,
ou plus exactement ce que nous appelons le signifiant. Il y a des in-
convénients à l'admettre, justement à cause de notre premier
principe. Le symbole a pour caractère de n'être jamais tout à fait
arbitraire; il n'est pas vide, il y a un rudiment de lien naturel entre
le signifiant et le signifié. Le symbole de la justice, la balance, ne
pourrait pas etre remplacé par n'importe quoi, un char, par exemple.

If we try to interpret this passage with the aid of Rudolf Engler's critical edition,[2] a number of ideas emerge, though what importance Saussure gave to each of these, and what he meant their relations with each other to be, is not very easy to make out. At least a few points stand out fairly clearly:

- that there are modes of expression based on completely natural signs (pantomime);
- that if the new science of semiology welcomes these, its main concern will still be with the systems based on the arbitrariness of the sign;
- that signs that are wholly arbitrary realize better than others the ideal of the semiological process; therefore linguistics should be the prime example for all branches of semiology;
- also that even if there is a certain natural expressiveness in some signs (such as formulae of politeness) they are nevertheless fixed by rule and it is the rule that counts; nevertheless also, on the other hand, that the term 'symbol' should not be used, because a symbol is not arbitrary, it could not be replaced by any other symbol.

What emerges from a study of the notes in Engler is a picture of some of these ideas as parenthetical and perhaps even to some extent tentative and provisional. Saussure asks himself how far semiology could extend its domain ('Où s'arrête la sémiologie? C'est difficile à dire d'avance.' – Engler, p. 154), and it seems that at least partly he thinks in terms of reluctantly going down a scale of decreasing arbitrariness. It is clear that Saussure pronounced a value judgment in favour of arbitrariness, in that he regards the systems based on arbitrary signs as more interesting for the semiologist to study than others. Saussure was wondering about the 'cut-off level' on the scale of decreasing arbitrariness where a system of signs would no longer be very interesting to semiologists.

It is possible that Saussure's value judgment about arbitrariness versus non-arbitrariness has influenced some recent attempts to determine the exact degree of arbitrariness of the signs in certain sign systems, not in the legitimate sense of making investigators more interested in the systems in which signs are more arbitrary, but rather in the misguided sense of making people anxious to prove as high a degree of arbitrariness as possible in any system of signs.[3]

Saussure confidently predicted that the new science of semiology had a right to existence; that its place was assured in advance (Mauro, p. 33). Today, with the rise of such schools as French structuralism in literary scholarship, and particularly since the first congress of the International Association for Semiotic Studies, held in Milan in 1974, many people think that Saussure's prophecy is coming true.

In the passage from the *Cours* cited above, Saussure, by mentioning them in the same context, linked the question of the extension of the domain of semiology and the question of the arbitrariness of signs. That link was prophetic because many of the new branches of semiotics proliferating at the moment inevitably sooner or later come up against the question of the degree of arbitrariness of signs. In fact, some of them not only come up against Saussure – they may also find it difficult to avoid the *physei-thesei* debate. The question of the boundaries of φύσις, nature, and νόμος, convention, was debated by the ancient Greeks in connection with language too, as in the *Cratylus*, and this question has been so basic through the ages that it actually seems possible to view the whole history of linguistics in terms of a pendulum swinging from one extreme on the *physei-thesei* continuum to the other, as Morton Bloomfield does in an essay in *Daedalus*.[4]

The very fact of the continued debate between naturalists and conventionalists could suggest that both are partly right and that language is a mixture of nature and convention. Even so, it remains to be determined what is the share of each. If Saussure's *arbitraire* is made into a dogma the sense of 'linguistic sign' should at least be strictly limited. It is therefore highly questionable to bring the idea of the *arbitraire* into a discussion of metaphor. This, however, does seem to happen. In

ON THE NATURE OF SIGNS USED IN CUCURBITIC METAPHORS

Derek Bickerton's 'Prolegomena to a Linguistic Theory of Metaphor', for instance, the author states quite bluntly: 'Meaning exists, if anywhere, only in the relationship speaker–language–hearer, not in any one of the three, and least of all in any connection between language and the extralinguistic universe.'[5] To illustrate this he has just given an example that, like those of Saussure, concerns sound, he points out that *le provoca un tinto?* means one thing to a Spaniard and another to a Colombian.

It is true that the sound sequence [laiən] for the idea of 'lion' in English is arbitrary. But to proceed from this to the idea that *the animal* 'lion' is chosen arbitrarily in the metaphor 'the man is a lion' is a very questionable jump, and an unjustified extension of the idea of the *arbitraire*. None the less, it seems as if some such idea did influence Bickerton's argument (pp. 38–9):

> This connection is subtle enough to have misled some very acute linguists. Bazell, for instance, remarks: 'Both *green wine* and *yellow wine* are combinations seldom or never to be found. But the reason is different for the former, where it is a question of lacking material motive, and for the latter, where it is a matter of syntactic convention' (1953, 83). Now by 'material motive' Bazell presumably means that 'there is no green wine in nature', and by 'syntactic convention', that wine which is (at least to speakers of what Whorf called SAE) optically yellow is habitually modified, across several languages, by the adjective white and its equivalents. But even leaving aside the fact that interpretation of the spectrum is a linguistic variable, this will not do. What of Portuguese *vinho verde*, or, nearer home, *yellow rat* (which is not a rat, either) or *green fingers*? Or take the following table:
>
> | | |
> |---|---|
> | iron-mine | +steel-mine |
> | iron ore | +steel ore |
> | ironworks | steelworks |
> | iron magnate | steel magnate |
> | iron production | steel production |
> | iron girder | steel girder |
> | iron determination | +steel determination |
> | iron will | +steel will |
> | iron discipline | +steel discipline |
>
> Bazell would presumably account for the non-occurrence of the first two items in the right-hand column, and the occurrence of the next four, by saying that while steel-mines and steel ore do not exist in nature, steelworks, steel magnates etc. do. But if he tried thus to account for the non-occurrence of the last three, he would be unable to account for the occurrence of the last three in the left-hand column. He would be obliged to treat these as metaphors, albeit somewhat moribund ones. But once he had done that, he would

> have to show why the last three in the right-hand column cannot similarly be treated.
> In fact we are better off if we forget about 'nature' and 'material motive' altogether.

We are not convinced that one is better off to forget about nature and material motive altogether. We do not believe that a theory of metaphor should ignore the question of the intrinsic suitability of the signs used.

We would define a metaphor as *a bisociation of two systems, whose focus is the alleged identicality (which is short for similarity) of two elements, one from each system.* Such bisociation will not take place unless there is an intrinsic reason in the suitability, one for the other, or both for each other,[6] of the two elements. This we believe to be true generally, but especially true in the case of metaphors making use of something from nature,[7] as nature is outside the control of speaking man.

Arguments such as Bickerton's lead to a theory that deals with only one aspect of metaphors, and the theory becomes somehow self-contained. Bickerton continues (p. 39):

> The non-occurrence of *steel-mines* is only accidentally connected with the non-occurrence of steel-mines; *yellow rats* occurs, though there are no yellow rats. If there were something which might be described as a 'steel-mine', just as there are some persons who might be described as 'yellow rats', *steel-mine* would occur, even in the absence of steel-mines. The reason why no such thing exists is simply that, in English at least, no specific attributes has been attached to *steel*.
> By 'specific attribute' is meant a particular quality, usually assumed to belong to the denotatum of a sign. Thus to *iron*, in English, is assigned the attribute 'hardness'. Natural as this may seem, it is in fact a fairly arbitrary process; hardness is only one of the attributes which iron might be supposed to possess (durability, weight, dark colour, etc.) and it possesses it to a lesser extent than many other substances, such as diamond, or, for that matter, steel itself. But to *diamond* has been attached the attribute 'value', perhaps also 'brightness'.

The argument moves at a level of great specificity. It may be that 'steel determination', 'steel will' and 'steel discipline' are impossible in English and should be starred. But *how* impossible are they? In relation to the communicative need of the person using the metaphor – who wants to depict the determination, will and discipline as strong – they may be impossible in one sense if 'iron' is prescribed by convention,

ON THE NATURE OF SIGNS USED IN CUCURBITIC METAPHORS

but nevertheless 'steel' is *more* possible in the context than, say, 'wax'; the difference being that wax is soft and steel hard.

Bickerton quotes the existence in other languages of a metaphoric use of steel as demonstration of the arbitrariness of the process (pp. 38-9):

> And the arbitrariness of the process is further demonstrated by the fact that it is not interlingual: *hierro* has no metaphorical value in Spanish, but *acero* has; even in loan-translations, *iron curtain* and *iron lung* are rendered as *telón de acero* and *pulmón de acero* respectively. Spanish simply attributes 'hardness' to steel rather than iron, thus reversing the English relationship.

But is this not rather a demonstration of the opposite? That 'steel' is possible in metaphors to suggest strength and hardness is indicated by its occurrence in Spanish (and other languages – there are also languages where both 'iron' and 'steel' are habitually used in metaphors).

That 'steel determination' will come into existence as a metaphor of a strong determination is more likely than that 'wax determination' will, simply because steel is harder and stronger than wax. We believe that a theory of metaphor should be probabilistic, not regulatorily descriptive – which is the same as prescriptive.

Bickerton stays within the rules and conventions of present-day English. However, it has often been pointed out that the distinctive feature of metaphors is their capacity to function as an innovating force in language. And when the boundaries of language are extended with the aid of metaphor, temporarily or lastingly, the outstandingly important fact is the interpretability of new metaphors the first time they are used. Their interpretability is closely related to their degree of intrinsic appropriateness. On the level of great specificity the present state of occurrence of 'iron will' and non-occurrence of '+steel-will' is governed by arbitrary convention; but on the level of lesser specificity, both the coming into existence of 'iron will' in the past, and the probability that as a metaphor of a strong will 'steel will' is more likely to come into existence in the future than 'wax will', are governed by the non-arbitrary principle of intrinsic suitability influencing probability.

It may be desirable not to restrict oneself entirely to a level of very great specificity. As Roger Brown writes in *Words and Things*:[8]

> The morpheme for *hot* stands for rage in Hebrew, enthusiasm in Chinese, sexual arousal in Thai and energy in Hausa. However, this disagreement does not suggest the operation of accidental factors since there is an undoubted kinship in the range of meanings. All

> seem to involve heightened activity and emotional arousal. No case
> was discovered in which the morpheme for *hot* named a remote,
> calm (in fact *cool*) manner.

This was predictable since anyone can see that heat induces speed and movement in nature whereas coldness induces slowness and repose. The predictability of new metaphors is intimately related to their interpretability. Bickerton's essay is synchronic (p. 50):

> So far we have considered only the synchronic component of a theory of metaphor. Such a theory, however, cannot be merely synchronic, otherwise it could neither account for the history of attribute-assignment (i.e. how countless expressions which must originally have seemed 'metaphorical' have now come to be accepted as virtually or completely 'literal') nor, what is perhaps more important, explain how countless other expressions, which may as yet not have occurred, may in the future pass through a similar process. For though in the present state of knowledge such a suggestion might seem wildly optimistic, the theory should have – if future processes prove to be modelled on past ones – at least some degree of predictive power.

It seems to us that for a theory of metaphor to have a predictive power it is necessary to root that predictability in assumptions of the speakers' and listeners' knowledge of nature rather than in their knowledge of convention. The metaphor 'the man is a lion' can be explained either as natural ('lions are brave') or conventional ('it is agreed that lions should be regarded as brave'), but for our skill in predicting, understanding and accepting new metaphors the former is more important.

One traditional view of metaphor stresses the principle of *similarity* involved – the man is similar to the lion in his courage, even though he is definitionally different in that he is a man and not a lion. In terms of our own way of thinking, we would like to put it like this: *there exist animals, and differences between these animals (in degrees of bravery, for instance), i.e. there is a system; and also there exist men, and differences between these men; and the metaphor 'the man is a lion' means that the position of the man among humans is analogous to that of the lion among animals.*

In a paragraph where he challenges the assumption that 'the interpretability of texts is mode-of-discourse free' Bickerton writes: 'Everyone accepts that context can affect interpretation. Few realise that we need not go outside language to account for this, (p. 37). We are not questioning Bickerton's argument at this specific point, but we are suspicious of theoretical treatises on the metaphor that do not 'go outside language'. Not to go outside may be just as arbitrary as not to go inside from the point of view of an objective inquiry into the function of this type of communication.

First of all we have to define the concept 'metaphor'. Bickerton's view is the dictionary view. But even in the case of the literal sense of 'dictionary' it can be observed that metaphors get into dictionaries only when they are dead, if even then. This means that metaphors are a matter of the sentence and the text as much as of the word. In our opinion the view of metaphor accepted by such works as Bickerton's is insufficient. The very fact that such treatises deal with the material in terms of the occurrence or non-occurrence of a certain expression means that the whole outlook is entirely within the *thesei* framework, since it is precisely a matter of convention whether an expression is regarded as existing in a language or not. In one sense any expression that you can think of in any language exists as soon as you have invented it and used it; and it exists as language for two or more people if it is understood; in other words, if it is interpretable. In another sense an expression exists in a language when it has been sanctioned by people who regard it as their task to determine the fitness of new expressions for the received code. In highly petrified languages such as Russian the split between these two views of what is thought to exist has become a very wide rift. In such languages not only are many incidental expressions refused admission to the status of language by the purists and traditionalists, but even expressions that have become recognizable stock items in casual spoken language are refused acceptance as part of the norm.

If the expression 'steel determination' is used in English by somebody in the sense 'strong determination' and understood by somebody as having that meaning, has it not then been a metaphor? The purist and the normative grammarian answer no, because to them language is above all convention and in this case convention prescribes 'iron will'.

But if a treatise on metaphor defines metaphor in terms of adherence or non-adherence to convention, that treatise cannot, by definition, make any contribution to the *physei–thesei* debate because it is entirely within the *thesei* framework and any argument would become circular. The very notational systems of such works, such as the starring of an expression, imply a *thesei* standpoint. It actually means that one restricts the definition of metaphors to those that become part and parcel of language – *i.e. of language as convention*. This definition is too narrow. First, these clichés have to come into existence at some point, and we would define them as being metaphors even the first time they are used. Second, we would also argue that a metaphor may be used only once and still quite clearly be a metaphor, in which case it cannot be explained as tradition, since it becomes a tradition only the second time it is used. We think that metaphors are incessantly invented, used, understood, and forgotten or remembered, as the case may be; a metaphor is better understood if it is more apt and it is in that case also more likely to be remembered and perhaps to become convention, even though very inept metaphors can also become convention and very expressive metaphors be lacking from the convention – which, again, does not mean that they are 'impossible' or unthinkable.

We think binarity should be rejected in the description of metaphors. Metaphoric expressions are not possible or impossible; they are more possible or less possible. Only if that part of nature or reality from which a metaphor is created is in itself clearly binary is a binary description justified. But in images of strength or hardness, for instance, there are infinite gradations between the two extremes of hardness and softness rather than a simple and absolute binary opposition; therefore 'steel determination' is 'possible' in the sense that it would probably be correctly understood by anyone happening to hear it, if it should happen to be used.

With metaphors there is an element of skill involved and this skill is not a matter of using metaphors either correctly or incorrectly; it is a matter of using metaphors as well as possible, and of metaphors there is the whole qualitative scale from very bad to very good ones. It is a distinguishing feature of metaphors that some are better than others. They are better if they comply with those intrinsic qualities that make them more expressive, and the foremost factor is the similarity between the element from one system and the element from the other. 'τὸ γὰρ εὖ μεταφέρειν τὸ τὸ ὅμοιον θεωρεῖν ἐστιν', says Aristotle[9] – 'to metaphorize *well* is to have an eye for resemblances' (our italics).

The conventionalist school of thought is primarily interested in what people *can* say. We, however, are primarily interested in what people *do* say, or *will* say. Binarity, which is the basis for the former attitude, has often been shown to exist in language as an ideal rather than in language as actually used by people. Acceptability tests have shown repeatedly how 'grammaticality' or 'acceptability' are often a matter of opinion – majority opinion or informed opinion – rather than an absolute and clear binarity opposition of possible/impossible. This is so with language in general, and very much so with metaphors.

ON THE NATURE OF SIGNS USED IN CUCURBITIC METAPHORS

We believe that metaphor is a dynamic, not a static, phenomenon. We are pleased to note that Paul Ricoeur in his book *La métaphore vive* takes the same view.[10]

Purists with a normative approach, such as the academies of various countries, have generally realized that metaphors are special and should be left outside their attempts to establish a stable and unified standard language. The aim of standardization is to ensure that people understand one another, and in the case of totally arbitrary signs it may be necessary to insist on conformity and strict convention in order to achieve this. But in the case of metaphors people will understand one another anyway, in so far as they share a knowledge of the nature (or reality) with the aid of which metaphors are created, and a similar perception of it. Thus, with metaphors, though it may be regarded as desirable, it is still not absolutely necessary that people share a convention as well.

With metaphors there is total anarchy in the sense that no convention can ever totally fetter the metaphorizer. It is the privilege of the metaphorizer, as of the poet and the philosopher, to say that which is not. Yet, precisely as in the case of the poet and the philosopher, there is method in the madness, and metaphors are tolerated and needed for the same reason as fiction and philosophy: all three are methods of cognitive exploration, and, we suspect, very closely related to each other. Free from the fetters of convention, metaphor is nevertheless not anarchy, because instead of order upheld by convention there is here order created by intrinsic suitability. Non-arbitrary signs do not need convention for order, whereas convention is the only thing that upholds order in the case of arbitrary signs. The conventionalists are very much oriented towards stasis, and therefore metaphor, which is a dynamic phenomenon, does not fit their world. But metaphors have a built-in system of stability that arbitrary signs lack: their tendency towards maximal suitability.

When cucurbitic metaphors are used there are probably cases when the interpretability rests almost purely on convention, and cases when it rests on a knowledge of both convention and nature. But we also think that in our material there were numerous cases when the thoughts of those using a cucurbitic metaphor (speakers and listeners, authors and readers) went straight to the real-life fruit or plant rather than to a literary or linguistic convention.

In the introduction we suggested that within language there are the two coexisting and contending forces of stability and lability. Thus the two young men, Hermogenes and Cratylus, who turn to Socrates in Plato's dialogue *Cratylus*, to have a difficult linguistic problem sorted out, have both got hold of part of the truth about language. Hermogenes maintains that there is no intrinsic connection between things and the names we give them; that we can change these names as we change the names of slaves at will; whereas Cratylus, who is a Heraclitan, grasps at language as a stable phenomenon in an unstable world. Socrates seems to lend his support to neither or to both, and although experts on the history of linguistics often warn against drawing too close parallels, there is doubtless some kinship between this attitude and that of Saussure who insisted on both the mutability and immutability of language (Mauro, pp. 104–13).

Metaphor is not bound by convention and should therefore belong to the 'lability' half of language. But though it often throws away the stability offered by convention it provides its own stability instead and it is therefore a very interesting phenomenon for literary authors. Authors can easily create new literary 'languages' in works of some length. This may even be 'language' quite literally, as in Richard Adams's *Watership Down*,[11] in which the language of rabbits is introduced gradually and absorbed and assimilated by the reader quite effortlessly. Thus language is characterized by its malleability in that an author can make anything mean anything through manipulation of the context. But in very short units, where there is little context, this is difficult; and indulging in lability – which is the same as individuality and novelty, as opposed to collectivity and habituality – involves the danger of not being understood. The enormous appeal of metaphors may be seen against this background. In naturally motivated signs, interpretability can be left to the audience's knowledge of nature or reality (i.e. whatever system is bisociated with the one under consideration). There will be stability; and interpretability will be assured; even though the speaker or writer abandons himself totally to lability in the form of individual inventive and innovative freedom.

In a metaphor such as 'the man is a lion', what is coupled with the man is *the word* 'lion' *only if the metaphor is dead.* As long as the metaphor is alive it is not the word but *the animal* lion that is coupled with the man. Some linguistic theories try to fit metaphor into the lexicon component of our linguistic skill, arguing that in the lexicon of our brains there is an entry for the word 'lion' saying something like 'wild beast in Africa', but then that there is also an additional entry, 'can also be used about a man'. We believe that such additional entries exist only in the case of dead metaphors, and that with normal metaphors the only entry in the lexicon is some such thing as 'wild beast in Africa' (for 'lion', and 'human male' for 'man'), and that if the metaphor 'the man is a lion' is alive it is *the animal lion* that is used to refer to the man rather than *the word 'lion'*. The *signifié* (*lion* the animal) of the *signifiant* (*lion* the word) has in turn become the *signifiant* (*lion* the animal) of another *signifié* (the lionlike man).

In other words, metaphor means that reality is used to refer to other reality. Nature *becomes* language. The normal relationship between language and reality is for language to refer to reality. But sometimes, also, language can refer to other language (*metalanguage*). And sometimes, also – the mirror-image of this – reality can refer to other reality (*metaphor*). Both of these latter cases – language referring to language and reality referring to reality – allow man to extend his knowledge and thought in a way that would be impossible if he stayed within the confines of language referring to reality.

It is this self-sufficiency of reality in metaphor, with reality referring to reality, that makes it possible to argue a thesis that could aptly be called 'On the Origin of Metaphors through Natural Selection'. The argument of natural suitability in our study is not an idea borrowed from Darwinism; it is Darwinism itself. In Darwinism the idea of natural suitability plays an important part. Ant-eaters all over the world tend to look alike. They usually have strong claws with which they can break the ant-hills, long tongues with which they can catch the ants and long snouts with which they can poke into ant-hills during their meals. Even if ant-eaters on different continents may have different ancestral origins they have developed in a direction which has made them similar, all because of the demands of natural suitability.

If your environment is the air then very simply you need something to fly with. Birds and insects have wings; bats, flying squirrels and flying fish may have found other solutions, but the flying apparatus was necessary for them all, because only beings that have something to fly with are suitable in the air environment.

Context is in literature what *environment* is in life, and if, in a certain context, a metaphor involving flight is suitable, then the metaphor, if it makes use of an animal, will make use of one which is capable of flying. This is so simple it should hardly require saying. That it nevertheless has to be said occasionally is all due to the mistake that some theories make of looking for the process of 'natural selection' in the collective slow development of language – in other words, in tradition. It is not there that the process of 'natural selection' takes place: natural selection takes place during a very short moment in the mind of an individual, namely the metaphorizer. In a flash of insight he perceives a natural suitability and creates the metaphor, using reality as language to refer to other reality.

The interpretability of new metaphors depends on the kinds of relations that exist between the elements in the two systems that are being bisociated, and on the audience's knowledge of these. If these relations are very clear the metaphor will also be clearly expressive. If, for instance, a pumpkin is clearly and dramatically different from other fruit in real life, the metaphor of calling a man a pumpkin will be clearly expressive of meaning since the analogy then demands that the man be as different from other men as a pumpkin is from other fruit.

Usually metaphors are used for clarity; they are used to make the audience see what it did not see before. But part of the technique is to make the metaphor startling, and being startling may well include an element of mystification. Difficult poets use difficult metaphors to try to put over difficult meanings. These authors exploit the natural instinct of people to attempt to see a meaning in any new metaphor. By frustrating expectations these subtle authors try to create something that is pregnant with meaning though it yields that meaning reluctantly. There is therefore no clear borderline between nonsense and metaphor. What would seem nonsense under different circumstances becomes meaningful literary metaphor when presented in accordance with certain literary conventions.

These metaphors are often regarded as the highest achievements of poetic invention, and partly because of this, and partly because of the challenge in interpreting them, literary scholars are very much attracted to them. The examples of metaphor that recur regularly in works on the theory of metaphor tend to be very strange, partly for these reasons, but also because they are normally used as test-cases or touchstones of the theories and are therefore often peripheral rather than representative. A different picture of metaphor emerges if one starts with the real-world object from which a metaphor (making use of real-world nature, for example) is created, and goes through the material along that dimension, as we have done in this study. Then metaphor seems a fairly simple thing.

When the Russians call 'a person of ruddy, healthy appearance' огу́рчик (affectionate dimunitive of огуре́ц) the case is quite clear.

ON THE NATURE OF SIGNS USED IN CUCURBITIC METAPHORS

With a sort of syllogistic reasoning the metaphorizer has observed that: (1) a cucumber is something intensively alive; (2) a certain man is intensely alive. It is a short step to proceed to the conclusion: the man is a cucumber. This establishes an analogy between a particular fruit and a particular man through the bisociation of two systems: those of plants and of men.

When Jacopo da Diacceto, on being put to the torture, unhesitatingly confessed: 'I wish to rid myself of this pumpkin of a body; we intended to kill the Cardinal' (Villari), his body, earlier – though similar to a pumpkin, since both were examples of life – was different since it was human; now it has become merely similar, and therefore worthless (cf. also Thurber, 'squashes', and Prou, 'coloquinte').

The abusive metaphor of 'pumpkin' (Galt), 'Kürbis' (Mrose), 'Kürbiss' (Goethe), 'pumpion' (Fletcher), 'Pompion' (Fletcher and Massinger [?]), 'melons' (Crane), etc., was rather general and took notice of several cucurbitic characteristics. The use was more specialized in Theopompus, Ruxton, Roth, etc., where the sex connotations were used positively; or in Jansson, Procopius, 'watermelon' for Negro, *Priapea*, Juvenal, Irenaeus and Anaxilas, where they were used negatively. Stupidity was hinted at in Tertullian and the Swabian saying, and short-livedness in Coleridge and Gauden.

In the *London Gazette* quotation, 'A piece of pure Gold in form of a Mellon', melon is called gold because gold and melons are both yellow. In John Hacket's 'But can that Nation pass over such a Triumph as this Entertainment, without Pumpian Words, and ruffling Grandiloquence?' 'pumpian words' and cucurbits are both characterized by excessive swollenness; and when a free-loader is called cucumber ('Σικύα') from the way he clings to parties he has shown himself to be similar to the cucurbitic plants – with their tendrils and their clinging and clutching propensities – in his need of the support of others.

Sex connotations helped by iconic appropriateness were found in 'kürbisfrau' (Verena Stefan), 'cucumis' (Plautus), 'pyntegræskar' (Jørgen Nash) and 'to sammenvoksede meloner' (Nash).

We found that cucurbitic symbolism tended not to exist, or not to survive, in parts of the world that lack the plants themselves. This suggests that cucurbitic metaphors are not convention, or if they be that the convention needs to be constantly or periodically revitalized by fresh observation of that part of nature from which the conventional metaphor in that case originally stems.

Whether you say 'What an absurd pumpkin!' about a pumpkin, or

ON THE NATURE OF SIGNS USED IN CUCURBITIC METAPHORS

'What an absurd man!' about a man depends on which you want to talk about, the pumpkin or the man; and that is a choice between real-world objects and is outside the realm of linguistics. But when you say 'What an absurd pumpkin!' about a man, the pumpkin is no longer a real-world object, but a sign in a system of meaning, and the investigation of its function should be regarded as part of linguistics, even though this should entail some sorting out of relations between real-world objects. The capability of users of these signs to grasp their meaning is dependent not only on knowledge of cucurbitic tradition, but also, and we think primarily, on knowledge of cucurbitic nature. The study of metaphor is therefore one area where the investigator cannot ultimately escape reality.

Conclusion

In a theory of literature that could adequately explain and account for the literary phenomena of the material presented in this study, the probabilistic principle would have to play a prominent role. The arguments of such a theory would have to be of the type that 'given such and such, it is likely that such and such will follow'.

Similarities in the usage of the word 'pumpkin' as a linguistic sign in the proper sense are based on similarity in the processes of memory. It is arbitrary convention and restricted to speakers of English. But in 'pumpkin' used as a sign in our wider sense in plant symbolism, similarities in usage are due not only to similarities in the processes of memory but also to similarities in the processes of perception. The similarity is interlingual and metachronic.

New metaphors are incessantly invented and new literary codes created by authors. How is it that new metaphors are understood, and how do readers acquire the key to new literary codes?

Confronted with a new system of meaning humans fall back on their guessing ability. But for their guesses to be informed rather than random there must be some factor influencing the guessing. What this factor may be in each case is an interesting question for the literary scholar. We thought that in the case of animal and plant symbolism the answer is obvious: the immutability of nature. We therefore decided to write our study on that theme.

In addition, in our desire not to compound the difficulty of understanding the mechanisms at work in literary signification with a choice of a material difficult *per se* – even *within* the field of plant and animal symbolism – we decided to write on the cucurbits, which are arguably the easiest family to deal with.

We assume that it must be one of the easiest because it is botanically very distinct. The degree of arbitrariness of signs in plant and animal

CONCLUSION

symbolism is influenced by two major factors. The first of these is variations in the strength of the instinct to symbolize, allegorize and assign attributes. During some periods this drive has been very strong and this, we think, influences the plant and animal symbolism of those periods. In the bestiaries of the Middle Ages the animals are sometimes given very inept roles. If the assignment of attributes becomes a game, and particularly when such a system begins to aim at completeness, similarity and natural motivation decrease and arbitrariness increases. This may happen in particular if attention is heavily focused on the tenor. If tenor becomes somehow primary, and symbolification at the same time is obligatory, then vehicles will be picked up with little regard to intrinsic suitability. If there are, for instance, ten things to be symbolized by something, and five vehicles are noticeably well suited for five tenors, the symbolizer will find vehicles for the remaining five too, even if it means doing some violence to natural appropriateness. Once established, systems like these may become codes, and if the spirit that created them is strong in the culture and period these arbitrary and conventional systems may extend far and survive for a long time. Another case is when the process of symbolification becomes an end in itself. Then plant and animal symbolism may be fairly arbitrary too, as in the *Cabbala*.

But probably the most important factor influencing the degree of arbitrariness in plant-signs is the degree of botanical difference between the real plant in question and other plants. The more different and distinct the plant, the more expressive of meaning will the plant-sign be.

The cucurbits are dramatically different from other plants and fruit. Therefore the degree of natural motivation in the cucurbit-sign is bound to be high. Cucurbits differ from other plants much more than, for instance, one flower usually differs from another. Therefore 'the language of flowers' tends to be convention to a higher degree and intrinsic appropriateness to a lesser degree than the language of cucurbits, even though some natural motivation is obvious, as in the case of the colour of flowers: white (lily) symbolizing death (pallor) or red (roses) symbolizing love (blushing), etc.

We started with the easiest plant family because we hoped that by doing so the material would seem convincing in its own right, even if our explications should fail to convince. It would have been difficult to argue convincingly at the beginning of this work that the pumpkin in *Cinderella* is a courtship symbol. But in the company of all its paradigmatic relatives, the pumpkin in *Cinderella* is easily, we think, recognized for what it is. Given the marriage to the prince later on in the story; given the antithesis between high and low; given the magic and the gold; given the naturally amiable temperament of Cinderella as contrasted with the artificial conventionality of her stepsisters and so on, it was probable that the pumpkin would creep in, and the pumpkin being connected with courtship or marriage in *Cinderella* is merely another example in literature of the tendency of these two things to be found together, as in Tolstoy, Kesey, Alemán, Lear, etc.

We hope that our study has in some way suggested something about the way the principle of probability works. There is, however, not much point in a very strict formalization of a literary theory involving probability as a chief guiding principle, at least not in the case of naturally motivated signs. We suspect that the 'intuitive' insight of a good reader or critic is largely based on an eye for resemblances and an ongoing calculation, weighing and judging of probabilities. But to turn this suspicion to any theoretical use in scholarship may be difficult. The probability principle that we have dealt with in this study was explained, we maintain, by the natural motivation of the signs. If, then, literature imitates life, and literature somehow is form, and life is content – how can one *formalize*, if *form* is dependent on *content*?

If it is impossible to understand one without understanding the other, the choice is either to let semiotics be diffused into an interesting but difficult 'semiotic of life' or, for purely practical reasons at least, to shy away from naturally motivated signs, and make arbitrary signs the chief domain of semiotics, as Saussure predicted they would be. It may be desirable to try out both of these alternatives. But that they *are* alternatives cannot be denied.

Thus we stand defeated. Form and content, convention and nature, are inextricably bound together. Drive nature out with a pitchfork; yet she will return.

Notes

Introduction

1 E.M. Forster, *Aspects of the Novel,* London: Edward Arnold, 1927, pp. 22-4.

2 See section on Carlyle, Part 1, p. 71.

3 Ina Loewenberg in 'Identifying Metaphors', *Foundations of Language,* vol. 12, pp. 315-38, 1975 (p. 338) writes:
> In philosophy, we often must try to persuade students that it is possible to talk about the world by (also) talking about language. I would like to persuade linguists that it is possible to talk about language by (also) talking about the world. In fact, in both cases, I believe it is necessary to do this.

We entirely agree with this and our arguments are based on the assumption that it is impossible to understand the signs we deal with without recognizing their dual allegiance; i.e., they function as language, but derive their meaning from nature.

4 Cf. Rulon Wells, 'Distinctively Human Semiotic', in *Essays in Semiotics* (*Essais de sémiotique*), ed. Julia Kristeva, *et al.*, pp. 95-119; in *Approaches to Semiotics,* ed. Thomas A. Sebeok, vol. 4. The Hague-Paris: Mouton, 1971, p. 96.

Please note, in this context, that we do not use the term 'symbol' for 'sign proper'. Our use of terminology may often differ - sometimes radically - from many standard works in the field, but we hope our usage will be self-explanatory.

5 Since we have found that geese, cows and donkeys always seem to find champions who wish to defend these beasts against the charge of stupidity, we must insist that geese, cows and donkeys are stupid, semiotically perceived. One must not be misled by the volume of the stories commenting on the cleverness of these animals, even though the bulk of these far exceeds that of the comments asserting their stupidity. The explanation is simple. It is not the ordinary but the exceptional that is interesting - thus the stories of surprised wonder at the discovery that geese, etc., do not really seem to be

stupid after all merely confirm the fact that what one generally *expects* is stupidity, and thus the rule holds. An imbecile who makes some intellectual progress and learns to read becomes the subject of many admiring comments, even though it is perfectly normal for people to know how to read. It is a matter of what was expected in the first place; and of geese, cows and donkeys very little is expected.

Geese are seen as stupid because they often walk in a line or a flock, following a leader whose decision where to take them often seems arbitrary, and who in addition seems to acquire his leadership by chance. Imitative habits contribute to the image of stupidity particularly strongly during this and the last few centuries since individualism is now regarded as a positive thing. Imitative animals have, however, probably always had some connotations of stupidity. The parrot speaks without understanding what it says, which is stupid. Geese, like sheep, follow their leader, which shows their inability to think for themselves. Geese have a funny way of walking – the Prussian way of marching was not named 'goose-step' by the English because they liked the phenomenon. The cackling of geese grates on the ear and their appearance is uncouth. The rounded labiality of the long vowel of 'goose' in English in intrinsically negative.

Even in cases when one might at first be misled into thinking that geese are honoured, on closer inspection they turn out to have their usual role. The geese on the Capitol saved Rome, but in the *Pro Sexto Roscio*, for instance, when Cicero names the prosecutors 'geese' it is obvious that he is playing on the negative sense of the word. It is good to have prosecutors as it is good to have watchdogs, and geese on the Capitol; but if the geese (by analogy the prosecutors) begin to cackle without reason we wring their necks. Cicero's analogy makes use of the inherent negative value of geese.

Part 1 'Pregnant Gourds' and 'Delirious Pumpkins': The Semiotic Matrix of Cucurbits

1 For taxonomical studies on the family see the works listed in the *New Encyclopaedia Britannica, Macropaedia* (15th ed.), vol. 5, p. 364.

For an ancient Greek comment on confusion see Athenaeus, *Deipnosophistae*, II.58f. Cf. also Viktor Hehn, *Kulturpflanzen und Haustiere in ihrem Übergang aus Asien*, Berlin: Gebrüder Borntraeger, 1911, pp. 314-26; and *Paulys Real-Encyclopädie der klassischen Altertumswissenschaft*, ed. Georg Wissowa, Stuttgart: J.B. Meltzer, 1893 – vol. 11, c. 2104 (*Kürbis*); vol. 7, c. 1946 (*Gurke*); vol. 15, c. 562 (*Melone*).

2 F. Woenig, *Die Pflanzen im alten Aegypten*, Leipzig: Verlag von Wilhelm Fridrich, 1886, pp. 200-7: 'Sie fehlt selten unter den Opfergaben und selten unter den Erfrischung bietenden Speisen, welche die Diener auf Tabulets zum Gastmahle herzutragen.' (p. 202). *Flaschenkürbis, Kalebasse* 2400 BC (p. 205).

See also Vivi Laurent-Täckholm, *Faraos blomster: En kulturhistorisk-botanisk skildring av livet i Gamla Egypten byggd pa verklighetens grundval och med bilder från de senaste årens grävningar*, Stockholm: Natur och kultur, 1964, pp. 162–6; see also p. 154.

3 On taxonomy, cultivation and the economic importance of cucurbits see Thomas W. Whitaker and Glen N. Davis, *Cucurbits: Botany, Cultivation and Utilization*, World Crops Books, London: Leonard Hill, 1962.

For ancient authors with descriptions, instructions for growing, recipes, medicinal use, etc., see e.g. Theophrastus, *Historia Plantarum*, I.11.4 and VII.3.5; Columella, *De Re Rustica*, XI.3.48ff; Pliny the elder, *Naturalis Historia*, XIX.23.64 and XX.2.3; Palladius, *Opus Agriculturae*, IV.9.6 and 16; Pliny the younger, *De Medicina*, 13; Gargilius Martialis, *Medicinae* 6, 15 and 16; Galenus, *Opera omnia*, ed. C.G. Kühn, Lipsiae: Cnobloch, 1823, vol. 6, p. 565; *Geoponica*, III.13.6 and V.11.1; Apicius, *De Re Coquinaria*, III.4–7; Dioscorides, *Materia Medica*, II.162–64 and IV.178. See also John Organ, *Gourds: Decorative and Edible for Garden, Craftwork and Table*, London: Faber & Faber, 1963.

4 Hugh C. Cutler and Thomas W. Whitaker, 'History and Distribution of the Cultivated Cucurbits in the Americas', *American Antiquity*, vol. 26, no. 4, April 1961, pp. 469–85. In the new world too the history of cucurbits in connection with human culture goes back several thousand years, the oldest dated 7000–5500 BC, and cucurbitas in agriculture about 4000 BC.

For further references to ancient European cucurbitic history see *Reallexikon der Vorgeschichte*, ed. Max Ebert, Berlin: Walter de Gruyter & Co., 1926, vol. 7, pp. 196–7.

5 Though now that the Japanese have discovered how to make wine from watermelons the competition will grow stiffer! The reason why cucurbits have not been used for wine-making before is probably not only technical; it is possible that the symbolic value of the fruits has played a role.

6 It fascinates man in the same way as the mustard seed or the acorn. Cf. Matt. 13:31–2.

For the growth of the acorn into an oak as a symbol of artistic creation, see Henry James's prefaces to the New York edition, *The Art of the Novel: Critical Prefaces*, introd. Richard P. Blackmur, New York: Scribner's 1962; first pub. 1934. James repeatedly refers to his *donnée* or idea as an acorn that grew and grew.

7 J.B. Friedreich, in his *Die Symbolik und Mythologie der Natur*, Würzburg: Verlag der Stachel'schen Buch- und Kunsthandlung, 1859, pp. 246–7, writes: So wählte man z.B. zur Beziehung der Kürze des dahin eilenden Lebens und der schnellen Vergänglichkeit seiner Freuden und Genüsse ein Rad, an welchem ringsherum Kürbisse herabhingen; zum Bilde der Nichtigkeit und der Täuschungen des Glückes und seiner Gunst, sowie aller scheinbaren Güter des Lebens, nahm man einen durch eine majestätische Fichte gestützten, auf deren Gipfel stolz ruhenden und darüber hinwegrankenden Kürbis, und gab ihm folgende Inschriften: 'cito nata cito pereunt', 'brevis

gloria', 'in momentaneam felicitatem'.
Friedreich refers to emblems and mottoes of the sixteenth century; cf. Arthur Henkel and Albrecht Schöne, *Emblemata: Handbuch zur Sinnbildkunst des XVI. und XVII. Jahrhunderts*, Stuttgart: J.B. Metzlersche Verlagsbuchhandlung, 1967, pp. 181, 331-2, 718.

8   Cf. Russian огу́рчик, affectionate diminutive of огуре́ц, person of ruddy, healthy appearance.

9   *John Milton's Complete Poetical Works: Reproduced in Photographic Facsimile*, comp. and ed. Harris Francis Fletcher, vol. 2, *The First Edition of Paradise Lost*, Urbana: The University of Illinois Press, 1945, p. 384.

10 In addition the German *Universal Lexicon aller Wissenschafte und Künste* Halle/Leipzig: Verlegts Johann Heinrich Bedler, 1732, vol. 20, c. 552, which takes a very negative view of cucurbits, as being the devil's plants, claims that the following prominent people have been victims of the plant (though presumably not from over-eating): the German emperors Friedrich III and Heinrich VII, the Italian king Rudolpho, and the popes Paul VII and Clemens VII.

11 Columella, *De Re Rustica*, XI.3.53; Pliny, *Naturalis Historia*, XIX.23.64. Augustus, who was more temperate and modest, made do with a more prosaic species of cucurbits for his Spartan breakfast: he used to eat 'cucumeris frustum' (cf. Suetonius, *Augustus*, 77).

12 Walter Harding, *The Days of Henry Thoreau*, New York: Knopf, 1970, pp. 89-90.

13 Erik Axel Karlfeldt, *Hösthorn*, in *Svalans Svenske Klassiker: Erik Axel Karlfeldt*, Stockholm: Albert Bonniers Förlag, 1965, p. 335.

14 On abundance and cucurbits in folk-literature see Stith Thompson, *Motif-Index of Folk-Literature, A Classification of Narrative Elements in Folktales, Ballads, Myths, Fables, Mediaeval Romances, Exempla, Fabliaux, Jest-Books and Local Legends*, rev. and enl. ed., vols 1-6, Copenhagen: Rosenkilde and Bagger, 1955-8, D981.11; *Magic pumpkin*, India: Thompson-Balys; Chinese: Eberhard FFC CXX 58, 67, 221. D1463.2.1. Magic pumpkin furnishes treasure. D1472.2.6. Magic pumpkin yields year's supply of rice. D1482.2. Magic pumpkin holds streams of oil. Cf. also A1433.2.1. *Silver coins from pumpkin* received from fishes. India: Thompson-Balys. See also D965.2. *Magic calabash (gourd)*. Chinese: Werner 347; Korean: Zong in-Sob 288; Africa (Ekoi): Talbot 27, 34, (Yoruba): Ellis 246, (Benga): Nassay 208 no. 33. D1463.2. Magic calabash furnishes treasure. D1470.1.4. Magic wishing-calabash. D1472.2.7. Magic calabash causes food to be furnished, etc.; also D1463.3. *Magic seed produces golden gourd seed*. Chinese: Graham, Eberhard FFC CXX 36f; and D973.1.1. *Rice-grains magically produced by gourd*. India: Thompson-Balys. For a story connecting the origin of gold with cucurbits, see Thompson A1432.2.1. *Gold comes from gourd received from fishes*. India: Thompson-Balys.

NOTES TO PAGES 17-18

This *Motif-Index* hereafter referred to as Thompson, with references given only in the form of the letter and the relevant number. Vol. 6, Index. 'Pumpkin', p. 617, 'Melon' and 'melons', p. 500, 'gourd' and 'gourds', p. 345. Works referred to listed in bibliography in Thompson, vol. 1.

15 The tradition of gourds as ornaments in frames is also influenced by a literary source; a disputed translation of some passages in the Old Testament; e.g. 1 Kgs. 6:18.

16 Wentworth and Flexner's *Dictionary of American Slang* gives two main senses of *melon*: '1 The total profit or monetary gain from a business or enterprise, whether legal or not; the spoils – 2 Fame, glory, or patronage obtained by a group, esp. a political party, to be distributed among the members (*Dictionary of American Slang*, comp. and ed. Harold Wentworth and Stuart Berg Flexner, London: Harrap, 1960).

17 *The Complete Works of Robert Browning,* with variant readings & annotations, ed. Roma A. King, Jr, *et al.*, vol. 3. Athens: Ohio University Press, 1971, p. 212. The monk he hates is a gardener. The use of melon also involves some cucurbitic connotations that we shall return to later on in this study.

18 Leitch Ritchie, *Wanderings by the Loire: with twenty-one engravings from drawings by J.M.W. Turner,* London: Longman, Green 1833, p. 63.

19 No. 2724/2. Note here that there is also a connection between cucurbits and alchemy. Cf. J.E. Cirlot, *A Dictionary of Symbols,* trans. Jack Sage. London: Routledge & Kegan Paul, 1971, pp. 266-7.

20 Evans-Pritchard relates how the Nuer, if they have no ox available for sacrifice, instead sacrifice a cucumber, and how on such occasions the cucumber is referred to as 'the ox'. Cucumber here functions as a symbol of the ox that it is a substitute for. Oxen, in turn, we take to mean 'something valuable'. Oxen are important to the Nuer, and if our contention is right that cucurbits, because of their biological nature, strike humans as intrinsically important, then the Nuer cucumber symbol has natural suitability for its role. E.E. Evans-Pritchard, *Nuer Religion,* Oxford: The Clarendon Press, 1956. pp. 128, 133, 141-2, 146, 184, 203, 205, 298. See also p. 254, and passages, *passim*, on symbolism.

21 Even in the fruit symbolism of gambling machines in British pubs the watermelon is often found at the top of the hierarchy.

22 For a brilliant study of figs, see William Rodgers Telford, *The Barren Temple and the Withered Tree: A redaction-critical analysis of the Cursing of the Fig-tree pericope in Mark's gospel and its relation to the Cleansing of the Temple tradition.* Diss. (Cantab.; to be published shortly by Sheffield University's Department of Biblical Studies, in the Dissertation Series attached to their new *Journal for the Study of the New Testament.* The same author has also written an essay (to be published later) on the symbolic role of figs in the Graeco-Roman world).

23 *The Poems of Tennyson,* ed. Christopher Ricks, London and Harlow: Longmans, 1969, p. 1278. This edition hereafter referred to as Ricks.

24 Bananas are soft; they are associated with monkeys; underdeveloped countries whose independence is threatened by multinational companies are called 'banana republics'; the skin of a banana is the traditional thing to slip on before vanishing into a manhole in street-scenes in early cinema comedy. In such expressions as the American 'I go bananas' the pejorative sense is reinforced by the sound of "bananas", with its initial labial consonant and its reduplication.

25 Denis Hills, *The White Pumpkin,* London: Allen & Unwin, 1975, p. 17.

26 Athenaeus, III, 74b. The etymology is uncertain. Scholars have tried to explain the word from Indo-European *teva-, designating, according to Hehn (loc. cit.) 'das Strotzende, Zeugungskräftige, Samenreiche'. He also wants to explain the reduplication in cucumis, cucurbita from this bulging growth. A more recent book on the subject, Jaques André, *Les mots à redoublement en Latin* (Paris: Editions Klincksieck, 1978), pp. 48–50, states: 'Le redoublement caractérise les plantes d'après leurs parties plus ou moins sphériques et volumineuses, racine et fruit'. André also lists examples of reduplication in words for cucurbits in several languages. Cf. also our comments on sound symbolism; Part 2, Chapter 3.

27 Athenaeus, III, 74c.

28 Λεξικὸν τῆς Νέας Ἑλληνικῆς Γλώσσης "Πρωίας", Ἐπιμέλεια: Γεωργίου Ζευγωλῆ, Ἔκδοσις Νεωτάτη (Ἀθῆναι: Ἐκδοτικὸς Οἶκος Σταμ. Π. Δημητράκου).

29 Athenaeus II. 59c. Cf. Organ, op. cit., p. 65: 'The Hawaiian chant such as the 'Pule Ipu" or "Prayer of the Gourds" offered by a Hawaiian father for his son, which in substance is a request for the offspring to become vigorous like a gourd vine, and a plea that any evil spirits which might pursue the boy shall become shut in the gourd, are quite common.'

30 Diphilus 98: ' Ἐν ἡμέραισιν αὐτὸν ἑπτά σοι, γέρον, / θέλω παρασχεῖν ἢ κολοκύντην ἢ κρίνον.' Cf. *Comicorum Atticorum Fragmenta,* ed. Theodor Kock, Leipzig: B.G. Teubner, 1888, vol. 2, p. 573 and (for Menander 934) vol. 3, p. 242.

31 Ll. 80–91; Ricks, pp. 843–4.

32 *Vitae Patrum,* III.50 (*Patrologia Latina,* LXXIII, c. 767).

33 The notion that cucumbers restrain sexual appetite is a typical result of the bifurcation of an idea from a common kernel of association (in this case with sex). Sometimes cucurbits are thought to induce sexual appetite, sometimes to restrain it, and occasionally both traditions coexist. In Chapter XXI of Boorde's *Dietary* cucumbers are thought to restrain veneriousness though the opposite tradition existed even at that time: 'Mylons doth ingender euyl humoures. Of gourdes, of cucŭbres & pepones. Gourdes be euyll of

nowrysshement, cucūbers, restrayneth veneryousnes or lassyuyousnes, or luxuryousnes. Pepones be in maner of lyke operacion: but the pepones ingenderyng euyll humours.' (*Hereafter foloweth a compendyous Regyment or a dyetary o Helth, made in Moūtpyllier, compyled by Andrew Boorde of Physycke Doctour, dedycated* etc.).

34 P. Dass, *Nordlands Trompet* (written during the last decades of the seventeenth century), ed. D.A. Seip, Oslo: H. Aschehoug, 1974, p. 12.

35 If 'cucumis' is explained as, e.g., the snake gourd, what happens to 'cresceret in ventrem'?

36 J. Conington and H. Nettleship, *The Works of Virgil*, London: Bell, 1898, vol. 1, p. 350.

37 The verb 'to belly' or 'to belly out' is in English used about swelling sails.

38 An illustration of the probability – not to say inevitability – with which pregnancy is associated with cucurbits is a recent article on pregnancy in a British feminist magazine in which the writer gets to the cucurbit as early as the third sentence of her article: 'My skin is unbelievably stretched into this large gourd...''Tessa Weare, 'Round in a Flat World', *Spare rib: A Women's Liberation Magazine*, no. 78, January 1979, p. 15; 'gourd' is repeated on p. 17.

39 For further parallels to the passage see e.g. *Copa* (in the *Appendix Vergiliana*), Ovid, *Metamorphoses*, IY 685 and Y 495.

40 Virgil, *Ländliche Gedichte*, ed. Johann Heinrich Voss, Altona: Johann Friedrich Hammerich, 1800, p. 772. There is of course a possibility that the scribe's change is merely an accidental error.

41 DuCange, *Glossarium Mediae et Infimae Latinitatis* (1678), Niort: L. Favre, 1883, vol. 2. p. 644.

42 There are speculations as to a Lombardic origin of the word. The precise etymological truth, however, is irrelevant here. What counts is that any sex-word and the words for the cucurbits are magnetically attracted to each other. Given half a chance, e.g. through phonetic similarity, folk-etymology, etc., the cucurbits will acquire the semantic role they are predestined for.

43 Athenaeus, II. 68d.

44 George Frederick Ruxton, *Life in the Far West* (Edinburgh and London: Blackwood, 1849), p. 266. The character who is speaking is enumerating all the wives he has had of various Indian nationalities, Blackfoot, Sioux, Shian, etc.

45 Benjamin Jonson, *Volpone: or The Foxe*, introd. and notes Arthur Sale, London: University Tutorial Press, 1951, p. 42: '...some yong woman must be streight sought out, /Lustie, and full of juice, to sleepe by him...' Full of juice is ambiguous but the two senses reinforce the same meaning.

46 Athenaeus, III. 73d.

47 *Priapea*, 63.12. The choice of cucurbits should not be explained here in terms of the conventional 'well being–garden-cliché' but rather in terms of Priapus's own nature.

48 Walafrid Strabo, *De Cura Hortorum* or *Hortulus*, vv. 99-280, *Monumenta Germaniae Historica, Poetae Latini Aevi Carolini*, ed. Ernst Dümmler, Berlin: Weidmann, 1884, vol. 2, pp. 339-41.

49 For fertility (with Virgil in mind) cf. vv. 133-5: 'totum venter habet, totum alvus, et intus aluntur/multa cavernoso seiunctim carcere grana,/quae tibi consimilem possunt promittere messem.'

50 Cf. Matt. 13:31; Mark 4:31; Luke 13:19.

51 Cf. Artemidorus Daldianus, *Onirocriticon*, I.67: 'πέπονες δὲ πρὸς μὲν τὰς φιλίας καὶ συμβιβάσεις εἰσὶν ἀγαθοί.'

52 The spiral as a symbol of cosmic procreation and eternity is old and widespread.

53 Cf. John 15:1 and 5.

54 Milton's *Paradise Lost* A New Edition, ed. Richard Bentley, London, 1732.

55 About half the editions have 'smelling'. For an additional comment on the epithet 'smelling' see also Pearce. Later commentators such as Hawkey or Major usually refer to Bentley and Pearce.

56 Milton, *Paradise Lost*, ed. Bentley, pp. 228-9.

57 John Milton, *Paradise Lost: Samson Agonistes; Lycidas*, annot. & biog. introd. Edward Le Comte, a Mentor Classic, New York and Toronto: The New American Library, 1961, p. 205.

58 Cf. Thompson, A1236.2. *Tribes emerge from melon.* Lao, Wa (Indo-China): Scott Indo-Chin. 286, 289. Cf. Organ, op. cit., p. 65 'Hawaiian mythology also claims that the universe developed from a gourd. . .'
It stands to reason that a fruit that is associated with the birth of children should be associated with the birth of mankind. Throughout the world, and throughout the ages, cucurbits are associated with pregnancy. Cf. e.g. Organ, op. cit., p. 64: 'In Malaya, for instance, an infusion of gourd leaves, with ashes from a wood fire, is used as a lotion for application to the abdomen during pregnancy.' Also A.F. Broun (comp.), *Catalogue of Sudan Flowering Plants: Giving short descriptions, a number of vernacular names and some economic and other uses*, Khartoum: El-Sudan Printing Press, 1906, pp. 34-6 for note of barren women taking the pulp of a cucurbit to stimulate pregnancy.

59 In this context see e.g. Prudence Andrew, *Mr Morgan's Marrow*, illus. Janet Duchesne, London: Collins, 1975.

60 '... he has the pleasure every evening of reading the newspaper, and abusing the ministers amongst his old customers, himself a customer; as well as of lending his willing aid in waiting and entertaining on fair-days and market-days, at pink-feasts and melon-feasts...' Mary Russell Mitford, *Our Village: Sketches of Rural Character and Scenery*, vol. 2, London: Whittaker, 1826, p. 4.

61 *The Poetical Works of John Greenleaf Whittier*, London: Macmillan, 1874, pp. 157-8.

62 *Funk & Wagnalls Standard Dictionary of Folklore, Mythology and Legend*, ed. Maria Leach, London: New English Library, 1975, p. 910.

63 *Benjamin Tompson: His Poems*, ed. Howard Judson Hall, Boston and New York: Houghton Mifflin, 1924, *New-England's Crisis*, p. 49.

64 Tompson was a classicist and must have been aware of the use of pumpkin in Seneca (see below).

65 For botanical evidence, cf. Paul Antin, *Saint Jérôme: Sur Jonas*, Paris: Les Editions du Cerf, 1956, p. 111, n.1; R.H. Harrison, *Healing Herbs of the Bible*, Leiden: E.J. Brill, 1966, pp. 21-2; and particularly *The Dictionary of the Bible: Dealing With its Language, Literature, and Contents Including the Biblical Theology*, ed. James Hastings, Edinburgh: T. & T. Clark, 1899, vol. 2, p. 256.

66 St Jerome *Commentarii in Ionam*, IV.6 (*Patrologia Latina*, XXV, c. 1117).

67 St Jerome, *Epistulae*, 112.21 (*Corpus Scriptorum Ecclesiasticorum Latinorum* LV, p. 392). Cf. *Originis Hexaplorum quae supersunt*, ed. Frederick Field, Oxford: Clarendon Press, 1875, to *Ionam*, IV.6 giving: 'Ο'. κολοκύνθη. Α. Θ. κικεῶνα. Σ. κισσόν.'

Jerome's claim, that he put 'hedera' in order to agree with the other translators, does not seem to be borne out by the facts. Symmachus is actually the only one who gives 'hedera'.

68 Cf. Hieronymus, *Commentarii in Ionam*, IV.6 (*Patrologia Latina*, XXV, c. 1148): 'Et revera in ipsis cucurbitis vasculorum, quas vulgo saucomarias vocant, solent apostolorum imagines adumbrare: e quibus et ille sibi non suum nomen assumpsit'; c. 1149; 'Ad personam vero Domini Salvatoris, ne penitus propter φιλοκολόκυνθον cucurbitam relinquamus, sic referri potest, ut illud commemoremus Isaiae:...' Cf. also Antin, op. cit., p. 109, nn. 3 and 5; and p. 112, n. 3.

69 Rufinus, *Apologia contra Hieronymum*, II.39 (*Corpus Christianorum* XX, p. 114).

70 Otto Mitius, *Jonas auf den Denkmälern des christlichen Altertums*, Freiburg: Verlag von J.C.B. Mohr, 1897.

71 ibid., p. 46. These, of course, are impossible botanical monstrosities.

72 Cf. Matt. 12:39; 16:4; Luke 11:29; cf. also Ambrosius, *Hexaemeron*, V.11.35.

73 Cf. *Kommentar zum Alten Testament,* ed. Wilhelm Rudolph, Gütersloh: Gütersloher Verlagshaus Gerd Mohn, 1971, vol. 13$_2$, p. 361, n.6a), where he says: 'Die nur hier vorkommende Pflanze ist nach HS der Kürbis (ebenso Luther), *was auch Hier. für richtig hält,* obwohl er sich aus Gründen, über die er sich im Kommentar verbreitet, in Vulg. für den Efeu entscheidet' (our italics; Rudolph misrepresents St Jerome's view). The confusion is still alive.

74 Cf. Uwe Steffen, *Das Mysterium von Tod und Auferstehung: Formen und Wandlungen des Jona-Motivs,* Göttingen: Vandenhoeck & Ruprecht, 1963, Plate V.

75 In writing his series of poems 'Dalmålningar på rim' Karlfeldt was influenced by the folk-painting of his native province Dalarna, as even the title indicates; and in this tradition again it is obvious that the source of inspiration for the ornamental plant that recurs so often in the paintings was Jonah.

76 In English a quick review shows the following: William Tyndale, *The Prophete Jonas* (translated from the Hebrew), 1531 (?): 'as it were a wild vine'; *Myles Coverdale,* 1535: 'The Bible that is the holy Scripture of the Oulde and newe Testament faithfully and newly translated out of Douche and Latyn into Englishe, "wylde vyne" ' (= *Thomas Matthew,* 1537); (cf. Luther's *'Jona ausgelegt'*); *Geneva* (exile-protest.), 1562, translated according to the Ebreve and Greke, and conferred With the best translations in divers langages: ' "f gourde", f which was a further meanes to couer him frõ the heat of the sunne, as he remained in his boothe'; *AV,* 1611, repeats *Geneva* with footnote; *RV,* 1885: 'gourd', Or Palma Christi. Heb. kikayon; *RSV,* 1952: 'plant^b', '^{b}Heb. qiqayon, probably the castor oil plant'; *Jerusalem Bible,* 1966: 'castor-oil plant'; *NEB,* 1970; 'a climbing gourd^b', '^{b} a climbing gourd or a castor-oil plant'; cf. also Martin Luther (ed.) 1534: 'kŭrbis'; cf. *Praelectiones in prophetas minores, Jona,* in *Werke* (Weimar: Hermann Böhlaus Nachfolger, 1897), vol. 13, p. 239; and *Praefatio in Ionam prophetam,* vol. 13, p. 257; and *Der Prophet Jona ausgelegt,* vol. 19, p. 243, in which he gives the reasons for his choice.

77 E.M. Clowes, *On the Wallaby through Victoria,* London: Heinemann, 1911, p. 30.

78 *Select Works of Ephrem the Syrian,* trans. J.B. Morris in *A Library of Fathers,* Oxford: J.H. Pàrker, 1847, p. 412. ('Rhythm the Third Concerning the Faith', ch. 15). For the original, təlāyē dṭməlî ettalmad akqarēh dəyawnân habbeḇ (our transliteration) cf. *Corpus Scriptorum Christianorum Orientalium, Scriptores Syri,* vol. 88, *Des Heiligen Ephraem des Syrers Sermones de Fide,* ed. E. Beck, Louvain: Secrétariat du CorpusSCO, 1961, p. 46 (*Serm.* VI, 223-4).

79 Samuel Taylor Coleridge, *The Piccolomini: Or, The First Part of Wallenstein. A Drama. Translated from the German of Schiller* in *The Complete*

Poetical Works, ed. B.H. Coleridge, Oxford: Clarendon Press, 1912, vol. 2, p. 700 (act IV, sc. VII). 'Jonah's Gourd' is not mentioned in the original. Schiller's *übernächtig* ('ein übernächtiges/Geschöpf der Hofgunst'; *Wallensteins Tod*, erster Aufzug, siebenter Auftritt) led Coleridge's thoughts to the Jonah's Gourd as a suitable image of fast growth with which he could fill the line.

80 Edward Earl of Clarendon, *The History of the Rebellion and Civil Wars in England, Begun in the Year 1641. With the* etc., Oxford: At the Theater, 1702-4, vol. 3, book XV, p. 492.

81 *The Complete Writings of William Blake: With Variant Readings*, ed. Geoffrey Keynes, London: Oxford University Press, 1966; *Jerusalem: The Emanation of The Giant Albion*, 1804, printed by W. Blake Sth Molton St Written and etched 1804-20, plate 66, 11. 78-84.

82 William Styron, *Lie Down in Darkness*, London: Hamish Hamilton, 1952, p. 392. Cucurbits may naturally symbolize life that is to be destroyed. In *The Day of the Jackal*, a film made in 1973 about a man hired to assassinate General de Gaulle, the assassin uses a watermelon as target in his shooting practice with the special gun which he intends to use as the murder weapon. The watermelon symbolizes the life he wishes to destroy.

83 William J. Scheick, 'Discarded Watermelon Rinds: The Rainbow Aesthetic of Styron's *Lie Down in Darkness*', *Modern Fiction Studies*, vol. 24, no. 2, Summer 1978, pp. 247-54; 253-4.

84 Sembene Ousmane, *Les bouts de bois de Dieu*, Paris: Presses Pocket, 1971; first published 1960, pp. 193-4.

85 OUIDA (De la Ramée) *Pascarèl, Only a Story*, vol. 1, London: Chapman & Hall, 1873, p. 6. The idea here is also strongly cyclical, since the gourd in turn is used to depict the life of the King Carnival who reigns supreme for a while, is then killed as a scapegoat, but though his nations burn him every year, he 'rises from his ashes, and they cry All hail! to him the next' (pp. 4-5).

86 Life easily suggests its opposite, death, and thus we find various symbolic expressions of their interconnection (cucurbits and graves, etc.). Cf. also Albertus Magnus who, in his *De Vegetabilibus*, says: 'Repit (cucurbita) autem anchis sicut vitis, et crescit subito, ita quod Hermes dicit, quod si cucurbita in cinere ossium humanorum oleo olivae irrigato planteturin loco umbroso, infra novem dies habebit florem et germen': *De Vegetabilibus*, VI. 312.

87 John Gauden, *A Sermon Preached In the Temple-Chappel, at the Funeral of the Right Reverend Father in God, Dr. Brounrig*, etc., London: Andrew Crook, 1660, p. 72.

88 See for instance John Kenneth Galbraith, *Money: Whence It Came, Where It Went*, London: André Deutsch, 1975.

89 Wentworth and Flexner mention a case of 'cucumber' for dollar in 1935. Vegetable or plant words for money are common in slang.

In John Vandercook's *Black Majesty* (the life of Christophe, king of Haiti) an anecdotal explanation is given:

> After the destruction of the plantations and the abolition of slavery, the black cultivators of Haiti had grown more and more dependent on wild produce. Their huts were made of mud and sticks and palm leaves. Food grew wild or with little urging. For utensils, bowls, spoons, and bottles, the blacks made use of the fruit of the gourd vine, dried in the sun, scraped clean of seeds, then cut into the requisite shapes. If there was such a thing as an irreplaceable necessity in the careless life of the peasants, it was the gourd, Christophe mused. Gourds were useful, but they soon wore out.
>
> Chief Christophe issued an arbitrary act which declared every green gourd in northern Haiti the property of the state. A new crop was just ripening and soldiers were sent to every commune to collect it. The peasants made no objection. Christophe was their master now and whatever he did was right.
>
> Gourd vines grew over many garden walls. Others had flung a rank, concealing tangle over the ruins of houses burned by Boukmann's rebels sixteen years before. Another sort grew on prim, round-headed little trees. Without regard for quality or ownership, Christophe's messengers took them all and a great procession of laden burros and high-piled farm carts brought them into Cap Haïtien. Before long 227,000 green gourds and calabashes were deposited in 'The Treasury'. Christophe put a value of twenty sous on each.
>
> The coffee crop was almost ripe. When the cultivators brought the dried berries into the capital, Christophe bought them at the current market rate and paid out his gourds, which by this time the peasants needed badly. Then he resold the coffee to European merchants for gold. Before the year was out the state of Haiti had a metal currency of absolute stability in circulation. To this day the standard coin of Haiti is called the *gourde*.

New York and London: Harper & Brothers, 1928, pp. 108-9: Whether or not there is any factual foundation for this anecdote does not really matter in our inquiry. True or not, the story testifies to the role of cucurbits in symbolizing riches. If the story is true the king's behaviour took account of symbolic appropriateness. If, again, it is fiction, then the inventors of the story did so.

90 According to the *Guinness Book of Records*, Colin Bowcock, of Willaston, Merseyside, is the current United Kingdom champion pumpkin grower, with a fruit of 209 lb 4 oz (94.913 kg) in 1976 (see plate XI). But a squash of 513 lb (232.69 kg) was grown by Harold Fulp, Jr, at Ninevah, Indiana, USA in 1977. Notable is also the watermelon weighing 197 lb (83.3 kg) grown by Ed Weeks of Tarboro, North Carolina, in 1975 (see plate XI). *Guinnes Book of Records*, 25th ed., ed. Norris McWhirter, Enfield: Guinness Superlatives, 1978, pp. 54-7. Gourds weighing more than 80 kilos and marrows weighing nearly 30 kilos also seem to figure in the records.

91 Athenaeus, III. 73e.

92 Cf. *Odyssey*, XI.576.

93 A further ramification of this is that cucurbits become symbolically appropriate as an ingredient or a tool in cures and remedies for swellings, cf. Organ, op. cit., pp. 64–5: 'Large fruits are also used as a poultice to the swollen leg of elephants, both treatments, of course, being homeopathic magic – the contact of a swollen fruit with a swollen body, such beliefs being common among primitive peoples.' Alternatively, of course, they are also appropriate in cures aimed at *introducing* a swelling; thus their use as a drug against barrenness, to introduce the swelling of pregnancy, is very widespread.

94 On enormous cucurbits and flood stories, cf. the relevant entries in Thompson, particularly A1029.4: *Flood: refuge in huge gourds* with seven rooms in each. India: Thompson-Balys.

95 In a curious twist of development the saying 'cool as a cucumber' can be used as a comparison describing almost itself as it were, at least in James Joyce: 'A nice salad, cool as a cucumber', *Ulysses*, New York: Random House, 1934, p. 169.

96 *The Complete Short Stories & Sketches by Stephen Crane,* ed. and introd. Thomas A. Gullason, Garden City, New York: Doubleday & Co., 1963, p. 505.

97 *The Rogve: or The Life of Guzman de Alfarache.* Written in Spanish by Matheo Aleman, Seruant to his Catholicke Maiestie, and borne in Sevill, London: printed for Edward Blount, 1622, Part Second, p. 59. Naturally it is significant that the subject is love (connection cucurbits–women–love).

Cf. Spanish, 'El melon y el casamiento ha de ser acertamiento' – choose a wife and a melon with great care.

98 John Galt, *Lawrie Todd; or, The Settlers in the Woods,* vol. 1, London: Henry Colburn and Richard Bentley, 1830, p. 90.

Apparently this was a Yankee cliché at the time; cf. Haliburton's *The Clockmaker; or The Sayings and Doings of Samuel Slick, of Slickville,* third series, London: Richard Bentley, 1840, p. 286. 'if that bean't pitikilar I am a punkin, and the pigs may do their prettiest with me. Didn't I tell you, Sam, nothin' could come up to a woman?'

Pumpkins, in New England, were also pig food, and this is another reason why pigs and pumpkins co-occur – in addition to the low symbolic value of both pigs and pumpkins – and the convenient alliteration; cf. John Palmer, *Journal of Travels in the United States of North America and in Lower Canada, Performed in the year 1817; containing* etc., London: Sherwood, Neely, and Jones 1818, p. 241.

99 Pasquale Villari, *The Life and Times of Niccolo Macciavelli,* trans. Linda Villari, new ed., vol. 2, London: T. Fisher Unwin, 1842, pp. 255–6.

100 Aristophanes, *Nubes*, 327.

101 The etymological connection between head, gourd, pot, etc. is labyrinthical but undoubtedly traceable; cf. Fr. 'tête', Lat. 'testa', Eng. 'crackpot', etc.
   On the connection between cucurbits and head, see also Thompson, Q551.3.3.1. *Punishment: melon in murderer's hand turns to murdered man's head*, Africa (Fulah): Equilbecq II. 205ff. no. 43.
   Of the numerous connections between head and cucurbits note for instance the use of gourds, as material for trepanning, in the skull surgery of South American Indian tribes (cf. Organ, op.cit., pp. 38–9). The material is suitable in every respect, also symbolically. Another case is that of head-hunters in southern Colombia using gourds as a tool when shrinking the heads of their enemies (cf. Organ, p. 42).

102 For an example of 'pumpkin-head' simply referring to size, see Israel Zangwill, *Children of the Ghetto*, London: White Lion Publishers, 1972, first published by William Heinemann in 1892, p. 30: '. . . (different sorts of children); with great pumpkin-heads, with oval heads, with pear-shaped heads; . . .'

103 Hermann Fischer, *Schwäbisches Wörterbuch*, Tübingen: Verlag der H. Laupp 'schen Buchhandlung, 1901.

104 David Lodge, *Language of Fiction: Essays in Criticism and Verbal Analysis of the English Novel*, London: Routledge and Kegan Paul, 1966, pp. 196 and *passim*.

105 On pumpkin-seeds see also Haliburton's *Clockmaker*. When the Yankee pedlar has just cheated a customer, he expresses his satisfaction thus: 'The next time you tell stories about Yankee pedlars, put the wooden clock in with the wooden punkin seeds, and Hickory hams, will you?' (p. 167). There is considerable antagonism in the book between the Yankee and the 'blue-noses' of Nova Scotia. *The Clockmaker; or, The Sayings and Doings of Samuel Slick, of Slickville*, Philadelphia, Lea & Blanchard, 1839.

106 Cf. H. Mrose in *Berliner philologischen Wochenschrift*, no. 12, 1914, p. 383. The connection between head and cucurbit is put to specialized use in southern France, where the saying 'to have a head like a *coucourbe*' means to have a headache.

107 P.G. Wodehouse, *Joy in the Morning*, London: Barrie & Jenkins, 1974, p. 9. See also p. 20 ('pumpkin-shaped head'). As is to be expected with a humorist, Wodehouse makes much of cucurbits in most of his books.

108 Cf. also 'stupidity', It. 'melonaggine'; and 'stupid talk', 'nonsense', mod. Gk. 'κολοκύθια' (pl. of 'τὸ κολοκύθι'). In American English Wentworth and Flexner give both 'gourd' and 'calabash' for head, but add that 'calabash' is obsolete.
   Cf. also Sp. 'no dársele a uno un pepino' = 'not to give a straw for something'; 'dar calabazas' = 'fail an exam'.

109 Denis Hills, op. cit., p. 92.

110 Athenaeus, II. 59c (Hermippus 79); Kock, *Comicorum Atticorum Fragmenta* vol. 1, p. 240; Plutarch, *Pericles*, 3.2, and Birt, *Rhèinisches Museum*, 46, 1891, p. 152.

111 Apuleius, *Met.* I.15; cf. Alexander Scobie, *Apuleii Metamorphoses: A Commentary*, Meisenheim am Glan: Verlag Anton Hain, 1975, p. 112; cf. also A. Otto, *Die Sprichwörter der Römer*, Leipzig: Teubner, 1890, p. 100.

112 F.A. Todd in *Classical Quarterly*, 1943, pp. 101-11; cf. below note on Petronius, *Satyricon*, 39.

113 Cf. Donatello's famous statue *Il Zuccone*, in e.g. H.W. Janson, *The Sculpture of Donatello*, Princeton: University Press, 1963, plate 15d.

114 Sir Samuel W. Baker, *The Nile Tributaries of Abyssinia: And the Sword Hunters of the Hamran Arabs*, London: Macmillan, 1867, p. 208.

115 Tertullianus, *De Anima*, 32:1; cf. J.H. Waszink, *Tertulliani De Anima*, Amsterdam: Meulenhoff, 1947, p. 385.

116 Tertullianus, *Adversus Marcionem*, IV.40.3; cf. A. Sonny, in *Archiv für Lateinische Lexicographie*, vol. 9, ed. E. Wölfflin, Leipzig: B.G. Teubner, 1898, p. 58.

117 In Chaucer's *The Canon's Yeoman's Tale*, 1. 794, for instance, *The Works of Geoffrey Chaucer*, ed. F.N. Robinson, 2nd edn, London: Oxford University Press, 1957, p. 216, 'cucurbites' are used as a name for laboratory vessels.

118 *Maison Rustique: or The Countrie Farme* etc., comp. Charles Steuens and John Liebault, trans. Richard Svrflet, London: Bouham Norton, 1600, p. 565. See also pp. 245-53 on cucumbers, gourds, melons and pompions; their uses, advice for growing and special observations. What the authors cite is still mostly ancient lore as, e.g., the following: 'A woman having her termes and walking by the borders of pompions, gourds, and cucumbers, causeth them to drie and die: but and if any of the fruite escape, it will be bitter' (p. 252). Though much of the advice is based on superstition and has only a symbolic role and no basis in reality, some of it is highly sophisticated, such as crop rotation (which is very important in this vegetable family, which is prone to root diseases), and drip irrigation.

119 The *Hermit in London; or Sketches of English Manners*, London: printed for Henry Colburn, 1819, vol. 3, p. 170; cf. p. 169; 'Mrs. - too is very corpulent, ...' and p. 170,

> Wheeling round, she had the trundle and rotundity of a well-hooped porter cask; and from betwixt her brawny shoulders issued a bump, which threw off her robe above the elbow, and so enlarged the circle around her, that no one would either wish or endeavour to circumvent or to circumvolate this tower of frippery.

NOTES TO PAGES 41-3

It is interesting to note how often unpleasant words occurring in passages where cucurbits are used derogatorily have the sound combination 'mp': qui*mp*e, bu*mp*, and, elsewhere in this study, lu*mp*. Since this sound combination is intrinsically unpleasant or funny in English, this opens up some interesting perspectives on the relation between these words and the word pu*mp*kin.

For one type of study in phonosemic correlations relevant in this context see Roger W. Wescott, 'Labio-Velarity and Derogation in English: A Study in Phonosemic Correlation', *American Speech*, vol. 46, nos. 1-2, Spring-Summer 1971, pp. 123-37, particularly p. 126, types four and three in the table. See also Part 2, Chapter Three.

120 Wentworth and Flexner list *melon-belly*, 'a man with a protuberant abdomen', though they add that the expression is not common.

121 *Salmagundi: or, The Whim-Whams and Opinions of Launcelot Langstaff, Esq and others* etc., vol. 1, London: J.M. Richardson, 1811, p. 102. Note Tucky's cucurbitic surname. The passage is violently anti-Negro. Cucurbit humour occurs frequently throughout *The Salmagundi Papers*.

122 Robert B. Todd (ed.), *The Cyclopaedia of Anatomy and Physiology*, London: Longman, Brown, Green, Longmans & Roberts, 1849-52, vol. 4, part 2, p. 1332, c. 1.

123 Athenaeus, II.68c and d.

124 George W. Harris, *Sut Lovingood. Yarns spun by a nat'ral born durn'd fool. Warped and Wove for public Wear*, New York: Dick & Fitzgerald, 1867, 'Blown up with Soda', p. 76.

125 Jerome K. Jerome, *Novel Notes*, London: The Leadenhall Press, 1893, p. 24. For a connection between an absurd activity – snoring – and cucurbits, see Wentworth and Flexner, who report that 'to saw gourds' once meant 'to snore' in American slang.

126 There is a close connection between poetry and magic since poetry in many cultures serves magic purposes. Thus, if pumpkin and magic are connected, pumpkin and poetry will also be, and consequently a modern compiler and editor calls his anthology of translated Red Indian poetry 'Shaking the Pumpkin', after a Senecan saying. Jerome Rothenberg, *Shaking the Pumpkin: Traditional Poetry of the Indian North Americas*, Garden City: Doubleday 1972. In this book see also p. 232 for sacred melons of the raingods; pp. 376-7 for big-bellied pumpkin; p. 385 for a Maya riddle ('Son, where it the old woman with buttocks seven palms wide, the woman with a dark complexion? It is a certain kind of squash') and for a variety of cucurbitic material, *passim*.

As to the pumpkin masks, it can be noted that cucurbitic masks have been very common among many tribes (see e.g. Organ, op.cit., p. 65, illustration no. 14 and *passim*). There is a persistent connection between magic and cucurbits.

It may be that another persistent connection, namely that between cucurbits and gambling (see e.g. Organ, op.cit., *passim*) is somehow related – the wheel of fortune and the cycle of life and death (life a gamble?) being perceived as similar.

127 Philip Thomson, *The Grotesque,* in *The Critical Idiom,* general ed. John D. Jump, vol. 24, London: Methuen, 1972, p. 28.

128 'The Courtship of the Yonghy-Bonghy-Bò', *The Complete Nonsense of Edward Lear,* ed. and introd. Holbrook Jackson, London: Faber and Faber, 1947, p. 237. Originally published as *Laughable Lyrics: A Fourth Book of Nonsense Poems, Songs, Botany, Music &c.,* 1877.

In the type of nonsense humour that children like (or at least are supposed to like) cucurbits predictably occur. A compiler of a recent book of this kind puts cucurbits into the very title of his book: *The Six-Million-Dollar Cucumber: A Bookful of zany Riddles about Birds and Beasts and Vegetables,* comp. E. Richard Churchill, London: Piccolo Pan Books, 1976. The riddle from which the title is derived is found on p. 71: 'What is green, has one bionic eye, and fights crime? The Six-Million-Dollar Cucumber'; see pp. 72 and 75 for further cucurbitic riddles.

In passing it can be noted that the title links cucurbits and money, adding yet another example to the cases in which cucumbers symbolize riches. Green paper dollar-notes occur together with a cucumber in the illustration on the cover. In fact there are many secondary cucurbitic connotations: prowess, magic, absurdity (link with physical deformity – humour in the reference to one artificial eye), etc.

129 P.G. Wodehouse, *Right Ho, Jeeves,* London: Herbert Jenkins, 1934, p. 251.

130 *The Correspondence of William Cowper,* ed. Thomas Wright, London: Hodder and Stoughton, 1904, 'Letter to Joseph Hill, Jan. 31, 1782,' vol. 1, p. 435. Cf. also the connection between lack of subjects and cucumbers in the expression 'cucumber-time' (see below).

The absolute insignificance of Cowper's life, as symbolized by the cucumber, is in turn taken up by C.S. Lewis, who was fascinated by it. Cf. Anne Arnott, *The Secret Country of C.S. Lewis,* London: Hodder and Stoughton, 1974, p. 89:

> Everything he read was significant to him. For example, because he found even the small details of life of interest, he records that the letters of the poet Cowper fascinate him, and this is because,
> > he had nothing – literally nothing – to tell anyone about; private life in a sleepy country town where Evangelical distrust of 'the world' denied him even such miserable society as the place would have afforded. And yet one reads a whole volume of his letters with unfailing interest. How his tooth came loose at dinner, how he made a hutch for a tame hare, what he is doing about his cucumbers – all this he makes one follow as if the fate of empires hung on it . . . .
>
> Because he too had this talent for seeing interest and significance in the

smallest things of life, his letters of this period are memorable. You could say he lived through each little event in his life with lively awareness. Nothing was unimportant.

The utterly ridiculous worthlessness of cucumbers is well expressed in the following famous cucumber-passage in Boswell: *The Journal of A Tour to the Hebrides with Samuel Johnson, Ll.D. by James Boswell, Esq.*, annot. Hester Lynch Thrale Piozzi, Bloomfield: Limited Editions Club, 1974, p. 212:

> By the by, Dr. Johnson told me, that Gay's line in the *Beggar's Opera*, 'As men should serve a cucumber,' &c. has no waggish meaning, with reference to men flinging away cucumbers as too *cooling*, which some have thought; for it has been a common saying of physicians in England, that a cucumber should be well sliced, and dressed with pepper and vinegar, and then thrown out, as good for nothing. – ' (Tuesday, 5th October).

131 *The Poetical Works of Robert Browning*, London: Smith, Elder & Co., 1897, vol. 2, pp. 658-9.

In Joseph Conrad's *Nostromo: A Tale of the Seaboard*, London: Dent, 1972, pp. 256-7, the woman who has 'adopted' the protagonist reproaches him, on her deathbed, because he only thinks of his reputation with others and does not see to it that he gets anything for himself. He remonstrates:

> Is it my fault that I am the only man for their purposes? What angry nonsense are you talking, mother? Would you rather have me timid and foolish, selling water-melons on the market-place or rowing a boat for passengers along the harbour, like a soft Neapolitan without courage or reputation?

Watermelons are used as a symbol of degradation or degeneration.

132 Whittier, op.cit., p. 157.

133 On pumpkins and carriages, see Thompson, D451.3.3 *Transformation: pumpkin to carriage*, Type 410, – Breton: Sébillot Incidents s.v. 'carousse'; Missouri French; Carrière; also F861.4.3, *Carriage from pumpkin*, Type 510 (Perrault's version).

134 Nathaniel Hawthorne, *The Scarlet Letter: A Romance*, introd. Douglas Grant, London: Oxford University Press, 1965, p. 96.

135 In Dickens's *Hard Times* the phoney self-made man Mr Bounderby, who always makes much of his supposedly humble origin, ostentatiously grows cabbages in the front garden of his fancy house. Dickens obviously disliked the excesses in the myth of the self-made man, a myth reinforced at this time by such books as Samuel Smiles's *Self-Help*, and wished to reduce this type of inverted snobbery to the absurd with Bounderby's act of showy cabbage symbolism.

136 Whittier, op.cit., p. 157.

137 Cf. Palmer, op.cit.; 'one or two dishes are peculiar to New England, and always on the table, toast dipped in cream and *pumpkin pie*' (p. 241).

138 Foote, 'Mayor of Garratt' in William Hone, *The Every-Day Book* etc., vol. 2, part 2, London: William Hone, 1827, c. 848.

139 Cf. Mrose, loc. cit. ref. to El-Correi, *Westermanns Monatschrift* 115.754. Thus cucurbits are also connected with inertia ('phlegmatisch'). Artemidorus states that inert people are called watermelons; Albert the Great: 'Est autem mala cucurbita melancholicis et phlegmaticis, et bona cholericis.' One is supposed to eat food with qualities opposite to those of one's own temperament (Artemidorus Daldianus, 1, 67; Albertus Magnus, *De Vegetabilibus*, VI.313).

140 Haliburton, *The Clockmaker*, 2nd series (Bentley), p. 153. The context is ironically humorous, pp. 139-40:
> Says I, I wish they had ahanged you, with all my heart; it's such critters as you that lower the national character of our free and enlightened citizens, and degrade it in the eyes of foreigners. The eyes of foreigners be d———! said he. Who cares what they think? – and as for these bluenoses, they ain't able to think. They ain't got two ideas to bless themselves with – the stupid, punkin-headed, consaited blockheads! – cuss me if they have. Well, says I, they ain't such an enlightened people as we are, that's sartain, but that don't justify you a bit; you hadn't ought to have stolen that watch. That was wrong, very wrong indeed. You might have traded with him, and got it for half nothin'; or bought it and failed, as some of our importin' marchants sew up the soft-horned British; or swapped it and forgot to give the exchange; or bought it and give your note, and cut stick afore the note became due. There's a thousand ways of doin' it honestly and legally, without resortin', as foreigners do, to stealing. We are a moral people, . . .

141 Washington Irving, *Rip Van Winkle and The Legend of Sleepy Hollow*, Philadelphia: Lippincott, 1923, pp. 73-148.
For an example enumerating some of the central characteristics of pumpkin, see Haliburton's *The Clockmaker*, 3rd series, (Bentley), pp. 153-4:
> No, says I, I'd be sure to lose, for I am the poorest shot in the world – Poorest shote, said he, you mean, for you have no soul in you. I believe you have fed on pumkins so long in Conne'ticut, you are jist about as soft, and as holler, and good-for-nothin', as they be: what ails you? You hante got no soul in you, man, at all.

142 *Tales by Nathaniel Hawthorne*, ed. Carl Van Doren, London: Oxford University Press, 1921, p. 133. In this connection, cf. Ital. 'zucconare', 'cut the hair very short.'

143 *A General History of Connecticut, From Its First Settlement* etc. 2nd ed., London, 1782, pp. 195-6. Among the advantages that the author lists is that those who have had their ears cut off as a punishment could not hide their shame.

144 Like cucurbitic words of abuse in general. 'Pumpkin-head' apparently came

so easily to mind in the seventeenth century that in T. Walkington's *The Optick Glasse of Hvmors: or The touchstone of a golden temperature* etc. (London: T.C. for Leonard Becket, 1614?), the English has 'pumpion headed' even though the Latin does not really warrant this translation (pp. 125–6):

> AErumnosique Solones/Obstipo capite & figentes lumine terram,/ Murmura cum secū & rabiosa silentia rodūt;/Atque exporrecto trutinantur verba labello:/AEgroti Veteris meditantes somnia gigni/De nihilo nihil, in nihilum nil posse reverti/" (Like pumpion headed Solonists they looke/The dull earth is their contemplation booke:/ They madly murmure in themselves for routh,/They heaue their words with leavers frō their mouth:/They musing dreā on th' antick axiome/ Nought's fram'd of nought, to nought ne ought may come.

The comment of course is on melancholy men. Though the translation of Persius, *Sat.* III.77, is wrong, the new expression 'pumpion headed Solonists', with its taste of oxymoron, may be thought better than the original.

145 Nathaniel Ward, *The Simple Cobler of Aggawam in America*, ed. P.M. Zall, Lincoln: University of Nebraska Press, 1969, p. 30.

146 *Tales by Nathaniel Hawthorne*, pp. 429–30: 'Get thee gone, my pretty pet, my darling, my precious one, my treasure; and if any ask thy name, it is Feathertop. For thou hast a feather in thy hat, and I have thrust a handful of feathers into the hollow of thy head, and thy wig too is of the fashion they call Feathertop, – so be Feathertop thy name!'

147 If you wish to give an idea of ridiculous softness, pumpkin pie is doubly appropriate, and triply appropriate if, as in the following example from Haliburton, a Yankee is speaking: 'As for a John Bull, or a Blue-nose, I never seed one yet that I couldn't walk right into like a pumpkin-pie. They are as soft as dough, them fellers' (*The Clockmaker*, 3rd series, Bentley, p. 182). See also p..252: 'He is as soft as dough, that chap, and your eyes are so keen they will cut right into him, like a carvin'-knife into a punkin' pie.'

148 On the tendency of similar symbolic elements to cluster, cf. also Thompson J2311.1.3.1, *Numskull believes he is dead when pumpkin falls on his head*. India: Thompson-Balys; also J2013.3, *A numskull ties a pumpkin to his leg at night so he shall know himself in the morning. Someone ties the pumpkin to another's leg and the numskull is not sure of his identity next morning* (Clouston Noodles 7); cf. also J1813.3, *Boiling pumpkin thought to be talking*. India: Thompson-Balys; also, for pumpkins involved in stories where one absurdity rebukes another, Thompson J1531.1. *The transformed golden pumpkin*. Borrower of golden pumpkin returns a brass pumpkin and claims that the gold has turned to brass. The lender takes the borrower's son and returns with an ape. He claims that the boy has turned into an ape. Köhler-Bolte I.533; India: Thompson-Balys.

149 Athenaeus, II. 59d.

150 Cf. Rudolf Helm, *Lucian und Menipp*, Leipzig/Berlin: B. G. Teubner, 1906, p. 378.

151 For a similar story ridiculing a man who questions the wisdom of nature's arrangements, see Thompson, J2571, 'Thank Fortune it wasn't a melon'. Man contends that melons should not grow on slender vines but on tall trees. He is hit on the nose by a falling nut. Is thankful it wasn't a melon. Italian Novella: Rotunda.

152 Charles Dickens, *The Mudfog Papers*, London: Richard Bentley & Son, 1880, 'Report of the Second Meeting of the Mudfog Association', pp. 114–15.

153 ibid., pp. 126–8.

154 Interpres Irenaei, *Adversus haereses*, I.11.4 (*Patrologia Graeca* VII, c. 567).

155 Interpres Irenaei, *Adversus haereses*, I.11.4.

156 S. Irenaeus, *Adversus Haereses*, ed. W.W. Harvey, Cantabrigiae: Typis Academicis, 1857, vol. 1, I.5.2-3.

157 The interpreter of dreams, Artemidorus Daldianus, in his *Onirocriticon* also understands the poetic adjective as a substantive, the fruit: 'πέπον γὰρ τὸ προςφιλέστατον οἱ ποιηταὶ καλοῦσι' (Artemidorus I.67).

158 *Pall Mall Gazette*, 4 September 1865, 16/2.

159 Otto Weinrich, *Senecas Apocolocynthosis*, Berlin: Weidmann, 1923, pp. 11-12.

160 Augustine, *De Moribus Manichaeorum*, II.16.39, *Patrología Latina*, XXXII, c. 1362.

161 Angelo de Gubernatis, *La Mythologie des Plantes*, Paris: C. Reinwald et Cie, Libraires Editeurs, 1878, vol. 2, p. 223.

162 ibid., p. 106.

163 Cf. Bächthold-Stäbli, *Handwörterbuch des deutschen Aberglaubens*, Berlin/Leipzig: Walter de Gruyter, 1932/3, vol. 5, c. 839.

164 Juvenal, *Satirae*, VI.365 (O_{4-6}); cf. F. Bücheler, *Rheinisches Museum*, 54, 1899, p. 486; M. Maas, *Archiv für lateinische Lexicographie* 11, 1900, p. 419; J.P. Postgate in *Classical Review*, 13, 1899, p. 206; and F. Leo in *Hermes*, 44, 1909, p. 600.

165 Procopius, *Anecdota*, 9.37; cf. Th. Birt, *Rheinisches Museum*, 46, 1891, p. 152.

166 One aspect of the connection between cucurbits and sex is their use as a contraceptive, a use that has a very long history. For the occurrences of σικύη and κολοκυνθίς in this connection in antiquity, cf. E. Littré (ed. and trans.), *Oevres completes d'Hippocrate*, Paris: J.B. Baillière et Fils, 1861,

vol. 10, p. 543 ('Courges'). A reason for choosing the cucurbit for this use may be its suitability for the purpose, but also one can make the general observation that whatever direction a use, a moral of a tale, semiotic subcategories of meaning, etc., may take, all these cluster round a common kernel, which stays the same – sex.

That cucurbits should have both bad and good semiotic value is thus no surprise. The basis stays the same so that even when they are denounced as the devil's plants in some texts, the author presumably recognizes the sex symbolism; it is just the attitude of the writer that varies.

Though cucurbitic fertility symbolism often refers specifically to femaleness (as fertility symbolism in general often tends to do since it is the women who give birth to children), this does not prevent such traditions as that of Greece and Roumania where pumpkin-seeds are eaten for virility. In Sembene Ousmane's *Les bouts de bois de Dieu* a conservative elderly woman severely criticizes the younger women for not making sure that the men eat and drink out of calabashes. Eating from plates will surely destroy their virility: 'Niakoro-la-vieille ne pouvait pas passer un aprèsmidi inactive. Tantôt elle ravaudait, tantôt elle réparait ou ornait des calebasses. "Je n'arriverai jamais à comprendre votre manque de goût, disait-elle aux autres femmes. Pourquoi ne vous souciez-vous pas de décorer vos ustensiles? Ne savez-vous donc pas que vos plats en fer affaiblissent la virilité des hommes?" ' (p. 17).

Similarly in Rwanda, Willfried van Eyen has found (personal communication) that the ceremonial drink of banana cider is always drunk out of a gourd. Drinking is an essential part of social life in Kinyarwandan culture. Whereas sorghum beer or Primus beer can be drunk out of jars or glasses, banana cider, which is traditionally a male drink, never given to women, is always drunk out of a gourd.

In this connection cf. also Jean Chevalier/Alain Gheerbrant, *Dictionnaire des symboles*, Paris: Robert Laffont, 1969, p. 248, for comments on the ambiguity of 'courge' as a symbol.

167 Plautus, *Casina*, 907–13.

168 For a connection between cucurbits and procreation see Matheo Aleman, *The Rogue: Or the life of Guzman de Alfarache*, trans. James Mabbe, introd. James Fitzmaurice-Kelly, vol. 1, London: Constable, 1924, p. 85: 'I call my selfe his sonne, and so I take my selfe to be: since that from that Mellon-bed* I was made legitimate by the holy right of Matrimony.' (Footnote: *'Agreeing with the phrase which we use to little children when we tell them that they were borne in their mothers Parsley-bed.') The custom of telling children that they come from a melon-patch seems to exist elsewhere too, e.g. in Israel.

For a connection cucurbit–birth and cucurbit–marriage, see Thompson T555.1.1. *Woman gives birth to pumpkin.* Chinese: Eberhard FFC CXX.77 and T555.2. *Queen gives birth to a gourd.* India: Thompson-Balys; cf. also T117.7 *Marriage to a gourd.* India: Thompson-Balys.

Another connection between cucurbits and sex is the occurrence of cucurbits in pregnancy tests in folk-medicine. In the Berlin papyrus, according to Laurent-Täckholm (p. 154), a woman (in ancient Egypt) is recommended to swallow a dose of watermelon mixed with milk from a woman who has given birth to a male child. If she throws up it is a sign of pregnancy. Cf. Hippocrates, *De Sterilibus*.

169 I, 1-13; Ricks, pp. 718-19.

170 *The Complete Poetical Works of James Whitcomb Riley*, pref. Donald Culross Peattie, Garden City, N.Y: Garden City Publishing Co., 1941, p. 254 (the whole poem 254-5).

171 John Updike, *Couples*, Harmondsworth: Penguin, 1971 (first pub. 1968), p. 166.

172 Robert Bridges, *Eight Plays, Nero, Parts I. & II. Palicio. Ulysses. Captives. Achilles. Humours. Feast of Bacchus* London: Bell J. and E. Bumpus, 1885 (?), p. 8.

173 Charles Merivale, *A History of The Romans under the Empire*, vol. 5, London: Longmans, 1856, p. 601.

174 *Athenaeum*, 8 July 1899, 71/3.

175 *The Spectator*, 15 October 1904, 559.1.

176 *Saturday Review*, 6 December 1884, 721/1.

177 Henry F. Chorley, *Memorials of Mrs. Hemans: With Illustrations of Her Literary Character from her Private Correspondence*, vol. 2, London: Saunders and Otley, 1836, p. 20.

178 *The Poems of Stephen Crane*, A Critical Edition, ed. Joseph Katz, New York: Cooper Square, 1971, p. 93.

179 J.W. Goethe, *Claudine von Villa Bella*, Act One, in *Werke*, Stuttgart/ Tübingen: J.G. Cotta'schen Buchhandlung, 1828, vol. 10, p. 224.

180 Dio Cassius, *Roman History*, LXIX.4.2.

181 Athenaeus, VI.257a.

182 *Rule a Wife, and have a Wife*, in *The Works of Francis Beaumont and John Fletcher*, Cambridge English Classics, vol. 3, act I, sc. I, p. 178.

183 *The Custom of the country*, in *Works of Beaumont and Fletcher*, vol. 1, act I, sc. 1, p. 316. Apart from abuse there is a link to lechery here in that the subject is sex, or, more precisely, the right of the seigneur.

184 John Hacket, *Scrinia Reserata: A Memorial Offer'd to the Great Deservings of John Williams, D.D. Who some time held the Places of* etc., London: Edw. Jones for Samuel Lowndes, 1693, Part I, p. 120.

185 *The Arden Edition of the Works of William Shakespeare: The Merry Wives of Windsor*, ed. H.J. Oliver, London: Methuen, 1971, p. 81, act III, sc. III,

35-6). 'Pumpion' occurs only once in Shakespeare, but then it is well applied. Falstaff is not only ridiculous, fat and absurd, but also a heavy drinker (connection to 'watery' and humidity). It seems that the only other cucurbit in Shakespeare is gourd, used in the meaning 'hollow dice', also in *The Merry Wives of Windsor*, I.iii, 84-5: (*The Riverside Shakespeare*, textual ed. G. Blakemore Evans, gen. introd. Harry Levin, Herschel Baker, Anne Barton, Frank Kermode, Hallett Smith, Marie Edel; essay on stage history Charles H. Shattuck, Boston: Houghton Mifflin, 1974):

>   *Pist.* Let vultures gripe thy guts! for
>   gourd and fullam holds,

Though the reference here apparently is to dice, nevertheless this idea may, by association, have grown out of the reference to Falstaff's belly which has again been the subject (p. 295, 58-62):

>   *Fal.*   I have writ me here a letter to her; and here another to Page's
>   wife, who even now gave me good eyes too, examin'd my
>   parts with most judicious iliads; sometimes the beam of her
>   view gilded my foot, sometimes my portly belly.
>   *Pist.* Then did the sun on dunghill shine.

There is of course another occurrence of 'pumpion' in Shakespeare if we count the passages in *Sir Thomas More* that are attributed to Shakespeare. In the relevant scene, the mob is about to stage a massacre of the foreigners in London. One argument in the scene – which, as Evans (following Chambers) notes, presents a strange mixture of humour and savagery – is that the foreigners introduce alien food and plants that can only be harmful. (Evans's modern version, p. 1687; cf. also pp. 1686 and 1698):

>   *Lincoln.*   They bring in strange roots, which is merely to the undoing
>   of poor prentices, for what's a sorry parsnip to a good heart?
>   *Williamson.* Trash, trash; they breed sore eyes and 'tis enough to infect
>   the city with the palsy.
>   *Lincoln.*   Nay, it has infected it with the palsy, for these bastards of
>   dung – as you know they grow in dung – have infected us, and
>   it is our infection will make the city shake, which partly comes
>   through the eating of parsnips.
>   *Clown.*   True, and pumpions together.

Evans comments (p. 1687):

> The concerted attack on the parsnip (and 'pumpion') which follows seems to be a purely comic ploy to make the 'reasons' of the commons appear even more absurd. In the first place, parsnips were not "straign (foreign) rootes"; in the second place, John Gerard in his *Herbal* (1597, p. 811) finds many virtues in the cultivated garden parsnip ("good for the stomache, kidneies, bladder and lungs"), though he admits it is "Somwhat windie". D's substitution of "a sorry" for "a watrie" is interesting, since parsnips were not according to Gerard, particularly watery. Also ('pumpions') pumpkins. Gerard also gives a good bill of health to pumpkins.

Evans's initial observation that the vegetable passage is meant to make the reasons of the mob absurd is obviously correct. But a couple of additional comments can be made. The argument that the plants engender evil humours, although absurd, is not totally without foundation, because the evidence on this point is contradictory. Though Gerard gives pumpkins a good bill of health, there were others who did not, cf. e.g. Boorde's dietary from the middle of the century.

The main point about the plants, however, is that they are comic; pumpkins are definitely and parsnips vaguely funny. The change from 'a watrie' to 'a sorry' parsnip is interesting. Could it be possible that when Shakespeare (?) wrote Lincoln's remark about strange roots he already had in mind the idea of using pumpkins to make the scene absurd? The prime association of 'pumpkin' for Shakespeare, as we know from the example in *The Merry Wives,* was to wateriness. Could it be that having already put down 'watrie', intending to go on with 'pumpion', the author got the idea of improving on the scene by having a milder lead-in of parsnips and saving pumpkins for the punch-line, and having the pumpkin punch-line spoken by the clown rather than by Lincoln which is far more appropriate? The only thing that speaks against this theory is the word 'rootes' at the beginning of Lincoln's remark.

186 Though not always. Since cucurbits are latently ridiculous, even the act of drinking out of a bottle may be regarded as humorous since bottles are made of gourds. In the *Towneley Plays* it is explicitly spelled out that 'It is an old by-worde,/It is a good bowrde, for to drynk of a gowrde, . . .' *The Towneley Plays,* ed. George England, side-notes and introd. Alfred W. Pollard. Early English Text Society, Extra Series, no. 71, 1897, London: Kegan Paul, Trench, Trübner, 1897, p. 115 (XII, 54, 481-3).

In Chaucer's *The Manciple's Prologue,* ed. F.N. Robinson, where 'bourde' is also rhymed with 'gourde', a draught of wine from a gourd is offered as a rite of reconciliation after a misunderstanding, which is now explained as having arisen from a jest: pp. 224-5.

187 Though for an example of a complex of heat, thirst, humour and cucurbits, see 'The Shamrock and the Palm,' ch. 10 in O. Henry, *Cabbages and Kings,* New York: McClure, Phillips, 1904, pp. 177-8:

> Johnny Atwood lay stretched upon the grass in the undress uniform of a Carib, and prated feebly of cool water to be had in the cucumber-wood pumps of Dalesburg. Dr. Gregg, through the prestige of his whiskers and as a bribe against the relation of his imminent professional tales, was conceded the hammock that was swung between the door jamb and a calabash-tree.

188 de Gubernatis, op. cit., p. 97.

189 Cf. ibid., p. 99.

190 Petronius, *Satyricon,* 39.12. Cf. Petronius, *Cena Trimalchionis,* ed. Martin Smith, Oxford: Clarendon Press, 1975, p. 91. Interesting in this respect is also Gargilius Martialis, *Medicinae,* 6: 'veteres medici de cucurbita ita senserunt ut eam aquam dicerent coagulatam'. For 'cucurbita' in the sense of 'cupping-glass', used to draw blood from the head in disorders of the brain,

cf. Juvenal, *Satirae*, 14.58 and the commentaries by L. Friedländer, Amsterdam: Verlag Adolf M. Hakkert, 1962, p. 500, and J.D. Duff, Cambridge: University Press, 1948, p. 417. Cf. also F.A. Todd, *Classical Quarterly*, 1943, pp. 101-11, who deals with the relevant passages in Petronius, Apuleius, Juvenal and the Apocolocynthosis. His suggestions do not seem convincing. He collects an important part of the classical Latin material, but he does nothing to avoid discrepancies in his readings. He presents piecemeal interpretations without any attempt to organize them into a coherent symbolic grammar.

Another book on cucurbits is Sheldon P. Stoff, *The Pumpkin Quest*, North Quincey: The Christopher Publishing House, 1978, which deals marginally with the symbolism of pumpkins. It is not relevant to our study.

191 Penelope Mortimer, *The Pumpkin Eater*, London: Hutchinson, 1962.

192 *The Poems of Emily Dickinson: Including variant readings critically compared with all known manuscripts*, ed. Thomas H. Johnson, Cambridge: The Belknap Press of Harvard University Press, 1955, Poem 445, vol. 1, pp. 344-5.

193 ibid., vol. 3, pp. 976-7.

194 Philip Roth, *Portnoy's Complaint*, London: Jonathan Cape, 1969, pp. 216-32: ' "The Pumpkin" is what I called her, in commemoration of her pigmentation and the size of her can. Also her solidity: hard as a gourd on matters of moral principle, beautifully stubborn in a way I couldn't but envy and adore' (p. 216). '*So sound*! Yes, that's what hypnotized – the heartiness, the sturdiness; in a word, her pumpkinness. My wholesome, big-bottomed, lipstickless, barefooted *shikse*, where are you now, Kay-Kay? Mother to how many? Did you wind up really fat? . . . In the meantime let me miss her substantiality a little. That buttery skin! That unattended streaming hair! And this is back in the early fifties, before streaming hair became the style! This was just *naturalness*, Doctor. Round and ample, sun-colored Kay! I'll bet that half a dozen kiddies are clinging to that girl's abundant behind (so unlike The Monkey's hard little handful of a model's ass!)' (p. 217). Conversion, p. 230. The other gentile girl in the novel is also characterized in sexual fruit-symbolism: 'The Monkey', eating a banana (p. 161).

195 *Daily News*, 10 March 1887, 3/1.

196 C. Astor Bristed, *The Upper Ten Thousand*, New-York: Stringer & Townsend, 1852, p. 216. This fits in well with the tendency of American slang words to be ambiguous.

In an expression such as 'to think pumpkins of oneself' = to think well of oneself (Eric Partridge, *The Penguin Dictionary of Historical Slang*, abr. Jacqueline Simpson, Harmondsworth: Penguin 1978), the two senses of the ambiguous sign can probably be assigned to different persons: presumably the person being talked about really thinks well of himself or herself (positive sense), but the talker perhaps thinks there is no foundation for that view (negative sense).

NOTES TO PAGES 68-73

197 *An Heroic Epistle to Sir William Chambers, Knight, Comptroller General of his Majesty's Works, And Author of a late Dissertation on Oriental Gardening: Enriched with explanatory Notes, chiefly extracted from that elaborate Performance,* London: J. Almon, 1773, p. 11. Characteristically, the lines occur in a parody, but characteristically, too, the subject of the controversy is the question whether man should improve on nature and impose abstractions on it; oriental gardening versus European; *Urbs in rure* or *Rus in urbe.* The author of the satiric poem and pamphlet is violently against Sir William's ideas.

    Cf. also 'The Melon-Seller' above. Wentworth and Flexner give 'pumpkin-roller' as a name for a farmer, and 'pumpkin' as a word for a small town or rural community; a rustic place; a town in the sticks.

198 *Daily News,* 29 November 1894, 6/3.

199 Stephen Crane, *The Complete Short Stories,* pp. 430-75.

200 There are exceptions. Cf. e.g. Partridge, *Penguin Dictionary of Historical Slang:* '*melon.* A new cadet: Royal Military Academy: from ca 1870; ob. Ex his greenness, as is 2, the Australian and New Zealand sense (late C. 19-20), a simpleton, a fool. Abbr. *paddy-melon,* a small kangaroo: Australian coll: from ca 1845.

201 Mark Twain, *Tom Sawyer & Huckleberry Finn,* introd. Christopher Morley, London: Everyman's Library, 1963, pp. 240 and 280.

202 Reprinted as a pamphlet in London in 1853.

203 Thomas Carlyle, *Critical and Miscellaneous Essays,* vol. 4 in *The Works of Thomas Carlyle,* Centenary Edition, vol. 29, London: Chapman and Hall, 1899, pp. 348-83.

204 'Thomas Carlyle on the Slave Question', pp. 24-36 in *The Prose Works of John Greenleaf Whittier,* vol. 2, *Literary Recreations and Miscellanies,* Boston: Houghton Mifflin, 1880.

205 Ralph Ellison, *Invisible Man,* Harmondsworth: Penguin, 1972 (first pub. 1952), p. 50.

206 ibid., p. 215. Though the 'moral' of the book drifts hither and thither, and even yams are discarded soon afterwards, the scene is a strong symbolization of one of the dominant themes of the novel. In a similar scene in Chapter 21 melons are involved (p. 370):
> Even down South they'd always shined their shoes. "Shined shoes, shoed shines", it rang in my head. On Eight Avenue, the market carts were parked hub to hub along the kerb, improvised canopies shading the withering fruits and vegetables. I could smell the stench of decaying cabbage. A watermelon huckster stood in the shade beside his truck, holding up a long slice of orange-meated melon, crying his wares with hoarse appeals to nostalgia, memories of childhood, green shade and summer coolness.

207 Alex Haley, *Roots: The Epic Drama of One Man's Search for His Origins*, London: Picador, 1977, p. 209.

208 E. A. El Maleh, 'Racisme: Les mots ne sont jamais innocents', *Le Monde*, 14-15 January 1979, p. 13.

209 Verena Stefan, *Autobiografische Aufzeichnungen: Gedichte, Träume, Analysen, Häutungen*, München: Verlag Frauenoffensive, 1975, p. 119.

210 Cf. Thompson H1047. *Task: bringing melon 12 cubits long with seed 13 cubits long.* India: Thompson-Balys.

211 In a frequency dictionary from the 1960s, Henry Kučera and W. Nelson Francis, *Computational Analysis of Present-Day American English*, Providence: Brown University Press, 1967, with a corpus of 1,014,232 words, 'pumpkin' and 'gourd' occurred twice ('half-gourd' once); 'watermelon' and 'melon' (and 'melon-like') were *hapax legomena*, and 'cucumber' did not occur at all. It is difficult to investigate statistically the frequency of words as rare as the names of the cucurbits. Nevertheless, it is obvious that the frequency of the names of the cucurbits in the comic authors we have studied is higher than the Kučera-Francis frequencies.

212 Lucian, *Verae Historiae*, II.37. Cf. Spanish 'calabaza' = 'lumbering old boat'. Cf. also Thompson F841.1.4. *Boat made of nutshells.* Breton: Sébillot Incidents s.v. 'coques', 'noix'; and F841.1.12. *Boat from gourd.* India: Thompson-Balys.

213 Lowell, like the other New England abolitionists of the mid-nineteenth century, argued that the natural course of history goes against slavery:
> Mr. Calhoun, who is made the chief speaker in this burlesque, seems to think that the light of the nineteenth century is to be put out as soon as he tinkles his little cow-bell curfew. Whenever slavery is touched, he sets up his scarecrow of dissolving the Union. This may do for the North, but I should conjecture that something more than a pumpkin-lantern is required to scare manifest and irretrievable Destiny out of her path. Mr. Calhoun cannot let go the apron-string of the Past. The Past is a good nurse, but we must be weaned from her sooner or later, even though, like Plotinus, we should run home from school to ask the breast, after we are tolerably well-grown youths. It will not do for us to hide our faces in her lap, whenever the strange Future holds out her arms and ask us to come to her.

(*Poems of James Russell Lowell*, London: Oxford University Press, 1912, p. 239).
> Lowell skilfully saddles his opponent with all the ridiculous, absurd, grotesque and comic associations by comparing his argument to a pumpkin-lantern and his attitude to childishness.

214 Ben Jonson, *Volpone: or The Fox*, introd. and notes Arthur Sale, London: University Tutorial Press, 1951, p. 29.

215 *The Poems & Letters of Andrew Marvell*, ed. H.M. Margoliouth, 2nd ed., vol. 1, Oxford: Clarendon Press, 1952, p. 49.

216 The occurrence of cucurbits in a riddle by Symphosius (fourth-fifth century) is a fair measure of the status of the cucurbits as household plants during late antiquity: 'Pendeo dum nascor; rursus, dum pendo, tumesco./ Pendens commoveor ventis et nutrior undis./Pendula si non sim, non sum iam iamque futura' (Raymond T. Ohl, *The Enigmas of Symphosius*, Philadelphia: University of Pennsylvania, 1928, pp. 74-7). Symphosius generally drew his subjects from the familiar, everyday world.

217 Cf. Orth in *Paulys Real-Encyclopädie*, vol. 7, cc. 1947-8. Actually, the assumption that cucurbits were not popular in the Middle Ages could well be questioned. There seems to be no climatological reason why we should think so. Certainly they were grown in the gardens of the monasteries as Walafrid Strabo's on Reichenau. The disproportionally great space he devotes to cucurbits in his poem would rather indicate that cucurbits were among the most prominent plants of the garden. At least they were the most prominent plants of his symbolic imagination. The cucurbits (cucumis, pepo, cucurbita, coloquentis) are also mentioned among the plants that Charlemagne ordered to be grown in the imperial 'villas' (*Caroli Magni Capitulare de villis imperialibus*, 70; *Patrologia Latina*, XCVII, c. 358). *The Geoponica* was compiled in the tenth century. Achmet's interpretations of dreams, known as *Apomasaris Apotelesmata*, which has a passage devoted specifically to cucurbits, is probably written before that, translated into Latin in 1160 and 1577. Albertus Magnus wrote his *De Vegetabilibus* in the middle of the thirteenth century.

218 For some additional material, especially on folk-lore and myth from the Far East, see Chevalier–Gheerbrant, *Dictionnaire des symboles*, pp. 133 and 248.

Part 2: Implications

Chapter 1 Is a literary work written by the author or by the readers?

1 Martin Heidegger, *Der Satz vom Grund*, Pfullingen: Verlag Günther Neske, 1957, p. 161. On these aspects of French structuralism, see Jonathan Culler, *Structuralist Poetics: Structuralism, Linguistics and the Study of Literature*, London: Routledge & Kegan Paul, 1975.

2 Claude Lévi-Strauss, *Le cru et le cuit*, Paris: Plon, 1964, p. 20.

3 Needless to say, survival of the fittest is a value judgment by the collective of reader-consumers that need not necessarily be the same verdict as that

NOTES TO PAGES 86-103

of an informed elite of evaluating literary critics – though they, too, establish a canon of 'world classics' through a mechanism that differs from this more in its degree of sophistication than in principle.

4 J. Stanley Lemons, 'Black Stereotypes as Reflected in Popular Culture, 1880-1920', *American Quarterly*, vol. 29, no. 1, Spring 1977, pp. 102-16.

5 In several languages, e.g. Hebrew or French, it is specifically only the female goose that is silly, not the male – 'gander' would not work as a word of abuse in the same way as 'goose'.

6 Of all the various theories on humour and comedy, that which stresses the role of the feeling of superiority is naturally only one, but we feel that there is some truth in most theories of the comic and accordingly in this one too.

7 In other similar postcards of the same period Negroes are associated with serious crimes of violence, but the violence is understood to be directed against other Negroes (see Lemons, op. cit.).

Chapter 2   *Does a literary work write itself?*

1 *Historia Augusta,* Clodius Albinus 11.3.

2 *Historia Augusta,* Carinus 17.3.

3 Aristotle, too, *Poetics* 1460 b 8ff, qualifies 'things as they were or are' with 'things as they are said or thought to be, or things as they ought to be'.

4 John Updike, *Rabbit Redux,* London: André Deutsch, 1972, pp. 378-9.

5 Jonathan Swift, *Gulliver's Travels,* introd. Harold Williams, Oxford: Basil Blackwell, 1941, p. 163.

6 Swift had a conservative suspicion of inventions and new methods. Some of the phenomena he ridicules – such as certain innovations in agriculture – have since become generally accepted. Today the satire is therefore most successful in those parts where it is less specific and more exaggerated and absurd, as in the cucurbit-and-excrement passage.

7 Jørgen Nash, *Galgenfuglen: Et romaneksperiment,* Copenhagen, Gyldendals tranebøger, 1967, p. 22.

8 Sven Holm, *Jomfrutur: En lille roman,* Copenhagen, Gyldendals tranebøger, 1977 (written in 1966).

9 Dennis Hills, *The White Pumpkin,* London: Allen & Unwin, 1975, p. 83. Cf. Organ op.cit., p. 40: 'In India too, the gourd is also of ancient use. In the past, gourds some three feet in length were frequently covered with

brightly painted coarse cloth and placed in the Maha-manta-pam, of the temple of the God Subrahmaniyam by women whose breasts were underdeveloped, as an ex-voto offering.'

10   George W. Harris, 'Sut Lovingood Reports What Bob Dawson Said, After Marrying a Substitute', in *Sut Lovingood's Yarns,* ed. M. Thomas Inge, New Haven: University Press, 1966, p. 280.

11   Λεξικὸν τῆς Νέας Ἑλληνικῆς Γλώσσης. For gourds used in beauty treatment by the Hausa women, see Organ, op. cit., p. 66.

12   Anne Bergman (personal comment).

13   A rapid survey of the merchandise in a High Street store of a leading British chemist's revealed that cucumber extract is an ingredient in many of the leading brands of beauty lotions, skin beautifiers and bath salts. One packet of bath salt, for instance, is sold with a colour picture of two splendid cucumbers and four cucumber-slices on the front, with the text: '*English Country Harvest: Cucumber Beauty Bath*'. The advertisement on the back of the packet reads: 'Come alive! Allow yourself a new sensation from our exciting range of Beauty Baths. Sprinkle the contents into your bath under running water and savour the fresh natural fragrance. Abandon yourself just once to this soft, sweet, luxurious world and the seed will be sown to experience this pleasure again and again. MADE IN ENGLAND BY JEAN SORELLE LIMITED.'

14   Even as to its negative connotations – 'calabash' in Igbo can also stand for 'stupidity'.
     For information on Igbo usage we are grateful to Father Emmanuel Ifesieh.

15   Mary Douglas, *Purity and Danger: An Analysis of Concepts of Pollution and Taboo,* London: Routledge & Kegan Paul, 1966, pp. 41–57. See also her *Implicit Meanings: Essays in Anthropology,* London: Routledge & Kegan Paul, 1975, esp. pp. 249ff.

16   It does not even – to stay within the factualistic frame of mind – matter whether parasites were known to the ancient Hebrew.

17   Cf. F.A. Todd, *Classical Quarterly,* 1943, pp. 101-11.

18   Cf. loc. cit.

19   Henry Rider Haggard, *King Solomon's Mines,* London and Glasgow: Collins, 1965, pp. 83–4.

20   Christina Rossetti, 'Goblin Market', *The Poetical Works of Christina Georgina Rossetti,* memoir and notes William Michael Rossetti, London: Macmillan, 1904, p. 5.

21   Jer. Taylor, *The Great Exemplar of Sanctity and Holy Life* etc., part III, London: Francis Ash, 1649, p. 21. The argument in the passage is that because of man's sins God has shortened human life repeatedly and had he gone on doing so this would have been the result.

22 For a guide to literature on this subject, see Thompson, J1772.1 ff.

23 René Goscinny and Albert Uderzo, *Astérix chez les Bretons*, Neuilly-sur-Seine: Dargaud Editeur, 1966, pp. 36–42. Goscinny and Uderzo are not the only ones who have noticed the suitability of a cucurbitic word for a football. Wentworth and Flexner report 'punkin' for football in a CBS radio network football broadcast in 1950.

24 The principle of 'symbols cluster' is also illustrated in the episode, since the mascot of one rugby team is a goose and that of the other a hen (p. 37).

   The principle of 'connotations cluster' has given rise to a distinct class of poems in which the author displays his mastery of 'lateral poetic thinking' in running through an inventory of all connotations he can think of on a subject. Whittier's 'The Pumpkin' (Part 1) was such an 'inventory poem'. Another is 'Περί ἀγγουρίου' by Ἰωάννης Βηλαρᾶς. The author praises the cucumber for being pleasurable to all the senses. In addition he gives a quick run-through of its medicinal properties, also managing to include references to its royal status, to gold (in an interesting word-play which equates green and gold) – plus, naturally, a fair amount of innuendo (''Απαντα, ἐπιμέλεια Γεωργίου Ἀχιλ. Βαβαρέτου, Ἀθῆναι: Ἐκδοτικός Οἶκος Πέτρου Δημητράκον Α.Ε., 1935, σελ. 168):

   Ἐπομένως τὸ ἀγγούρι φέρει ἄκραν ἡδονήν,
   Εἰς τὰς τέσσαρας αἰσθήσεις, δίδει τέρψιν ἱκανήν.
   Ἔχει χάριτας μεγάλας, ὑπέρ κάθε ἄλλο τί,
   Ὄμμα, ὄσφρησιν καί γεῦσιν, καί ἀφήν εὐχαριστεῖ.
   Εἶν' γλυκύτατον στήν γεῦσιν, εἰς τήν ὅρασιν τερπνόν,
   Εἰς τήν ὄσφρησιν εὐῶδες καί εἰς τήν ἀφήν ψυχρόν.
   Διουρητικόν τόν σπόρον ἔχει καί δροσιστικόν,
   Τό δέ ἔσωθεν ὑγρόν του εἶν ἀντιφλογιστικόν.
   Εἰς τήν ἄκραν φέρει πλῆθος ἀκανθίδια λεπτά,
   Τά ὁποῖα στάζουν δρόσον, χείρ ἐγγίζουσα αὐτά.
   Εἰς τήν κορυφήν ἕν ἄνθος, ὡς κορῶνα του φορεῖ,
   Ἐπειδή καί ὑπέρ πάντα τά λοιπά ὑπερτερεῖ.
   Ἔχει σχῆμα τηλικοῦτον, εἶν' λεπτόν, μακρόν, γλισχρόν,
   Σκῆπτρον βασιλέως μοιάζει, χρυσοπράσινον, λαμπρόν,
   Ἕν ἐλάττωμα δέ ἔχει, δύσπεπτον εἰς μερικούς,
   Πλήν κατ' ἐξοχήν εἰς ἄκρον βλάπτει τούς καχεκτικούς.

25 Mateo Alemán, *Primera y segvnda parte de Gvzman de Alfarache*, Madrid, 1661 (first pub. 1599), p. 250. Alemán's metaphor became a simile in Mabbe's translation ('I am like a Melon-mongers Knife').

26 Cf. *Don Quijote*, II, xxxii: '– Eso juro yo bien – dijo Sancho: – cuchillada le hubieran dado, que le abrieran de arriba abajo como una granada, o como a un melón muy maduro' (Miguel de Cervantes Saavedra, *Don Quijote de la Mancha*, ed. Martín de Riquer, London: Harrap, 1950, p. 804).

   In Henry James's tale, 'A Tragedy of Error' (1864) there is an interesting conversation between the heroine and a man whom she hires to assassinate her husband. This man has been a sailor, and the conversation turns to the cruelty of the Spaniards of South America who kill very easily and think nothing of it (in Maqbool Aziz, ed., *The Tales of Henry James,* Vol. 1, (1864-1869), London: Faber & Faber, 1973, p. 12):

> 'How odd!' said Madame Bernier, with a shrill kind of laugh.
> 'A man who owed you a grudge of this kind would just come up and stab you, I suppose, and think nothing of it?'
> 'Precisely. Drive a knife up to the hilt into your back, with an oath, and slice open a melon with it, with a song, five minutes afterward.'

27 Edgar Wallace, *The Angel of Terror,* London: Pan Books, 1962, pp. 117-18; slashing incident, p. 113.

28 See Ralf Norrman, 'Techniques of Ambiguity in the Fiction of Henry James: With Special Reference to *In the Cage* and *The Turn of the Screw', Acta Academiae Aboensis,* ser. A, vol. 54, no. 2, Åbo: Åbo Akademi, 1977, p. 90 and *passim.*

29 E.g. Northrop Frye, *Anatomy of Criticism: Four Essays,* Princeton: University Press, 1971 (first pub. 1957), *passim.*

30 Richard Brautigan, *In Watermelon Sugar,* London: Jonathan Cape, 1970, p. 1.

31 The author succeeds fairly well in Book 2, 'inBOIL', but not so well in Book 3, 'Margaret'. In Book 3 the bad guys are more convincing than the good guys.

Chapter 3 *Sign and signification*

1 Even in a greengrocer's display of fruit the pumpkins may have some consciously contrived semiotic significance and be given preferential treatment and a prominent position for the sake of their advertisement value rather than for their sales potential.

2 A. Karkavitsas, *He Ligere,* Histias Publishing Co., Athens, 1896, p. 22.

3 On life and cucurbits cf. Thompson E711.2.1. *Soul in calabash* (gourd). Africa (Hottentot): Bleck 55 No. 24; N.A. Indian (Seneca): Curtin-Hewitt RBAE XXXII 572 No. 116 E765.3.2. Life bound up with calabash. 'cucumber' p. 182.

4 James Thurber, 'The Cane in the Corridor', *The Thurber Carnival,* written and illus. James Thurber, Harmondsworth: Penguin, 1962, p. 45.

5 Suzanne Prou, *Méchamment les oiseaux,* Paris: Calmann-Lévy, 1971, p. 121.

6 An X-rated film version of *Cinderella* has recently been released in Britain. Pumpkins figure prominently in the posters advertising the film.

7   An especially tricky variation of this is when the inclusive concept and one of the subcategories bear the same name as in English *man* (Ger. 'Mensch'), subcategories *man* ('Mann') and *woman* ('Frau'). This category needs a shelf of its own in a library of studies in ambiguity.

8   Ken Kesey, *Sometimes a Great Notion,* London: Magnum Books, 1976, pp. 156–69 and *passim*; see also Thompson, H611.1. *Melons ripe and overripe analogous to girls ready for marriage.* Iraq: H335.2. Suitor task: *cutting open magic gourd.* Indo-Chinese: Scott Indo-Chinese 290; C31.1.5. *Tabu: opening gourd in which star-wife is kept.* When curious girls do so, she flies up to sky. S. Am. Indian (Camacoco): Métraux MAFLS XL 48.

9   Tolstoy, L.I., *Sobraniye Sochineniya, Tom Dvenadstati,* ('Collected Works', vol.12), ed. I. I. Akopovoi, I. K. Gudziya, I. I. Guseva, M. B. Khrapchenko, Moscow: Editions 'Khudozhyestvenoye Literatura', 1964, p. 150.

10 Charles Dickens, *Nicholas Nickleby,* ed., introd. and notes Michael Slater, Harmondsworth: Penguin, 1978 (first pub. 1839), p. 567.

11 See Slater's note, p. 972.

12 To reinforce a negative use of a cucurbit as a symbol of marriage (i.e. of a hateful marriage), an author can even activate the 'human vegetable' connotations that we exemplified in Chapter 3 with passages from James Thurber and Suzanne Prou. In the Swedish translation of President Sadat's autobiography (Anwar al-Sadat, *Mitt liv, mitt land: En självbiografi,* trans. (from the American manuscript) Gunnar Ruud, Stockholm: Rabén & Sjögren, 1978, p. 83), the author explains in Chapter 3 why he felt he had to divorce his first wife:

> God knows I did not have anything against my wife as a person, but I simply had to do something about the matter before it was too late. If I go on living with this woman, I argued, I shall end up as a typical Egyptian civil servant, who when work is over for the day, goes home to his family, maybe with a watermelon under his arm, and then goes out again in the afternoon to the local café to play a game of backgammon, and returns home in the evening. Next morning: back to work again. A man without anything to urge him on, with no visions that can come true. Merely an existence for its own sake. There would be no goal in my existence, no sense of a mission – only because of my wife.
>
> I began to realize that she really stood in my way, that something really had to be done to avoid the otherwise inevitable disappointment.

(Our translation is from the Swedish back into English).

This passage does not appear in the English edition (Anwar el-Sadat, *In Search of Identity,* London: Collins, 1978). If the passage was deleted (after it was too late to change the Swedish version) as the result of second thoughts, one can easily see why.

A usage similar to Sadat's can be studied in an article by Jill Tweedie,

'Her policies will be forgotten, her sex remembered forever', in *The Guardian*, 26 April 1979, p. 11. Ms Tweedie debates whether women ought to vote for a woman politician because she is a woman even though they may not agree with her opinions. In the course of her article Ms Tweedie writes:

> Girls – who begin so smart, who outdistance their brothers so easily – mysteriously fade at about age fifteen and turn, like Cinderella's carriage, into pretty pumpkins waiting for a Prince to reactivate them. Why? Because, as all the experts agree, they have no image upon which to model themselves, no active figureheads at whom they may point.

In this usage a whole range of connotations are activated. There are the 'lovely-woman-as-cucurbit' connotations; the 'ready-for-marriage' connotations, and in general all those positive connotations in which cucurbits are thought of in connection with sex, female beauty, etc. But the author mixes these with a negative view by also bringing in the stupidity connotation and in fact even the 'vegetable-existence' connotation. Apparently this ambivalence in the symbolism perfectly matches some kind of ambivalence in the contents of the article. The traditional views on women are being questioned, values are being investigated. What has been thought good is perhaps bad in the light of a new view and what has been thought bad may perhaps be good. This fluidity of values seeks a corresponding type of symbolism in which traditional stable symbolic meaning is destroyed or refashioned.

13 M. Aleman, *Primera y segunda parte de Guzman de Alfarache*, Madrid, 1661, p. 397. Cf. 'dar calabazas', 'reject a lover'.

14 Tove Jansson, *Pappan och havet*, Helsingfors: Almqvist & Wiksell, 1975 (first pub. 1965), pp. 144–6 and *passim*.

15 *The Poetical Works of John Keats*, ed. H.W. Garrod, 2nd ed., Oxford: Clarendon Press, 1958, p. 273.

16 *The Poetical Works of Christina Georgina Rossetti*, London, Macmillan, 1904, p. 1.

17 Sylvia Plath, *Fiesta Melons*, introd. Ted Hughes, Exeter: Rougemont Press, 1971, pp. 14–15.

Chapter 4 Independent creation versus tradition

Chapter 5 On the nature of signs used in cucurbitic metaphors

1 Ferdinand de Saussure, *Cours de linguistique générale*, pub. Charles Bally and Albert Sechehaye in collaboration with Albert Riedlinger, critical ed. Tullio de Mauro, Paris: Payot, 1972, p. 100.

2   Ferdinand de Saussure, *Cours de linguistique générale,* ed. Rudolf Engler, Wiesbaden: Otto Harrassowitz, 1967, fascicule 2, pp. 153-5. The literature on the *arbitraire* is voluminous. For a brief survey, see de Mauro, pp. 442-9; for further references, see E.F.K. Koerner, *Bibliographia Saussureana, 1870-1970: An annotated, classified bibliography on the background, development and actual relevance of Ferdinand de Saussure's general theory of language,* Metuchen: The Scarecrow Press, 1972, pp. 127-79; also his *Contribution au débat post-saussurien sur le signe linguistique: Introduction générale et bibliographie annotée,* The Hague: Mouton, 1971.

See also Robert Godel, *Les sources manuscrites du Cours de linguistique générale de F. de Saussure,* Geneva: Droz, 1957.

3   Another factor also influences these attempts to emphasize arbitrariness. There is a tendency for people always to regard the signs of their own semiotic systems as inherently 'natural'. Having discovered that this is fallacy, it is tempting to generalize the discovery to a universal theory of semiotic relativity and make arbitrariness a dogma, in the initial enthusiastic desire to share with one's readers the discovery that systems may vary.

4   Morton Bloomfield, 'The Study of Language', *Daedalus* (Summer 1973); *Language as a Human Problem,* Proceedings of The American Academy of Arts and Sciences, vol. 102, no. 3, pp. 5-13.

5   Derek Bickerton, 'Prolegomena to a Linguistic Theory of Metaphor', *Foundations of Language,* vol. 5, no. 1, February 1969, pp. 34-52. We have chosen this article to represent the kind of approach that we think is inadequate and we are not arguing against the article as such but against the school of thought that it represents.

6   It has often been thought that there is some sort of order in the relationship of the two systems — and thus between the two elements — and this has given rise to such terminological distinctions as that of Richards between 'vehicle' and 'tenor'. There seems to be some truth in this, but if the idea is accepted that there is such a structure in some, most or all metaphors, the 'order' is, of course, relative, not absolute. Which system is the starting-point, or hierarchically superior, varies. The thrust of a cucurbitic metaphor may be anthropomorphic, as when you call a pumpkin 'king of the garden'; or phytomorphic, as when you call a man 'pumpkin'. But there may be cases when the connection is anthropo-phytomorphic or phyto-anthropomorphic, and actually it is debatable whether it is not the case in *all* metaphors that both systems influence each other. In that case 'the man is a lion' does not mean only that the man has courage, but that he has animal-like courage.

7   I.e. using a system from nature, such as the system of plants, as one of the systems in the bisociation.

The term 'bisociation' has been used by Arthur Koestler in several books for a number of mental processes (including metaphor) that are, in his view, closely related. See e.g. Arthur Koestler, *Insight and Outlook,* New York and London: Macmillan, 1949 or *The Act of Creation*, New York: Macmillan, 1964.

8   Roger Brown, *Words and Things*, Glencoe, Ill.: The Free Press, 1958, p. 146.

9   Aristotle, *Poetics*, XXII.9-10. We think that those modern commentators who translate 'to metaphorize well is to see the similar in dissimilars' are true to the spirit of Aristotle's text even though the word 'dissimilar' is not in the Greek.

10 Paul Ricoeur, *La métaphore vive*, Paris: Editions du Seuil, 1975. For a comprehensive and suggestive treatment of the phenomenon of metaphor, as well as for further references, see this work. See also Warren A. Shibles, *Metaphor: An Annotated Bibliography and History*, Whitewater: The Language Press, 1971.

11 Richard Adams, *Watership Down*, London: Rex Collings, 1972.

Works cited

Achmet, *Apomasaris Apotelesmata*.
Adams, Richard, *Watership Down*, London: Rex Collings, 1972.
Albertus Magnus, *De Vegetabilibus*, VI.
Alemán, Mateo, *Primera y segvnda parte de Gvzman de Alfarache*, Madrid, 1661.
Alemán, Mateo, *The Rogue: or The Life of Guzman de Alfarache*, trans. James Mabbe, Introduction by James Fitzmaurice-Kelly. London: Constable 1924, vol. 1.
Alemán, Mateo, *The Rogve: or The Life of Guzman de Alfarache*, trans. James Mabbe, London: Printed for Edward Blount, 1622, Part Second.
Alfons, Sven, *Symbolister 2 Giuseppe Arcimboldo: En biografisk och ikonografisk studie. Tidskrift för konstvetenskap XXXI*. Pub. Ragnar Josephson, Malmö: Allhems Förlag, 1957.
Ambrosius, *Hexaemeron*, V.
André, Jaques, *Les mots à redoublement en Latin*, Paris: Editions Klincksieck, 1978.
Andrew, Prudence, *Mr Morgan's Marrow*, illus. Janet Duchesne. London: Collins, 1975.
Antin, Paul. *Saint Jérôme: Sur Jonas*, Paris: Les Éditions du Cerf, 1956.
Apicius, *De Re Coquinaria*, III.
Apuleius, *Metamorphoses*, I.
Aristophanes, *Lysistrata*.
Aristophanes, *Nubes*.
Aristotle, *Poetics*, XXI and XXII.
Arnott, Anne, *The Secret Country of C.S. Lewis*, London: Hodder & Stoughton, 1974.
Artemidorus Daldianus, *Onirocriticon*, I.
Athenaeum, 8 July 1899.
Athenaeus, *Deipnosophistae*, III and VI.
St Augustine, *De Moribus Manichaeorum*, II (*Patrologia Latina*, XXXII).
Baker, Samuel W., Sir, *The Nile Tributaries of Abyssinia: And the Sword Hunters of the Hamran Arabs*, London: Macmillan, 1867.
Beaumont, Francis and Fletcher, John, *The Custom of the country*. vol. 1 of *The Works of Francis Beaumont and John Fletcher*. Cambridge English Classics, 1625.

WORKS CITED

Beaumont, Francis, and Fletcher, John, *Rule a Wife, and have a Wife*, vol. 3 of *The Works of Francis Beaumont and John Fletcher*, Cambridge English Classics, 1623.

Beck, E. (ed.), *Des Heiligen Ephraem des Syrers Sermones de Fide*, vol. 88 of *Corpus Scriptorum Christianorum Orientalium, Scriptores Syri*, Louvain: Secrétariat du Corpus SCO, 1961.

Bickerton, Derek, 'Prolegomena to a Linguistic Theory of Metaphor', *Foundations of Language*, 5, no. 1, February 1969, pp. 34–52.

Birt, Th., *Rheinisches Museum*, 46, 1891.

Blake, William, *The Complete Writings of William Blake: With Variant Readings*, ed. Geoffrey Keynes, London: Oxford University Press, 1966.

Bloomfield, Morton, 'The Study of Language', *Daedalus*, Summer 1973, 'Language as a Human Problem', *Proceedings of The American Academy of Arts and Sciences*, 102, no. 3, pp. 5–13.

Boorde, Andrew, *Dietary*.

Boswell, James, *The Journal of A Tour to the Hebrides with Samuel Johnson, Ll.D. by James Boswell, Esq.*, annotated by Hester Lynch Thrale Piozzi, Bloomfield: Limited Editions Club, 1974.

Brautigan, Richard, *In Watermelon Sugar*, London: Jonathan Cape, 1970.

Bridges, Robert, *Eight Plays. Nero, Parts I. & II. Palicio. Ulysses. Captives. Achilles. Humours. Feast of Bacchus*, London: George Bell & Sons and J. and E. Bumpus, 1885 (?).

Bristed, Astor, C., *The Upper Ten Thousand*, New York: Stringer & Townsend, 1852.

Broun, A.F. (comp.), *Catalogue of Sudan Flowering Plants: Giving short descriptions, a number of vernacular names and some economic and other uses.* Khartoum: El-Sudan Printing Press, 1906.

Brown, Roger, *Words and Things*. Glencoe: The Free Press, 1958.

Browning, Robert, *The Complete Works of Robert Browning*, with variant readings and annotations, ed. Roma A. King, Jr, *et al.* Athens: Ohio University Press, 1971, vol. 3.

Browning, Robert, *The Poetical Works of Robert Browning*, London: Smith, Elder, 1897, vol. 2.

Bücheler, F., *Rheinishes Museum*, 54, 1899.

Bächthold-Stäbli, *Handwörterbuch des deutschen Aberglaubens*, Berlin/Leipzig: Walter de Gruyter, 1932/3, vol. 5.

Carlyle, Thomas, *Critical and Miscellaneous Essays*, vol. 4 of *The Works of Thomas Carlyle*, Centenary Edition, vol. 29. London: Chapman & Hall, 1899.

Cassius, Dio, *Roman History*, LXIX.

de Cervantes Saavedra, Miguel, *Don Quijote de la Mancha*, ed. Martín de Riquer. London: Harrap, 1950.

Charlemagne, *Caroli Magni Capitulare de villis imperialibus*, 70 (*Patrologia Latina*, XCVII).

Chaucer, Geoffrey, *The Canon's Yeoman's Tale*. In *The Works of Geoffrey Chaucer*, ed. F.N. Robinson, 2nd ed. London: Oxford University Press, 1957.

WORKS CITED

Chaucer, Geoffrey, *The Manciple's Prologue*. In *The Works of Geoffrey Chaucer*, ed. F.N. Robinson, 2nd ed. London: Oxford University Press, 1957.

Chevalier, Jean and Gheerbrant, Alain, *Dictionnaire des symboles*. Paris: Robert Laffont, 1969.

Chorley, Henry F., *Memorials of Mrs Hemans: With Illustrations of Her Literary Character from her Private Correspondence*, vol. 2, London: Saunders & Otley, 1836.

Churchill, E. Richard (comp.), *The Six-Million-Dollar Cucumber: A Bookful of zany Riddles about Birds and Beasts and Vegetables*, London: Piccolo Pan Books, 1976.

Cicero, *Pro Sexto Roscio*.

Cirlot, J.E., *A Dictionary of Symbols*, trans. Jack Sage, London: Routledge & Kegan Paul, 1971.

Clarendon, Edward, Earl of, *The History of the Rebellion and Civil Wars in England, Begun in the Year 1641*. Oxford: At the Theater, 1702-1704, vol. 3, book XV.

Clowes, E.M., *On the Wallaby through Victoria*. London: Heinemann, 1911.

Coleridge, Samuel Taylor, *The Piccolomini: Or, The First Part of Wallenstein. A Drama. Translated from the German of Schiller*. In *The Complete Poetical Works*, ed. B.H. Coleridge, vol. 2. Oxford: Clarendon Press, 1912.

Columella, *De Re Rustica*, XI.

Conington, J. and Nettleship, H., (eds.), *The Works of Virgil*, vol. 1, London: George Bell, 1898.

Conrad, Joseph, *Nostromo: A Tale of the Seaboard*, London: J.M. Dent, 1972.

Copa, In *Appendix Vergiliana*.

Crane, Stephen, *The Complete Short Stories & Sketches by Stephen Crane*, ed. and introd. Thomas A. Gullason. Garden City: Doubleday, 1963.

Crane, Stephen, *The Poems of Stephen Crane*, a critical edition by Joseph Katz. New York: Cooper Square Publishers, 1971.

Culler, Jonathan, *Structuralist Poetics: Structuralism, Linguistics and the Study of Literature*. London: Routledge & Kegan Paul, 1975.

Cutler, Hugh C., and Whitaker, Thomas W., 'History and Distribution of the Cultivated Cucurbits in the Americas', *American Antiquity*, 26, no. 4 April 1961, pp. 469-85.

Daily News, 10 March 1887.

Daily News, 29 November 1894.

Dass, Petter, *Nordlands Trompet*, ed. D.A. Seip. Oslo: H. Aschehoug, 1974.

Dickens, Charles, 'Report of the Second Meeting of the Mudfog Association', in *The Mudfog Papers*. London: Richard Bentley & Son, 1880.

Dickens, Charles, *Nicholas Nickleby*, ed., introd. and notes Michael Slater. Harmondsworth: Penguin, 1978.

Dickinson, Emily, *The Poems of Emily Dickinson: Including variant readings critically compared with all known manuscripts*, ed. Thomas H. Johnson, vols. 1 and 3. Cambridge: The Belknap Press of Harvard University Press, 1955.

Dictionary of American Slang, comp. and ed. Harold Wentworth and Stuart Berg Flexner. London: Harrap, 1960.

WORKS CITED

The Dictionary of the Bible: Dealing With its Language, Literature etc., ed. James Hastings, vol. 2. Edinburgh: T. & T. Clark, 1899.

Dioscorides, *Materia Medica*, II and IV.

Douglas, Mary, *Purity and Danger: An Analysis of Concepts of Pollution and Taboo*. London: Routledge & Kegan Paul, 1966.

Douglas, Mary, *Implicit Meanings: Essays in Anthropology*. London: Routledge & Kegan Paul, 1975.

DuCange, *Glossarium Mediae et Infimae Latinitatis* (1678). Niort: L. Favre, 1883.

Ellison, Ralph, *Invisible Man*. Harmondsworth: Penguin, 1972.

Evans-Pritchard, E.E., *Nuer Religion*. Oxford: The Clarendon Press, 1956.

Field, Frederick (ed.), *Originis Hexaplorum quae supersunt*. Oxford: The Clarendon Press, 1875.

Fischer, Hermann, *Schwäbishes Wörterbuch*, Tübingen: Verlag der H. Laupp'schen Buchhandlung, 1901.

Fletcher, Angus, *Allegory: The Theory of a Symbolic Mode,* Ithaca and London: Cornell University Press, 1964.

Foote, 'Mayor of Garratt', in William Hone, *The Every-Day Book* etc., vol. 2, Part II. London: William Hone, 1827.

Forster, E.M., *Aspects of the Novel*, London: Edward Arnold, 1927.

Friedreich, J.B., *Die Symbolik und Mythologie der Natur*. Würzburg: Verlag der Stachel'schen Buch- und Kunsthandlung, 1859.

Frye, Northrop, *Anatomy of Criticism: Four Essays*, Princeton University Press, 1971.

Funk & Wagnalls Standard Dictionary of Folklore, Mythology and Legend, ed. Maria Leach. London: New English Library, 1975.

Galbraith, John Kenneth, *Money: Whence It Came, Where It Went*, London: André Deutsch, 1975.

Galenus, *Opera omnia*, ed. C.G. Kühn, vol. 6. Lipsiae: Cnobloch, 1823.

Galt, John, *Lawrie Todd: or, The Settlers in the Woods*, vol. 1. London: Henry Colburn & Richard Bentley, 1830.

Gargilius Martialis, *Medicinae*.

Gauden, John, *A Sermon Preached In the Temple-Chappel, at the Funeral of the Right Reverend Father in God, Dr Brounrig*, etc., London: Andrew Crook, 1660.

Geoponica, III and V.

Godel, Robert, *Les sources manuscrites du Cours de linguistique générale de F. de Saussure*, Geneva: Droz, 1957.

Goethe, J.W., *Claudine von Villa Bella* Act One, in *Werke*, vol. 10. Stuttgart/Tübingen: J.G. Cotta'schen Buchhandlung, 1828.

Goscinny, René, and Uderzo, Albert, *Astérix chez les Bretons*, Neuilly-sur-Seine: Dargaud Éditeur, 1966.

de Gubernatis, Angelo, *La Mythologie des Plantes*, vol. 2. Paris: C. Reinwald et Cie, Libraries Editeurs, 1878.

Guinness Book of Records, ed. Norris McWhirter, 25th ed. Enfield: Guinness Superlatives, 1978.

Hacket, John, *Scrinia Reserata: A Memorial Offer'd to the Great Deservings of John Williams, D.D. Who some time held the Places of* etc., Part I. London: Edw. Jones for Samuel Lowndes, 1693.

WORKS CITED

Haggard, Henry Rider, *King Solomon's Mines,* London and Glasgow: Collins, 1965.
Haley, Alex, *Roots: The Epic of One Man's Search for His Origins,* London: Picador, 1977.
Haliburton, *The Clockmaker; or The Sayings and Doings of Samuel Slick, of Slickville,* 3rd ser. London: Richard Bentley, 1840.
Haliburton, *The Clockmaker; or* etc. Philadelphia: Lea & Blanchard, 1839.
Harding, Walter, *The Days of Henry Thoreau,* New York: Knopf, 1970.
Harris, George, W., *Sut Lovingood. Yarns spun by a nat'ral born durn'd fool. Warped and Wove for public Wear,* New York: Dick & Fitzgerald, 1867.
Harris, George W., 'Sut Lovingood Reports What Bob Dawson Said, After Marrying a Substitute', in *Sut Lovingood's Yarns,* ed. M. Thomas Inge, New Haven: Yale University Press, 1966.
Harrison, R.H., *Healing Herbs of the Bible,* Leiden: E.J. Brill, 1966.
Hawthorne, Nathaniel, *The Scarlet Letter: A Romance,* introd. Douglas Grant. London: Oxford University Press, 1965.
Hawthorne, Nathaniel, *Tales by Nathaniel Hawthorne,* ed. Carl Van Doren. London: Oxford University Press, 1921.
Hehn, Viktor, *Kulturpflanzen und Haustiere in ihrem Übergang aus Asien,* Berlin: Gebrüder Borntraeger, 1911.
Heidegger, Martin, *Der Satz vom Grund,* Pfullingen: Verlag Günther Neske, 1957.
Helm, Rudolf, *Lucian und Menipp,* Leipzig/Berlin: B. G. Teubner, 1906.
Henkel, Arthur, and Schöne, Albert, *Emblemata: Handbuch zur Sinnbildkunst des XVI. und XVII. Jahrhunderts,* Stuttgart: J.B. Metzlersche Verlagsbuchhandlung, 1967.
Henry, O., 'The Shamrock and the Palm', In *Cabbages and Kings,* New York: McClure, Phillips, 1904.
The Hermit in London: or, Sketches of English Manners, vol. 3. London: Printed for Henry Colburn, 1819.
An Heroic Epistle to Sir William Chambers, Knight, Comptroller General of his Majesty's Works, And Author of a late Dissertation on Oriental Gardening: Enriched with etc., London: J. Almon, 1773.
Hills, Denis, *The White Pumpkin,* London: Allen & Unwin, 1975.
Hippocrates, *De Sterilibus.*
Historia Augusta.
Holm, Sven, *Jomfrutur: En lille roman,* Copenhagen: Glydendals tranebøger, 1977.
Homer, *Odyssey,* XI.
Horace, *Epistulae,* I.
S. Irenaeus, *Adversus Haereses,* ed. W.W. Harvey, vol. 1. Cantabrigiae: Typis Academicis, 1857.
Interpres Irenaei, *Adversus haereses,* I (*Patrologia Graeca,* VII).
Irving, Washington, *Salmagundi: or, The Whim-Whams and Opinions of Launcelot Langstaff, Esq and others* etc., vol. 1. London: J.M. Richardson, 1811.
Irving, Washington, *Rip Van Winkle and The Legend of Sleepy Hollow,* Philadelphia: Lippincott, 1923.
James, Henry, *The Art of the Novel: Critical Prefaces,* introd. Richard P. Blackmur. New York: Scribner's, 1962.

WORKS CITED

James, Henry, 'A Tragedy of Error', ed. Maqbool Aziz. *The Tales of Henry James, Volume One, 1864-1869*, London: Faber & Faber, 1973.
Janson, H.W., *The Sculpture of Donatello*, Princeton University Press, 1963.
Jansson, Tove, *Pappan och havet*, Helsingfors: Almqvist & Wiksell, 1975.
St Jerome, *Commentarii in Ionam*, IV (*Patrologia Latina*, XXV).
St Jerome, *Epistulae*, 112 (*Corpus Scriptorum Ecclesiasticorum Latinorum*, LV).
Jerome, Jerome K., *Novel Notes*, London: The Leadenhall Press, 1893.
Jonson, Benjamin, *Volpone: or The Foxe*, introd. and notes Arthur Sale. London: University Tutorial Press, 1951.
Joyce, James, *Ulysses*, New York: Random House, 1934.
Juvenal, *Satirae*, VI and XIV.
Juvenal, *Satirae*, comm. J.D. Duff. Cambridge: University Press, 1948.
Juvenal, *Saturae*, comm. L. Friedländer. Amsterdam: Verlag Adolf M. Hakkert, 1962.
Καρκαβίτσας, Α., Ἡ Λυγερή, Ἐν Ἀθήναις: Τυπογραφεῖον τῆς "Ἑστίας", 1896.
Karlfeldt, Erik Axel, *Hösthorn*, in *Svalans Svenske Klassiker: Erik Axel Karlfeldt*, Stockholm: Albert Bonniers Förlag, 1965.
Keats, John, *The Poetical Works of John Keats*, ed. H.W. Garrod, 2nd ed. Oxford: The Clarendon Press, 1958.
Keble, John (trans.), *Five Books of S. Irenaeus' Against Heresies*, in *A Library of Fathers*, Oxford: James Parker, 1872.
Kesey, Ken, *Sometimes a Great Notion*, London: Magnum Books, 1976.
Kock, Theodor (ed.), *Comicorum Atticorum Fragmenta*, vols. 2 and 3. Leipzig: B.G. Teubner, 1888.
Koerner, E.F.K., *Contribution au debát post-saussurien sur le signe linguistique: Introduction générale et bibliographie annotée*. The Hauge: Mouton, 1971.
Koerner, E.F.K., *Bibliographia Saussureana, 1870-1970: An annotated, classified bibliography on the background, development and actual relevance of Ferdinand de Saussure's general theory of language*, Metuchen: The Scarecrow Press, 1972.
Koestler, Arthur, *Insight and Outlook*, New York and London: Macmillan, 1949.
Koestler, Arthur, *The Act of Creation*, New York: Macmillan, 1964.
Kučera, Henry and Francis, W. Nelson, *Computational Analysis of Present-Day American English*, Providence: Brown University Press, 1967.
Laurent-Täckholm, Vivi, *Faraos blomster: En kulturhistorisk-botanisk skildring av livet i Gamla Egypten byggd på verklighetens grundval och med bilder från de senaste årens grävningar*, Stockholm: Natur och kultur, 1964.
Lear, Edward, *The Complete Nonsense of Edward Lear*, ed. and introd. Holbrook Jackson. London: Faber & Faber, 1947.
Legrand, Francine Claire, and Sluys, Félix, *Giuseppe Arcimboldo et les Arcimboldesques*, Aalter: André de Rache, 1955.
Lemons, J. Stanley, 'Black Stereotypes as Reflected in Popular Culture, 1880-1920'. *American Quarterly*, 29, no. 1, Spring 1977, pp. 102-16.
Leo, F., *Hermes*, 44, 1909.
Lévi-Strauss, Claude, *Le cru et le cuit*, Paris: Plon, 1964.

WORKS CITED

Λεξικὸν τῆς Νέας Ἑλληνικῆς Γλώσσης, "Πρωΐας", ἐπιμέλεια, Γεωργίου Ζευγωλῆ, Ἔκδοσις Νεωτάτη. Ἀθῆναι: Ἐκδοτικὸς Οἶκος Σταμ. Π. Δημητράκου.

Littré, E. (ed. and trans.), *Oeuvres complètes d'Hippocrate*, vol. 10. Paris: J.B. Baillière et Fils, 1861.

Livy, *Ab Urbe Condita Liber*, I.

Lodge, David, *Language of Fiction: Essays in Criticism and Verbal Analysis of the English Novel*, London: Routledge & Kegan Paul, 1966.

Loewenberg, Ina, 'Identifying Metaphors', *Foundations of Language*, 12, 1975, pp. 315-38.

London Gazette, no. 2724/2, 1691.

Lowell, James Russell, *Poems of James Russell Lowell*, London: Oxford University Press, 1912.

Lucian, *Verae Historiae*, II.

Luther, Martin, *Praelectiones in prophetas minores, Jona*. In *Werke*, vol. 13. Weimar: Hermann Böhlaus Nachfolger, 1897.

Maas, M., *Archiv für lateinische Lexicographie*, 11, 1900.

El Maleh, E.A., 'Racisme: Les mots ne sont jamais innocents', *Le Monde*, 14-15 January 1979.

Marvell, Andrew, *The Poems & Letters of Andrew Marvell*, ed. H.M. Margoliouth, 2nd ed. vol. 1. Oxford: The Clarendon Press, 1952.

Merivale, Charles, *A History of The Romans under the Empire*, vol. 5. London: Longman, Brown, Green and Longmans, 1856.

Milton, John, *Paradise Lost* (new ed.), ed. Richard Bentley, London, 1732.

Milton, John, *The First Edition of Paradise Lost*, vol. 2 of *John Milton's Complete Poetical Works: Reproduced in Photographic Facsimile*, comm. and ed. Harris francis Fletcher. Urbana: University of Illinois Press, 1945.

Milton, John, *Paradise Lost; Samson Agonistes; Lycidas*, annot. and biog. introd. Edward Le Comte. New York and Toronto: The New American Library, 1961.

Mitford, Mary Russell, *Our Village: Sketches of Rural Character and Scenery*, vol. 2. London: Geo. B. Whittaker, 1826.

Mitius, Otto, *Jonas auf den Denkmälern des christlichen Altertums*. Freiburg: Verlag von J.C.B. Mohr, 1897.

Morris, J.B. (trans.), *Select Works of Ephrem the Syrian*, in *A Library of Fathers*, Oxford: J.H. Parker, 1847.

Mortimer, Penelope, *The Pumpkin Eater*, London: Hutchinson, 1962.

Mrose, H., *Berliner philologischen Wochenschrift*, no. 12, 1914.

Nash, Jørgen, *Galgenfuglen: Et romaneksperiment*, Copenhagen: Gyldendals tranebøger, 1967.

The New Encyclopaedia Britannica: Macropaedia, 15th ed., vol. 5.

The New Yorker, 1 November 1976.

Norrman, Ralf, 'Techniques of Ambiguity in the Fiction of Henry James: With Special Reference to *In the Cage* and *The Turn of the Screw*', *Acta Academiae Aboensis*, ser. A, 54, no. 2. Åbo: Åbo Akademi, 1977.

Ohl, Raymond T., *The Enigmas of Symphosius*, Philadelphia: University of Pennyslvania, 1928.

WORKS CITED

Organ, John, *Gourds: Decorative and Edible for Garden, Craftwork and Table*, London: Faber & Faber, 1963.
Otto, A., *Die Sprichwörter der Römer*, Leipzig: Teubner, 1890.
OUIDA [De la Ramée], *Pascarèl. Only a Story*, vol. 1. London: Chatman and Hall, 1873.
Ousmane, Sembène, *Les bouts de bois de Dieu*,Paris: Presses Pocket, 1971.
Ovid, *Metamorphoses*, IX, X and XI.
Pall Mall Gazette, 4 September 1865.
Palladius, *Opus Agriculturae*, IV.
Palmer, John, *Journal of Travels in the United States of North America and in Lower Canada, Performed in the year 1817; containing* etc., London: Sherwood, Neely and Jones, 1818.
Parshall, Peter W., 'Albrecht Dürer's *St. Jerome in His Study*: A Philological Reference', *The Art Bulletin*, 53, no. 3, September 1971, pp. 303-5.
Partridge, Eric, *The Penguin Dictionary of Historical Slang*, abr. Jacqueline Simpson. Harmondsworth: Penguin, 1978.
Paulys Real-Encyclopädie der klassischen Altertumswissenschaft, ed. Georg Wissowa. Stuttgart: J. B. Meltzer, 1893-.
Peter, S., *A General History of Connecticut, From Its First Settlement*, etc., 2nd ed. London, 1782.
Petronius, *Cena Trimalchionis*, ed. Martin Smith. Oxford: The Clarendon Press 1971.
Petronius, *Satyricon*.
Plath, Sylvia, *Fiesta Melons*, introd. Ted Hughes. Exeter: The Rougemont Press, 1971.
Plautus, *Casina*.
Plato, *Cratylus*.
Pliny the elder, *Naturalis Historia*, XIX and XX.
Pliny the younger, *De Medicina*.
Plutarch, *Pericles*.
Postgate, J. P., *Classical Review*, 13, 1899.
Priapea.
Procopius, *Anecdota*.
Prou, Suzanne, *Méchamment les oiseaux*, Paris: Calmann-Lévy, 1971.
Prynne, William, *A Gagge* for *Long-Hair'd Rattle-Heads* who revile all civill Round-heads', 1644(?).
Reallexikon der Vorgeschichte, ed. Max Ebert, vol. 7. Berlin: Walter de Gruyter & Co., 1926.
Ricoeur, Paul, *La métaphore vive*, Paris. Éditions du Seuil, 1975.
Riley, James Whitcomb, *The Complete Poetical Works of James Whitcomb Riley*, pref. Donald Culross Peattie. Garden City: Garden City Publishing Co., 1941.
Ritchie, Leitch, *Wanderings by the Loire: with twenty-one engravings from drawings by J. M. W. Turner*, London: Longman, Rees, Orme, Brown, Green, and Longman, 1833.
Rossetti, Christina, *The Poetical Works of Christina Georgina Rossetti*, memoir and notes William Michael Rossetti. London: Macmillan, 1904.
Roth, Philip, *Portnoy's Complaint*, London: Jonathan Cape, 1969.

Rothenberg, Jerome, *Shaking the Pumpkin: Traditional Poetry of the Indian North Americas*, Garden City: Doubleday & Company, 1972.
Rudolph, Wilhelm (ed.), *Kommentar zum Alten Testament*, Gütersloh: Gütersloher Verlagshaus Gerd Mohn, 1971. Vol. 13$_2$.
Rufinus, *Apologia contra Hieronymum*, II (*Corpus Christianorum*, XX).
Ruxton, George Frederick, *Life in the Far West*, Edinburgh and London: William Blackwood and Sons, 1849.
el-Sadat, Anwar, *In Search of Identity*, London: Collins, 1978.
al-Sadat, Anwar, *Mitt liv, mitt land. En självbiografi*, trans. Gunnar Ruud. Stockholm: Rabén & Sjögren, 1978.
Saturday Review, 6 December 1884.
de Saussure, Ferdinand, *Cours de linguistique générale*, ed. Rudolf Engler, vol. 2. Wiesbaden: Otto Harrassowitz, 1967.
de Saussure, Ferdinand, *Cours de linguistique générale*, pub. Charles Bally and Albert Sechehaye in collaboration with Albert Riedlinger: critical ed. Tullio de Mauro. Paris: Payot, 1972.
Scheick, William J., 'Discarded Watermelon Rinds: The Rainbow Aesthetic of Styron's *Lie Down in Darkness*', *Modern Fiction Studies*, 24, no. 2, summer 1978, pp. 247-54.
Schulz, Wolfgang, 'Lambert Doomer als Maler', *Oud Holland*, 92, no. 2, 1978.
Scobie, Alexander, *Apuleii Metamorphoses: A Commentary*, Meisenheim am Glan: Verlag Anton Hain, 1975.
Seneca, *Apocolocynthosis*.
Shakespeare, William, *The Arden Edition of the Works of William Shakespeare: The Merry Wives of Windsor*, ed. H. J. Oliver. London: Methuen, 1971.
Shakespeare, William, *The Riverside Shakespeare*, textual ed. G. Blakemore Evans; gen. introd. Harry Levin, *et al.* Boston: Houghton Mifflin, 1974.
Shibles, Warren A., *Metaphor: An Annotated Bibliography and History*. Whitewater: The Language Press, 1971.
Sonny, A., in *Archiv für lateinische Lexicographie*, E. Wölfflin, vol. 9. Leipzig: B. G. Teubner, 1898.
The Spectator, 15 October 1904.
Stefan, Verena, *Autobiografische Aufzeichnungen: Gedichte, Träume, Analysen, Häutungen*. München: Verlag Frauenoffensive, 1975.
Steffen, Uwe, *Das Mysterium von Tod und Auferstehung: Formen und Wandlungen des Jona-Motivs*. Göttingen: Vandenhoeck & Ruprecht, 1963.
Steuens, Charles, and Liebault, John (comps), *Maison Rustique: or The Countrie Farme* etc., trans. Richard Svrflet. London: Bouham Norton, 1600.
Stoff, Sheldon P., *The Pumpkin Quest*, North Quincey: The Christopher Publishing House, 1978.
Strabo, Walafrid, *De Cura Hortorum* or *Hortulus*, vol. 2 of *Monumenta Germaniae Historica, Poetae Latini Aevi Carolini*, ed. Ernst Dümmler. Berlin: Weidmann, 1884.
Styron, William, *Lie Down in Darkness*, London: Hamish Hamilton, 1952.
Suetonius, *Augustus*.
Swift, Jonathan, *Gulliver's Travels*, introd. Harold Williams. Oxford: Basil Blackwell, 1941.

WORKS CITED

Taylor, Jer., *The Great Exemplar of Sanctity and Holy Life* etc., part III. London: Francis Ash, 1649.
Telford, William Rodgers, *The Barren Temple and the Withered Tree* etc. Diss. (Cantab.).
Tennyson, Alfred, *The Poems of Tennyson*, ed. Christopher Ricks. London & Harlow: Longmans, Green, 1969.
Theophrastus, *Historia Plantarum*, I and VII.
Tertullianus, *Adversus Marcionem*, IV.
Tertullianus, *De Anima*.
Thompson, Stith, *Motif-Index of Folk-Literature* etc., vols. 1–6. Copenhagen: Rosenkilde and Bagger, 1955-8.
Thomson, Philip, *The Grotesque*, in *The Critical Idiom*, gen. ed. John D. Jump, vol. 24. London: Methuen, 1972.
Thurber, James, 'The Cane in the Corridor', in his *The Thurber Carnival*, Harmondsworth: Penguin, 1962.
Tietze-Courat, E., *Dwarfs and Jesters in Art*, London: Phaidon, 1957.
Todd, F.A., *Classical Quarterly*, 1943, pp. 101-11.
Todd, Robert B. (ed.), *The Cyclopaedia of Anatomy and Physiology*, vol. 4, part 2. London: Longman, Brown, Green, Longmans & Roberts, 1849-52.
Tolstoy, L.I. *Sobraniye Sochineniya, Tom Dvenadstati*, ('Collected Works', vol. 12), ed. I.I. Akopovoi, I.K. Gudziya, I.I. Guseva, M.B. Khrapchenko, Moscow: Editions 'Khudozhyestvenoye Literatura', 1964.
Tompson, Benjamin, *Benjamin Tompson: His Poems*, ed. Howard Judson Hall, Boston and New York: Houghton Mifflin, 1924.
The Towneley Plays, ed. George England, side-notes and introd. Alfred W. Pollard. Early English Text Society, Extra Series, no. 71. London: Kegan Paul, Trench, Trübner & Co., 1897.
Twain, Mark, *Tom Sawyer & Huckleberry Finn*, introd. Christopher Morley. London: Everyman's Library, 1963.
Universal Lexicon aller Wissenschafte und Künste, vol. 20. Halle/Leipzig: Verlegts Johann Heinrich Bedler, 1732.
Updike, John, *Couples*, Harmondsworth: Penguin, 1971.
Updike, John, *Rabbit Redux*, London: André Deutsch, 1972.
Vandercook, John W., *Black Majesty: The Life of Christophe King of Haiti*, New York and London: Harper, 1928.
Βηλαρᾶς, Ἰωάννης. Ἅπαντα. Ἐπιμέλεια Γεωργίου Ἀχιλ. Βαβαρέτου. Ἀθῆναι: Ἐκδοτικός Οἶκος Πέτρου Δημητράκου Α.Ε., 1935.
Virgil, *Georgics*, IV.
Virgil, *Ländliche Gedichte*, ed. Johann Heinrich Voss. Altona: Johann Friedrich Hammerich, 1800.
Villari, Pasquale, *The Life and Times of Niccolo Macciavelli*, trans. Linda Villari (new ed.), vol. 2. London: T. Fisher Unwin, 1842.
Vitae Patrum, III.
Walkington, T., *The Optick Glasse of Hvmors: or The touchstone of a golden temperature* etc., London: T.C. for Leonard Becket, 1614 (?).
Wallace, Edgar, *The Angel of Terror*, London: Pan Books, 1962.

WORKS CITED

Ward, Nathaniel, *The Simple Cobler of Aggawam in America*, ed. P.M. Zall. Lincoln: University of Nebraska Press, 1969.

Waszink, J.H., *Tertulliani De Anima*, Amsterdam: Meulenhoff, 1947.

Weare, Tessa, 'Round in a Flat World', *Spare Rib: A Women's Liberation Magazine*, no. 78, January 1979.

Weinrich, Otto, *Senecas Apocolocynthosis*, Berlin: Weidmann, 1923.

Wells, Rulon, 'Distinctively human Semiotic', in *Essays in Semiotics/Essais de sémiotique*, ed. Julia Kristeva *et al.*, vol. 4. *Approaches to Semiotics*, ed. Thomas A. Sebeok, pp. 95-119. The Hague-Paris: Mouton, 1971.

Wescott, Roger W., 'Labio-Velarity and Derogation in English: A Study in Phonosemic Correlation', *American Speech*, 46, nos. 1-2, Spring-Summer 1971, pp. 123-37.

Westermanns Monatschrift, 115.

Whitaker, Thomas W., and Davis, Glen N., *Cucurbits: Botany, Cultivation and Utilization*, World Crops Books. London: Leonard Hill, 1962.

Whittier, John Greenleaf, *The Poetical Works of John Greenleaf Whittier*, London: Macmillan, 1874.

Whittier, John Greenleaf, 'Thomas Carlyle on the Slave Question', in *The Prose Works of John Greenleaf Whittier*, vol. 2: *Literary Recreations and Miscellanies*. Boston: Houghton Mifflin, 1880.

Wilenski, R.H., *Modern French Painters*, 4th ed. London: Faber & Faber, 1963.

Wodehouse, P.G., *Joy in the Morning*, London: Barrie & Jenkins, 1974.

Wodehouse, P.G., *Right Ho, Jeeves*, London: Herbert Jenkins, 1934.

Woenig, F., *Die Pflanzen im alten Aegypten*, Leipzig: Verlag von Wilhelm Fridrich, 1886.

Wright, Thomas (ed.), *The Correspondence of William Cowper*, vol. 1. London: Hodder and Stoughton, 1904.

Zangwill, Israel, *Children of the Ghetto*, London: White Lion Publishers, 1972.

Translations

i   But behold my gourd,/its elevation and vigour! /Ever higher it sprouts,/ grows royal and huge,/a cucumber of cucumbers all/from the countries where the sun dwells.

ii   Cucumbers grow in gardens when the moon is full, and their growth is as visible as that of sea-urchins.

iii   It is truly much more wholesome than a pumpkin.

iv   ... and [how] the gourd, winding in the grass, swells into a belly ....

v   It is believed that conception is aided by the [woman] carrying a [cucumber] seed, if it has not touched the ground.

vi   One has to be on one's guard so that a woman is admitted as little as possible to that place in which either cucumbers or gourds are sown. For almost by her contact will the shoots of the young plants wither. If, however, she on top of it has her period, she will kill the young plants even by looking at them.

vii   *Cucurbitare,* to dishonour by adultery another's wife; esp. of a vassal who dishonours his master's wife, and inflates her belly like a pumpkin, i.e. makes her pregnant.

viii   She is more yielding than a melon to me.

ix   Munching a cucumber, woman, weave thy cloak!

x   I am called the wooden guard of pumpkins.

xi   Just so the aspiring pumpkin, rising from an insignificant seed, casts huge shadows with the shields of its leaves, ...

xii   Now who can worthily admire its fruits hanging everywhere down from its branches?

xiii   At this point a certain Cantherius of the venerable family of the Cornelians, or, as he himself boasts, a descendant of Asinius Pollio, is in Rome recently said to have accused me of sacrilege, because I translated ivy instead of gourd: he was, you see, afraid that if ivies were growing up instead of gourds Jonah would lack a place to have a drink privately and in the shadow.

xiv	We have dealt with this matter at full length in the commentary on the prophet Jonah. Suffice it now to say that in that passage in which the seventy translators gave 'gourd' and Aquila with the rest 'ivy', that is [a rendering of] קיקיון, the Hebrew has 'kikeion' [a plant], which the Syrians commonly call 'kikeia'. It is, however, a kind of bush that has broad leaves like the vine, and when once it has been planted it shoots up into a small tree without any support of poles and props, which both gourds and ivies need, holding itself upright by its stem. If I had wanted, therefore, to translate word for word and give 'kikeion', nobody would have understood; if I had put 'gourd', I would have said that which is not in the Hebrew. I put 'ivy' in order to agree with the other translators.
xv	Now then, after four hundred years, the truth of the law comes forth to us; it has been bought for money in the synagogue. When the world is grown old and everything hastens to the end let us even put it on the tombs of our ancestors, so that it may be known to them too, who read a different version, that Jonah did not have the shadow of a gourd but of an ivy; and again, when it so pleases the legislator, not an ivy but some other bush.
xvi	Houdia M'Baye did not have the same presence of mind and the jet hit her face knocking her head back like a blow from a giant's fist. She opened her mouth to cry out but the water plunged into her throat. In the roar of the hoses one could not hear the ridiculous little snapping of the cartilage in her neck. Houdia M'Baye flapped with her arms as if trying to get hold of the air, as drowning people do; then her hands seized at her blouse tearing it to pieces, and she fell on her side, half-naked, her shrivelled breasts resembling gourds left in the sun in the hot season.
xvii	And I beheld a cucumber, son of glorious Earth, lying in the vegetable market. It lay stretched out over nine tables.
xviii	Now you must see them [the goddesses] unless your eyes are running with gourds.
xix	What a big head he has. As big as a pumpkin!
xx	Why do you call his body bread, and not rather a pumpkin, which Marcion had instead of a heart.
xxi	Don't you see that Leagrus, of Glaucon's grand line, the stupid, silly Cuckoo, wanders about with legs like a seedless [eunuch] melon.
xxii	[His] ankles were swollen larger than a melon.
xxiii	There is a kind of first beginning, royal, before and above comprehension, a power before and above substance, rolling itself ever onward. Now with this exists a power, which I call a gourd: and with this gourd is a power, which also I call perfect emptiness. This gourd, and perfect emptiness, being one thing, emitted, without emitting it, a fruit, in all respects visible, eatable and sweet, which fruit their speech calls a Cucumber. But with this fruit is a power of the same tendency with it, which also I call a Pompion. These powers, the gourd, and the perfect emptiness,

TRANSLATIONS

and the cucumber, and the pompion, emitted the rest of the multitude of Valentinus' delirious pompions. [*Five Books of S. Irenaeus' Against Heresies,* trans. John Keble in *A Library of Fathers,* Oxford: James Parker, 1872, pp. 27-8].

xxiv Oh, you nonsense-talking sophists!

xxv Oh weaklings, base reproaches to your name, Achaean women, and men no more.

xxvi They allow these [people] to desecrate the food and admit them to the table, and they give orders to wash the vessels that ought to be smashed, when Pumpkin drinks or the bearded Chelidon.

xxvii Ol: I was afraid she had a sword; I started searching, to make sure she didn't have one, and while I did that I got hold of the hilt. But on consideration she had no sword, because a sword would have been cold.

Cl: Speak out.

Ol: But I am so ashamed.

Cl: Was it perhaps a radish?

Ol: No it wasn't.

Cl: A cucumber then?

Ol: Good heavens no; no vegetable at all. But one thing is certain; that whatever it was, no blight had ever touched it. It was well-grown, whatever it was.

xxviii Be off and draw your gourds! You have no idea what this is all about. ([Hadrian] happened just then to pride himself on such a drawing).

xxvix in the mirror two pale brown smooth gourds bent over the wash basin. white little hairs appeared in the sun in the countryside. Cloe laughed out loudly. hedgehog-breasts! she murmured, gourdhedgehog, hedgehoggourd . . . she thought of the banned oval and round forms. the womb a gourdfruit, . . .

xxx one year ago she had had her hair cut quite short. she had wanted once more to feel the shape of her head and her bare face (and she had hoped thereby to reduce the street-molestations). her hair had become stronger and thicker. it had grown quickly. now she was able to brush it out of her face again. she thought of the woman she had been a year ago and the woman the year before that and –

Sheddings of the skin.

This is the year of the gourdwoman! she rose and went to her room. no more the would-like-to-be-slim-woman, the if-only-I-had-flat-breasts-woman . . . .

xxxi Bear in mind that I came from a raw and heavy peasant world with rural theories of this and that, which did not at all match the culture of the metropolitans. For her the streets were broad garden paths, and the rows of houses greenhouses.

– Every evening I go down and water the cobblestone flowers, she said, and it was obvious that when she spoke she totally lived the part. But this strange empathy was undeniably titillating for my strict sense of reality. Now, afterwards, I am well able to see how ridiculous my objections were, since it was obviously in accordance with the truth, when she claimed that her arms were cucumbers, her mouth a tomato, her eyes plums and on certain occasions gooseberries. It would never have occurred to my girlfriend back in Jutland to say that her behind was two melons grown together. When I asked Lis Nemesis Jensen what in that case her breasts were, she unbuttoned her blouse and said:

– They are a woman's ornamental gourds.

It suddenly occurred to me that, in a recent letter to my beloved, I had myself written that her breasts were two turtle-doves.

xxxii Naturally you were upset at the very sight and instinctively checked whether the bra-strap had burst. But it wasn't you who had dropped the vegetables.

xxxiii I am neither happy nor sad. I am scarcely alive. I vegetate, stretched out all day long like a creeping plant. Sometimes, to complete the resemblance, it seems to me that leaves shoot out of me, here and there, that I reach for the objects around me with tendrils rather than hands. My head swells like a gourd: I reflect; I study the present and the past.

xxxiv Yes, so these jerseys and curls and bustles caught me. And it was easy to catch me, for I was brought up in the conditions in which amorous young people are forced like cucumbers in a hot-bed.

xxxv Consider marriage; what is it if not a gamble, just as for one who buys a melon: for each good one there are a hundred gourds or pumpkins.

xxxvi The seahorses swam forth and stood up on the threshold of the sea, the water reached their knees.

It's me! It's me! they both answered and giggled themselves half dead.

Aren't you going to save me? asked one of them. Tiny little fat sea-cucumber, do you look at my portrait every day? Do you?

He isn't a sea-cucumber, said the other one reproachingly. He's a tiny little mushroom who's promised to save me if the wind starts blowing. He's a little mushroom who finds seashells for his mother. Isn't it charming! Charming!

The Moomin troll's eyes grew hot.

Index

acceptability, *see* grammaticality
Achmet, 200
Adams, Richard, 164
Albertus Magnus, 182, 190, 200
Alemán, Mateo, 37, 101, 116, 139, 171, 193, 203
Alfred, King, 30
ambiguity, 65-7, 78, 107, 112, 115, 120, 123, 125-41, 145, 146-8, 193, 197, 205, 206
Ambrosius, St, 181
analogy, 30, 84, 124, 160, 166, 167, 173, 205
Anaxilas, 42, 167
Andersen, Hans Christian, 52, 99
André, Jaques, 177
animal symbolism, 6, 170; bear, 49, 53; bull, 203; chicken, 34, 88-91, 108; cow, 7, 172-3, 199; cuckoo, 42; dog, 75, 78; dog-whelp, 63; donkey, ass, 7, 108, 113, 172-3; dove, 102, 103; ephemeron, 112; fish, 29; fly, 32, 97, 112; fox, 178, 199; goat, he-, 101; goat, scape-, 182; goose, 6-7, 172-3, 201, 203; hedgehog, 76; hen, 203; horse, 70; jackal, 182; lion, 7, 115, 157, 160, 164, 165, 207; monkey, ape, 177, 191, 197; ox, 176; oyster, 95; parrot, 173; pig, 37, 44, 71, 136, 137, 184; pink(-feast), 180; rabbit, 98, 101, 113; rat, 46, 48, 157, 158; sheep, lamb, 42, 113, 173; trout, 121
Antin, Paul, 180
antithesis, 19-20, 21, 26, 35, 44, 45, 46, 51, 54, 55, 61, 62, 65, 66, 86, 96, 98, 108-12, 115, 171

anthropomorphia, 207
anthropo-phytomorphia, 207
Apicius, 174
Apuleius, 40, 197
arbitraire du signe, 5, 6, 7, 84, 130, 131, 146, 147-8, 154-68, 169, 206-8
Aristophanes, 22, 37, 52
Aristotle, 162, 201, 208
Arnott, Anne, 188
Artemidorus Daldianus, 179, 190, 192
Athenaeum, 194
Athenaeus, 18, 22, 52, 62, 173, 177, 178, 184, 186, 187
Augustine, St, 28, 55, 78, 129
autobiography, 91
auxiliary symbolism and semiotic economy, 52
Aziz, Maqbool, 204

Bächthold-Stäbli, 192
Baker, Samuel W. Sir, 40
Bally, Charles, 154
Beck, E., 181
Bentley, Richard, 24-6
Bergman, Anne, 202
Bergson, Henri, 50, 207
Bible: Baruch, 66; Deuteronomy, 106; Job, 45; John, 179; Jonah, 20, 24, 27-32, 47, 56, 60, 111, 112, 151, 152, 181, 182; Kings, 176; Leviticus, 106; Luke, 179, 181; Mark, 176, 179; Matthew, 133, 174, 179, 181; Numbers, 19, 20, 110, 152
Bible versions: Aquila, 28, 180; *Authorised version (AV)*, 181;

INDEX

Bible versions: (cont.)
    Coverdale, Myles, 181; Geneva, 181; Jerusalem Bible, 181; Matthew, Thomas, 181; New English Bible (NEB), 20, 66, 110, 181; Revised standard version (RSV), 27, 181; Revised version (RV), 181; the Septuagint, 28, 29, 30, 180; Symmachus, 180; Theodotion, 180; Tyndale, William, The Prophet Jonas, 181; Vetus Latina (early Latin versions), 28, 29, 30, 78; the Vulgate, 28, 29, 30, 78, 181
Bickerton, Derek, 157-61
binarity, 162
Birt, Th., 186, 192
bisociation, 158, 164, 166, 167, 207
Blackmur, Richard P., 174
Blake, William, 32
Bloomfield, Morton, 156
Boorde, 101, 177-8, 196
Boswell, James, 188
Brautigan, Richard, 121-3, 204
Bridges, Robert, 60
Bristed, Charles Astor, 67, 115, 197
Broun, A. F., 179
Brown, Roger, 159-60
Browning, Robert, 17, 43, 44, 120, 198
Bücheler, F., 192

Cabbala, the, 170
Campani, Ferdinando Maria, 101
caricature, 39, 77
Carinus, 15, 95, 146-7
Carlyle, Thomas, 4, 69-72, 125
Caroli Magni Capitulare de villis imperialibus, 200
de Cervantes Saavedra, Miguel, 203
Chaplin, Sir Charles, 38, 51
Chaucer, Geoffrey, 186, 196
Chevalier, Jean and Alain Gheerbrant, 193, 200
chiastic inversion, 118-23
choice, see selection and choice
Chorley, Henry F., 194
chronology, 7-8, 146-8
Churchill, E. Richard, 188
Cicero, 60, 173
Cinderella, 45-6, 101, 120, 121, 132, 170-1, 204, 206
Cirlot, J. E., 176

classicism, see romanticism and classicism
Clodius Albinus, 15, 95, 146
Clowes, E. M., 31
Coleridge, Samuel Taylor, 31-2, 167
Columella, 16, 22, 101, 174
communicative need, 6
competence, 83, 92
Conington, J., 21
connotations cluster, 114, 203
Conrad, Joseph, 189
Cooper, James Fenimore, 49
cosmetics, see folk-medicine
cosmogonies, 26, 63-4, 179
Cowper, William, 44
Crane, Stephen, 36, 43, 61-2, 68-9, 117, 167
cryptography, 150
cucumber-sacrifice among the Nuer, 176
cucumber-time, 54, 188
cucurbitic connotations (cross references refer within this entry): absurdity, 27, 36, 42, 44, 47, 52, 54, 61, 65, 66, 67, 68, 71, 92, 97, 98, 100, 114, 122, 123, 134, 167, 168, 188, 189, 195, 196, 199; abundance, 14, 15, 17, 19, 26, 35, 71, 78; alchemy, 176; baldness, and hair style, 38, 40, 46, 49-51, 53, 58, 76, 100, 107, 129, 137, 190, 191, 197; belly, 21, 60, 145, 178, 179, 187, 195; birth-control, 59, 101, 192, breasts, 34, 76, 77, 102, 103, 104, 199, 202; castration, 74, 101; celibacy, 20, 133; chastity, 20, 101, 103, 133; comedy, see humour; courtship, and marriage, 46, 67, 101, 105, 125, 132, 133, 134, 135, 136, 137, 138, 139, 170, 171, 178, 184, 193, 205, 206; cyclicity, 14, 15, 29, 56, 64, 110, 174-5, 182; death, see life and death; defloration, see droit du seigneur; dicebox, see gambling; droit du seigneur, and defloration, 101, 194; emptiness, and hollowness, 13, 34, 38, 51, 52, 53, 54, 55, 60, 190, 191, 195; eyes, 37, femininity, 22, 51, 53-4, 56, 59-60, 65, 67, 74,

225

INDEX

76, 89, 101, 102, 122, 130, 131, 132, 184, 186, 193, 206; fertility, 14, 18, 19, 22, 26, 27, 35, 49, 56, 64, 71, 113, 131, 176, 179, 184, 193; friendship, 23, 179; gambling, dice-box, gambling-machines in British pubs, etc., 107, 117, 176, 187, 195, 205; gluttony, 15, 20, 92, 94, 95, 96, 147; gold, 18, 46, 47, 48, 55, 115, 116, 167, 171, 175, 183, 191, 203; grotesqueness, 42–3, 47, 134, 199; hair style, *see* baldness; head, 28, 36, 37, 38, 39, 40, 41, 42, 44, 48, 49, 50, 51, 52, 53, 55, 58, 61, 69, 99, 100, 113, 114, 127, 129, 145, 185, 190, 191, 196; heart, 40; hollowness, *see* emptiness; homosexuality, 56, 76, 101, 147; humour, ridicule, comedy, 35, 44, 49, 57, 60, 69, 71, 77, 78, 89, 92, 93, 100, 101, 107, 114, 128, 141, 177, 185, 187, 189, 190, 195, 196, 199, 201; immobility, *see* inertia; incest, 72, 101; inertia, passivity, immobility phlegma, 48, 71, 78, 90, 190; insensitivity, 36; lechery, 101, 194; legs, 36, 41, 137, 184; life and death, 19, 29, 30, 31, 32, 33, 34, 36–7, 63–4, 65, 66, 96, 97, 108–10, 111, 112, 115, 116–17, 121–3, 128, 170, 174–5, 176 (Nuer), 176 (Mark), 182, 188, 189, 204, 205, 206; lightness, 51, 52, 99, 120, 125, 191; marriage, *see* courtship; masculinity, *see* virility; masturbation, 98, 101; menstruation, *see* moon; money, *see* riches; moon, and menstruation, 18, 64, 101, 186; Negro, 34, 40, 41, 42, 47, 67, 69–75, 87–91, 98, 101, 107–8, 114, 115, 167, 183, 187, 201; obesity, 41, 67, 92, 98, 137, 140, 142, 145, 186, 195, 197; parasitism, 62, 167; passivity, *see* inertia; phlegma, *see* inertia; physical deformity, 36, 41, 42, 55, 60, 68–9, 74, 137, 188; *podex*, 102, 103, 104, 187, 197; pregnancy, 21, 41, 64, 101, 105, 106, 145, 178, 179, 184, 193; procreation, 179, 193; prostitution, 101, 144–5; prudery, 134, 135; resurrection, 23, 29–31, 56, 64; riches, money, value, 18, 19, 35, 46, 47, 67, 71, 90, 106, 175, 176, 182, 183, 188, 191; ridicule, *see* humour; royalty, *see* social status; sex, 20, 37, 42, 51, 56, 57, 58, 59, 68, 75–6, 90, 91, 92, 97, 98, 101, 102, 103, 104, 111, 113, 115, 116, 130, 131, 133, 134, 136, 146, 159, 167, 177, 178, 192, 193, 195, 197, 203, 204, 206; snoring, 187; social status, upper-classness, royalty, 14, 17, 27, 44, 45, 54, 55, 61, 62, 67, 77, 120, 151, 171, 175, 182, 183, 193, 203; softness, 22, 37, 189, 190, 191; spiral, 23, 179; sterility, 64, 101, 131, 176, 179, 184, 194; stupidity, 28, 37, 38, 39, 40, 42, 51, 52, 53, 54, 55, 60, 63, 64, 67, 89, 99, 108, 113, 114, 134, 135, 145, 167, 172–3, 185, 189, 190, 198, 202, 206; summer, *see* sun; sun, summer, 14, 16–17, 18, 32, 34, 47, 54, 58, 70, 76, 100, 109, 110, 122, 181, 197; swelling, 36, 37, 41, 60, 142, 167, 184, 187, 200; transport, cucurbitic means of, 46, 47, 77, 121, 189, 199, 206; unfaithfulness, 22, 64, 65, 91, 101, 133; upper-classness, *see* social status; value, *see* riches; virginity, 63, 103; virility, masculinity, 51, 75, 98, 105, 130, 131, 193, 194; vitality, 14, 15, 19, 35, 68, 69, 128, 167, 177, 204; waist, 42, 104; wateriness, 26, 36, 63, 64, 68, 92, 93, 108 ff, 187, 195, 196, 200; worthlessness, 35, 189, 190

cucurbits, biology of, 5, 14, 174
cucurbits, cultivation of, 174
cucurbits, cultural history of, 14, 174, 183
cucurbits, economy of, 5, 16, 174, 183
cucurbits, and musical instruments, 14, 34, 38, 41, 59–60, 63, 101
cucurbits, names of, ἀγγούρι, 57, 102, 125, 203; ἀγγούρια, 19; ἀγγουριά, 19; ἄγγουρος, 125; *agurk* (Dan. and Norw.), 54, 103, 141; *calabaça* (Port.), 139; calabash, 13, 34, 38, 39, 106, 147,

226

cucurbits, names of, (cont.)
175, 183, 185, 193, 196, 202, 204;
calebasse (Fr.), 114, 193; *calabaza*
(Sp.), 39, 185, 199, 206; cantaloup,
117, 141; *citrouille* (Fr.), 39;
citrullo (It.), 39; *cocomero* (It.),
39; *coloquentis* (Lat.), 200; *coloquinte* (Fr.), 128-9, 167; *cornichon*
(Fr.), 39; *coucourbe* (Occitanian),
185; *courge* (Fr.), 193; crook-neck,
47; cucumber, *cucūber*, *cucūbre*,
8, 13, 14, 15, 16, 17, 18, 20, 22,
36, 41, 44, 48, 53, 54, 57, 62, 66,
100, 102, 105, 108, 110, 125, 132,
134, 135, 137, 138, 139, 140, 141,
142, 147, 167, 176, 177, 183, 184,
186, 188, 189, 196, 199, 202, 203,
204; *cucumis* (Lat.), 13, 21, 22, 24,
53, 57, 102, 167, 175, 177, 178,
200; *cucurbita* (Lat.), 13, 22, 23,
24, 28, 29, 30, 31, 40, 53, 78, 98,
107, 111, 129, 177, 180, 182, 190,
196, 200; *Flaschenkürbis* (Germ.),
173; gherkin, 14; gourd, *gourde*,
gowrde, 13, 14, 15, 24, 26, 31, 32,
34, 35, 38, 39, 41, 42, 44, 47, 58,
59, 60, 63, 64, 74, 77, 97, 103,
104, 107, 112, 139, 173, 174,
175, 176, 177, 178, 179, 181, 182,
183, 184, 185, 186, 187, 193, 195,
196, 197, 199, 201, 202, 204, 205;
gourde (Fr., incl. Am. Fr.), 18, 34,
35, 39, 183; *gurka* (Sw.), 16, 140;
Gurke (Germ.), 54, 141, 173; *Kalebasse* (Germ.), 173; καρποῦξι, 39;
κολοκύντη (κολοκύνθη), 19, 28,
30, 39, 40, 54, 55, 60, 62, 108,
111, 129, 180; κολοκύθια, 185;
κολοκυνθίς, 192; κολοκύντιος, 57;
komkommer (Dutch), 54; кратуна
(Bulgarian), 39; *Kürbis, Kürbiss*
(Germ.), 38, 39, 48, 51, 55, 62, 76,
102, 167, 173, 174, 181; *kurbits*
(Sw.), 16-17; *kurkku* (Fin.), 141;
marrow, 103, 134, 135, 138, 139,
141, 179, 183; *mellone* (It.), 39;
melo (Lat.), 55; *melon* (Dan.), 102,
167; *melon* (Fr.), 39, 75; *melón*
(Sp.), 132, 139, 184, 203; melon,
mellon, mylon, 13, 14, 15, 16, 17,
18, 19, 20, 22, 25, 27, 33, 34, 36,
37, 39, 40, 41, 44, 45, 47, 48, 53,
59, 61, 62, 68, 69, 72, 78, 95, 96,
97, 101, 102, 103, 104, 105, 108,
109, 110, 111, 116, 117, 120,
132, 139, 141, 142, 143, 144, 147,
167, 176, 179, 184, 185, 186, 187,
192, 193, 198, 199, 203, 204, 205;
melonaggine (It.), 185; *Melone*
(Germ.), 173; musk-melon, 14, 15,
18, 78, 95, 141; огурец (Russian),
133, 166, 175; огурчик (Russian),
166, 175; *pepino* (Sp.), 139, 185;
pepo (Lat.), 13, 23, 40, 42, 53,
129, 141, 200; πέπων, 39, 54,
179, 192; pepone, 177, 178;
peponella (It.), 39; *Peponer*
(Norw.), 21; pompeon, 62, 151;
pompion, 27, 43, 63, 167, 186;
pumkin, 50, 190; pumpian, 63,
167; pumpion, 63, 92, 167, 191,
195; pumpkin, 5, 7, 13, 14, 15, 17,
18, 19, 22, 26, 27, 36, 37, 39, 40,
42, 43, 45, 46, 47, 48, 49, 50, 51,
52, 53, 54, 55, 56, 58, 59, 60, 61,
64, 65, 66, 67, 69, 70, 71, 74, 75,
77, 78, 92, 93, 98, 99, 100, 101,
103, 105, 109, 113, 121, 124,
125, 127, 128, 129, 131, 141,
142, 144, 145, 147, 166, 167,
168, 169, 170, 171, 173, 175,
176, 180, 183, 184, 187, 189,
190, 193, 196, 197, 198, 199,
203, 204, 206, 207; punkin, 48,
58, 68, 69, 73, 74, 89, 101, 115,
184, 190, 191, 203; *pyntegraeskar*
(Dan.), 102, 167; *sandio* (Sp.),
39; σικύα (σικύη), 62, 167, 192;
σίκυος (σικυός), 18, 22, 36, 42;
squash, 14, 41, 128, 141, 167,
183, 187; тиква (Bulgarian),
39; *tvrda tikva* (Croatian), 39;
watermelon, 13, 14, 15, 16, 19,
20, 32, 33, 34, 67, 68, 69, 72,
73, 88, 89, 90, 96, 101, 102,
108, 110, 115, 121, 122, 123,
132, 139, 145, 167, 174, 176,
182, 183, 189, 190, 194, 198,
199, 205; *zucca* (It.), 39; *zuccone* (It.), 39, 186
cucurbits, as taboo subject, 1, 35, 72, 127
cucurbits, and wine-making, 174
Culler, Jonathan, 200
Cutler, Hugh C. and Thomas W. Whitaker, 174

INDEX

Daily News, 197, 198
Darwinism, 86, 165–6
Dass, Petter, 21
Day of the Jackal, 96
Delphic oracle, 107
desert, 19–20, 31, 96, 109, 110, 110, 111, 144
Dickens, Charles, 53, 134–9, 189
Dickinson, Emily, 65–6
dictionary, and lexicon, 161, 164–5
Dio Cassius, 62
Dioscorides, 174
Diphilus, 19
Donatello, 186
Doomer, Lambert, 101, Plates IV and V
Douglas, Mary, 106, 202
dreams, and stream-of-consciousness, 111, 144–5, 179, 200
du Cange, *Glossarium*, 22, 101
Dümmler, Ernst, 179
Duff, J. D., 197

Ebert, Max, 174
Edward Earl of Clarendon, 182
elegant variation, 93
Ellison, Ralph, 72, 101, 102, 129, 198
emblems, 175
England, George, 196
Engler, Rudolf, 155
Ephraem Syrus, 31
Epicrates, 52
ethnic vituperation, 48–9, 67 ff, 75–6
ethographia, 125
etymology, 145, 178, 185
euthanasia, 127–8
Evans, Blakemore, 195
Evans-Pritchard, E. E., 176
Eyen, Willfried van, 193

faction, 87, 88
feminism, 76–7, 101, 178
Field, Frederick, 180
film, 38, 68, 77, 96–7, 101, 177, 182, 204
filter-model of literary autogenesis, 86 ff, 96
Fischer, Hermann, 185
Fletcher, Harris Francis, 175
Fletcher, John, 63, 167
Fletcher and Massinger, 63, 101, 167
Floris, Frans, 101
folk-medicine, medicinal use, cosmetics, 14, 105, 130, 131, 174, 178, 184, 193, 202, 203
folk-painting in Dalarna, Sweden, 151, 181
Forster, E. M., 4
Frankenstein, Dr, 147
French structuralism, 83–4, 156
Friedländer, L., 197
Friedreich, J. B., 174
Frost, Robert, 107
Frye, Northrop, 204
Funk & Wagnalls Standard Dictionary of Folklore, Mythology and Legend, 180

Galbraith, John Kenneth, 182
Galenus, 174
Galt, John, 37, 167
Gargilius Martialis, 174, 196
Garrod, H. W., 206
Gauden, John, 167, 182
Geoponica, 174, 200
Gerard, John, 195
Godel, Robert, 207
Goethe, J. W., 62, 167
Goscinny, René, 114
grammaticality and acceptability, 162
Grant, Douglas, 189
Gubernatis, Angelo de, 192, 196
guessing ability, 169
Guinness Book of Records, 9, 94, 183
Gullason, Thomas A., 184

Hacket, John, 167, 194
Haggard, Henry Rider, 109, 111, 152
Haley, Alex, 73–4, 87–91, 101
Haliburton, Thomas Chandler, 48, 184, 185, 190
Hall, Howard Judson, 180
Halloween, 42–3, 65, 98
Harding, Walter, 175
Hardy, Oliver, 38
Harris, George Washington, 42, 104
Harrison, R. H., 180
harvest feasts, melon parties, Thanksgiving, etc., 16, 26–7, 47, 132, 180
Harvey, W. W., 192
Hastings, James, 180
Hawthorne, Nathaniel, 16, 46, 49, 52, 66, 99, 120, 125, 142, 191

228

Hehn, Viktor, 173, 177
Heidegger, Martin, 84
Helm, Rudolf, 192
Henkel, Arthur and Albrecht Schöne, 175
Henry, O., 196
hermeneutics, 106
Hermippus, 40
Hermit in London, 41, 142, 186
Heroic Epistle to Sir William Chambers etc., An, 198
hierarchy of fruits, 18, 98, 176
heightened clichés, 38
Hills, Denis, 18, 74-5, 103, 186
Hippocrates, 105, 192, 194
Historia Augusta, 95-6, 146-7
Hogarth, William, 38
Holm, Sven, 103, 132
homeopathy, 184
Homer, 36, 54
Hone, William, 190
Horace, 171
Hughes, Ted, 206

iconic signs, 6, 92, 167
Ifesieh, Father Emmanuel, 202
imitation, 149-50, 152-3; for imitation in the Aristotelian sense, see mimesis
independent creation, 61, 62, 85, 93, 149-53
indexical signs, 6
inevitability, see probability
Inge, M. Thomas, 202
interlanguage, 3
intrinsic appropriateness, see naturally motivated signs
inventory poem, 203
Irenaeus, 13, 53, 129, 167
irony, 4
Irving, Washington, 41, 49, 104, 124
Islam, 87-8

jack-o'-lantern, see masks
Jackson, Holbrook, 188
James, Henry, 38, 119-20, 174, 203-4
Janson, H. W., 186
Jansson, Tove, 101, 139-41, 167
Jerome, Jerome K., 42, 113
Jerome, St, 28, 181
Johnson, Samuel, 188
Johnson, Thomas H., 197
Jonson, Ben, 22, 77

Joyce, James, 101, 103-4, 142, 144, 145, 184
Jump, John D., 188
Juvenal, 56, 101, 167, 197

Karkavitsas, A., 125
Karlfeldt, Erik Axel, 16-17, 55, 100
Katz, Joseph, 194
Keats, John, 142
Kesey, Ken, 132, 133, 139, 171
Keynes, Geoffrey, 182
King, Roma A. Jr, 176
Kock, Theodor, 177, 186
Koerner, E. F. K., 207
Koestler, Arthur, 207
Kristeva, Julia, 172
Kučera, Henry and W. Nelson Francis, 199
Kühn, C. G., 174

labiality, 141, 142, 143, 173, 177, 187
lability of language, 6, 164
Laurel, Stan, 38, 51
Laurent-Täckholm, Vivi, 173, 194
Leach, Maria, see Funk & Wagnalls
Lear, Edward, 43, 101, 171
Le Comte, Edward, 179
Lemons, Stanley, 89
Leo, F., 192
Lévi-Strauss, Claude, 84
Lewis, C. S., 188
lexicon, see dictionary
Λεξικὸν τῆς Νέας Ἑλληνικῆς Γλώσσης "Πρωΐας,, , 28, 202
'lie-model' of literary autogenesis, 86 ff, 96
Littré, E., 192
Livy, 21
locus amoenus, 23
Lodge, David, 38
Loewenberg, Ina, 172
London Gazette, 18, 167
Longus, 76
Lowell, James Russell, 66, 199
Lucian, 77
Luther, Martin, 181

Maas, M., 192
Mabbe, James, 37, 116, 193
Madonna, the, 127
magic, superstition, witchcraft, 42-3, 45-6, 49, 52, 63, 77, 114,

INDEX

125, 171, 175, 177, 184, 186, 187, 188, 205
Maison Rustique, 101, 186
Maleh, E. A. El, 75–6
Margoliouth, H. M., 200
Marvell, Andrew, 78
masks, facial, 42–3, 47, 66, 98, 187, 199
Matron, 8, 36
Maupassant, Guy de, 118–9
Mauro, Tullio de, 154–5, 156, 164, 207
maximal appropriateness, 94–108, 111, 112, 113, 154–68
Maya, 187
melon parties, *see* harvest feasts
Menander, 19
Merivale, Charles, 60
metaphor, 5, 69, 70, 93, 115, 121, 122, 154–68, 169, 172, 203, 206–8
Milton, John, 15, 24–7, 63, 97
mimesis, 87, 95–7, 117–18, 171; *for imitation in the Horatian sense, see* imitation
Mitford, Mary Russell, 180
Mitius, Otto, 180
Moretum, 21
Morse code, 6
Mortimer, Penelope, 64, 101
Mrose, H., 167, 184, 190

Nash, Jørgen, 102, 167
naturalism, 61
naturally motivated signs, and intrinsic appropriateness, 4, 5, 6, 85, 86, 87, 91, 92, 93, 148, 254–8, 169–71, 206–8
new criticism, 2
New Encyclopaedia Britannica, 173
Nixon, Richard Milhouse, 77, 78, 129
nonsense, 43, 188
Norrman, Ralf Georg, 204
numskull, 113

Ohl, Raymond T., 200
Oliver, H. J., 194
Organ, John, 174, 177, 179, 184, 185, 187, 201
Origines, 180
Otto, A., 186
OUIDA, 34
Ousmane, Sembène, 34, 193
Ovid, 21, 23, 178

oxymoron, 46, 140, 191

Palladius, 174
Pall Mall Gazette, 54
Palmer, John, 184, 189
paradigmatic relations, 2–7, 93, 96, 99, 112, 113, 121, 170
parody, 54, 58–9, 68, 77, 101, 198
Partridge, Eric, *The Penguin Dictionary of Historical Slang*, 197, 198
Paulys Real-Encyclopädie der klassischen Altertumswissenschaft, see Wissowa
Pavlov, Ivan, 78
'Peanuts', 77, 129
Peattie, Donald Culross, 194
Perrault, 45–6, 101, 121, 189
Persius, 191
Peter S., 49–50, 100, 190
Petronius, 64, 186, 197
phenomenology, 147, 151
Philippon, Charles, 39
phonology, 124
phonosemic correlations, *see* sound symbolism
physei-thesei debate, the, 156–68
phyto-anthropomorphia, 207
phytomorphia, 207
Piozzi, Hester Lynch, 188
plant and vegetable symbolism: apple, 78, 95, 147, 203; arrowroot, 71; artichoke, 39, 122, 127; banana, 18, 52, 177, 193, 197; beans, 38, 39, 122, 134; beanstalk, 36; black-eyed peas, 73; breadfruit, 73; cabbage, 39, 46, 48, 77, 115, 116, 127, 128, 189, 196, 198; carrot, 122; castor-oil plant, 27, 181; cherry, 142; cinnamon, 71; coconut, 39; coffee, 71, 183; cucurbits, *see cucurbitic entries*; daisy, 128; fig, 18, 75–6, 95, 176; fir-tree, 174; garlic, 20, 110; gooseberry, 102; grape and vine, 14, 18, 23–4, 46, 58, 78, 95, 98; groundnut, 73; heart of palm, 73; ivy, *hedera, Efeu*, κισσός, 23–4, 28, 29, 30, 31, 78, 180, 181; kanjo, *see sub-entry for* okra; leek, 20, 110; lemon, 39; lettuce, 122; lily, 19, 71, 108–9, 170; mango, 73, 96; mushroom, 112, 140; mustard seed, 23, 174; nec-

plant and vegetable symbolism (cont.)
 taren, 78; nut, peanut, 39, 77
 115, 116, 142, 192, 199; oak,
 acorn, 77, 174; okra, 73; olive, 182;
 onion, 20, 110, 122, 138; orange,
 78; palm, 183; parsley, 193; parsnip, 195, 196; peach, 18, 39; pear,
 18, 39; pepper, 71; pine, 121;
 plum, 18, 102; potato, 39, 48, 122,
 127; *qiqayon, ciceia, ciceion,
 kikayon,* κικεών, ן''ק'ק, 27-31,
 129, 180; raspberry, 142; rose, 124,
 170; sago, 71; so-so, *see sub-entry
 for* black-eyed peas; sugar, 71;
 thistle, 101; tomato, 102; turnip,
 39, 43, 127; turnip-radish, 138;
 yam, 73, 129, 198
Plate I, 124
Plate II, 127
Plate III, 127
Plate IX, 88
Plate XI, 183
Plath, Sylvia, 142-3
Plato, the comic poet, 41-2
Plato, the philosopher, 156, 164
Plautus, 57, 102, 167
Pliny the elder, 16, 22, 101, 174
Pliny the younger, 174
Plutarch, 186
Pope, Alexander, 93
positivism, 106
pragmatism, 86
predetermination, *see* probability
Priapea, 23, 167
probability, predictability, inevitability, predetermination, 19, 20, 64, 109, 110, 114, 159, 160, 169, 171, 178
Procopius, 56, 101, 167
Propertius, 21, 24, 25
Prou, Suzanne, 128-9, 167, 205
Prudence, Andrew, 179
Prynne, William, 50-1
puritans, 46, 49-52, 100, 129

racism, 74-6
realia, 4, 5, 7
Realphilologie, 106
reduplication, 141, 177
Richards, I. A., 207
Ricks, Christopher, 177
Ricoeur, Paul, 163, 208
Riley, James Whitcomb, 58-9, 101, 129

Riquer, Martín de, 203
Ritchie, Leitch, 17
Robinson, F. N., 186, 196
Roeg, Nicholas, 96
romanticism and classicism, 93
Rossetti, Christina, 111, 142, 144
Rossetti, William Michael, 202
Roth, Philip, 67, 101, 103, 167, 197
Rothenberg, Jerome, 187
Rudolf, Wilhelm, 181
Rufinus, 28-9, 78, 129
Ruxton, G. F., 22, 101, 167

Sadat, Anwar al-, 205
Sale, Arthur, 178, 199
satire, 54-60, 77, 99, 101
Saturday Review, 194
Saussure, Ferdinand de, 3, 8, 84, 147, 154-6, 164, 171, 207
Scarry, Richard, 95
Scheick, William J., 33
Schiller, Friedrich, 31-2
Scobie, Alexander, 186
Sebeok, Thomas A., 172
Sechehaye, Albert, 154
Seip, D. A., 178
selection and choice, 86, 87, 91, 93, 95, 97, 107, 108, 168
semiotic economy and auxiliary symbolism, 99, 100, 101, 107, 108, 114
'semiotics of life'-model of literary autogenesis, the, 87 ff, 96
Seneca minor, the Roman author, 54-62, 101, 120, 151, 152, 180, 197
Seneca, Red Indian nation, 187
Servius, 21
Shakespeare, William, 63, 92, 101, 194-6
Shibles, Warren A., 208
signifiant, 165
signifié, 165
signs proper, 6, 172
similar yet different, similarity and difference, 115-23, 139, 150, 160, 167, 169-71
situation-of-choice, 90-1, 107-8
slang, 115, 143, 176, 183, 187, 197, 198, 203
Slater, Michael, 205
Smiles, Samuel, 189
Smith, Martin, 196

231

INDEX

Sonny, A., 186
sound symbolism and phonosemic correlations, 46, 75, 141-4, 154, 173, 177, 187
Spectator, The, 194
stability of language, 6, 164
Stefan, Verena, 76-7, 101, 102, 167
Steffen, Uwe, 181
Steuens, Charles and John Liebault, *see Maison Rustique*
Stoff, Sheldon P., 197
stream-of-consciousness, *see* dreams
Styron, William, 32-4, 115
Suetonius, 175
superstition, *see* magic
Swift, Jonathan, 99-100, 201
symbols cluster, 50, 68, 101, 112-15, 141, 191, 203
Symphosius, 200
syntagmatic relations, 93, 95, 99, 113

tailor, 48, 54
Tain, The, 100
taxonomy, 173, 174
Taylor, Jer., 202
teleology, 149
Telford, William Rodgers, 176, 179
Tennyson, Alfred Lord, 18, 19, 32, 58, 97-8, 100, 101, 109
Tertullian, 40, 167
Thanksgiving, *see* harvest feasts
Theophrastus, 174
Theopompus, 22, 67, 101, 167
Thompson, Stith, 175, 184, 185, 189, 191, 192, 193, 199, 203, 204, 205
Thomson, Philip, 43
Thoreau, Henry David, 16
Thurber, James, 128, 167, 205
Tiberius, 16
Todd, F. A., 186, 197, 202
Todd, Robert B., 187
Tolstoy, Count Leo, 132-3, 139, 171
Tompson, Benjamin, 27, 120, 151, 152
Towneley Plays, 196
tradition, 8, 14, 31, 61, 62, 78, 79, 84, 91, 149-53
trepanning, 185
Triçanku, 56
Twain, Mark, 69

Tweedie, Jill, 205-6

Uderzo, Albert, 114
Universal Lexicon aller Wissenschafte und Künste, 175
Updike, John, 59-60, 98, 101, 129

Valentinus, the gnostic, 53, 129
Vandercook, John, 183
Van Doren, Carl, 190
vegetable symbolism, *see* plant symbolism
vehicle and tenor, 170, 207
velarity, 141
Βηλαρᾶς', Ιωάννης, 203
Villari, Pasquale, 167, 184
Virgil, 13, 21-3, 24, 101
Vitae Patrum, 20, 101, 177
Voss, Johann Heinrich, 178

Walafrid Strabo, 23-4, 56, 79, 98, 200
Walkabout, 96
Walkington, T., 191
Wallace, Edgar, 117-18
Ward, Nathaniel, 51-2
Waszink, J. H., 186
Weare, Tessa, 178
Weinrich, Otto, 54-5
Wells, Rulon, 172
Wentworth, Harold and Stuart Berg Flexner, *Dictionary of American Slang*, 176, 183, 185, 187, 197, 203
Wescott, Roger W., 187
Whitaker, Thomas and Glen N. Davis, 174
Whittier, John Greenleaf, 27, 45-6, 47-8, 72, 101, 203
Williams, Harold, 201
Wissowa, Georg, *Paulys Real-Encyclopädie*, 173, 200
witchcraft, *see* magic
Wodehouse, P. G., 39, 44, 185
Wölfflin, E., 186
Woenig, F., 173
Wright, Thomas, 188

Yankee, 16, 47, 48-9, 184, 185, 191

Zall, P. M., 191
Zangwill, Israel, 185

For Product Safety Concerns and Information please contact our EU
representative GPSR@taylorandfrancis.com
Taylor & Francis Verlag GmbH, Kaufingerstraße 24, 80331 München, Germany

www.ingramcontent.com/pod-product-compliance
Lightning Source LLC
Chambersburg PA
CBHW071822300426
44116CB00009B/1407